SOULS UNDER SIEGE

SOULS UNDER SIEGE

STORIES OF WAR, PLAGUE, AND CONFESSION IN FOURTEENTH-CENTURY PROVENCE

NICOLE ARCHAMBEAU

CORNELL UNIVERSITY PRESS
Ithaca and London

First published 2021 by Cornell University Press

Library of Congress Cataloging-in-Publication Data
Names: Archambeau, Nicole, author.
Title: Souls under siege : stories of war, plague, and confession in fourteenth-century Provence / Nicole Archambeau.
Description: Ithaca, [New York] : Cornell University Press, 2021. | Includes bibliographical references and index.
Identifiers: LCCN 2020021651 (print) | LCCN 2020021652 (ebook) | ISBN 9781501753664 (hardcover) | ISBN 9781501753671 (ebook) | ISBN 9781501753688 (pdf)
Subjects: LCSH: Delphina, of Signe, 1284–1360. | Healing–Religious aspects–Christianity–History–To 1500. | War and society–France–Provence–History–To 1500. | Plague–France–Provence–History–To 1500. | Penance–History–France–Provence–To 1500. | France–Social life and customs–1328–1600.
Classification: LCC DC33.2 .A73 2021 (print) | LCC DC33.2 (ebook) | DDC 944.9/025—dc23
LC record available at https://lccn.loc.gov/2020021651
LC ebook record available at https://lccn.loc.gov/2020021652

For my parents, Peter and Carol Archambeau,
who showed me the power of stories

Contents

Illustrations

Acknowledgments

Over the course of writing this book I have accrued many debts. I thank Sharon Farmer at UC Santa Barbara for suggesting I take a look at the canonization inquest of Delphine de Puimichel. Sharon's insightful advice and critique of this project from its early stages to its present form have been indispensable. I am grateful for the advice and guidance I received at UCSB, particularly from Anita Guerrini, Carol Pasternak, Cynthia Brown, Ed English, Carol Lansing, and Debra Blumenthal.

My research in France was supported by the Camargo Foundation and was greatly helped by Sylvain Piron, Marie-Claude Leonelli, and Michael Osborne, among many others. I owe a debt to the archivists at the Archives départmentales des Bouches-du-Rhône and du Vaucluse and at the municipal archives in Apt, Provence.

The threads of this project came together over many years. At UCLA, Elinor Ochs supported my continued research in anthropological linguistics, while Simon Teuscher introduced me to methods of exploring medieval legal documents. My work in the history of emotions was shaped by a colloquium hosted by Damien Boquet and Piroska Nagy and attended by Daniel Lord Smail, Barbara Rosenwein, and others. At the 2009 NEH Summer Seminar, "Disease in the Middle Ages," I benefited from the expert guidance of Monica Green and Walton Schalick and from the knowledgeable and lively participants and instructors. At the 2012 NEH Summer Institute, "Networks and Knowledge: Synthesis and Innovation in the Muslim-Christian-Jewish Medieval Mediterranean," hosted by the Mediterranean Seminar, Peregrine Horden and Fernando Salmón helped me rethink my project in useful ways. This institute has allowed me to continue to work with the interdisciplinary and innovative Mediterranean Seminar, led by Sharon Kinoshita and Brian Catlos. In fall 2014, the Shelby Cullom Davis Center, led by Philip Nord, hosted fellows studying the aftermath of catastrophe. I am grateful for the insights of this exceptional group.

I owe sincere thanks to the American Council of Learned Societies, which supported my work through their New Faculty Fellowship Award program.

Through this program, I was able to work with Warren Brown and Jean-Laurent Rosenthal, among many others, at the California Institute of Technology and explore the collections at the Huntington Library.

While finishing this book, I was hired as an assistant professor in History at Colorado State University. I found a supportive atmosphere there and received advice and support from Ann Little, Ruth Alexander, and others.

This book has gone through many drafts and has benefited from diverse conversations and the attention of careful and generous readers of full drafts and sections. I am especially indebted to John Arnold and Sharon Farmer for their willingness to read drafts and engage the ideas in this project. I benefited from the comments of Ann Carmichael, William Chester Jordan, Erika Milam, Michael Gordin, Peregrine Horden, Anthony Grafton, Peter Potter, Mahinder Kingra, the anonymous reviewers, and participants in the California Medieval Seminar. I appreciate the advice of Daniel Lord Smail, Mary Carruthers, and Monica Green. Their insight and willingness to share their time and knowledge made this book better.

I deeply appreciate the support and patience of my husband, Patrick. He has heard these stories many times and still listens.

Abbreviations

ADBR	Archives Départmentales des Bouches-du-Rhône
ADV	Archives Départmentales de Vaucluse
BL	British Library
MGH	Monumenta Germaniae Historica
PL	Patrilogia Latina

A Note on Names

The spelling of names is not consistent across books and articles about Delphine and her entourage. Even her name varies, with André Vauchez and Gérard Veyssière using "Delphine" and others, like Paul Amargier, Florian Mazel, and Pierre-André Sigal, using "Dauphine." In this book, as in my earlier articles and book chapters, I've followed André Vauchez and used "Delphine." For most other names, I follow a Provençal pattern.

In some cases, however, the Provençal spelling is not feasible. For example, the French spelling of Bishop Philippe Cabassole's name has become the norm. So to be consistent with other publications, I have used the French spelling. I also use the French spelling of certain notaries' names to be consistent with how they appear in archival guides. For other names, like Francis Petrarch, Francis Meyronne, and Mary Magdalene, I use the English spelling, since these names vary according to the language of the author. There are individual names throughout the book that may appear in different ways in different publications. If pertinent, I indicate other spellings in a footnote.

In terms of place-names, I have used French spellings unless there is not a single, clear modern referent for the place indicated.

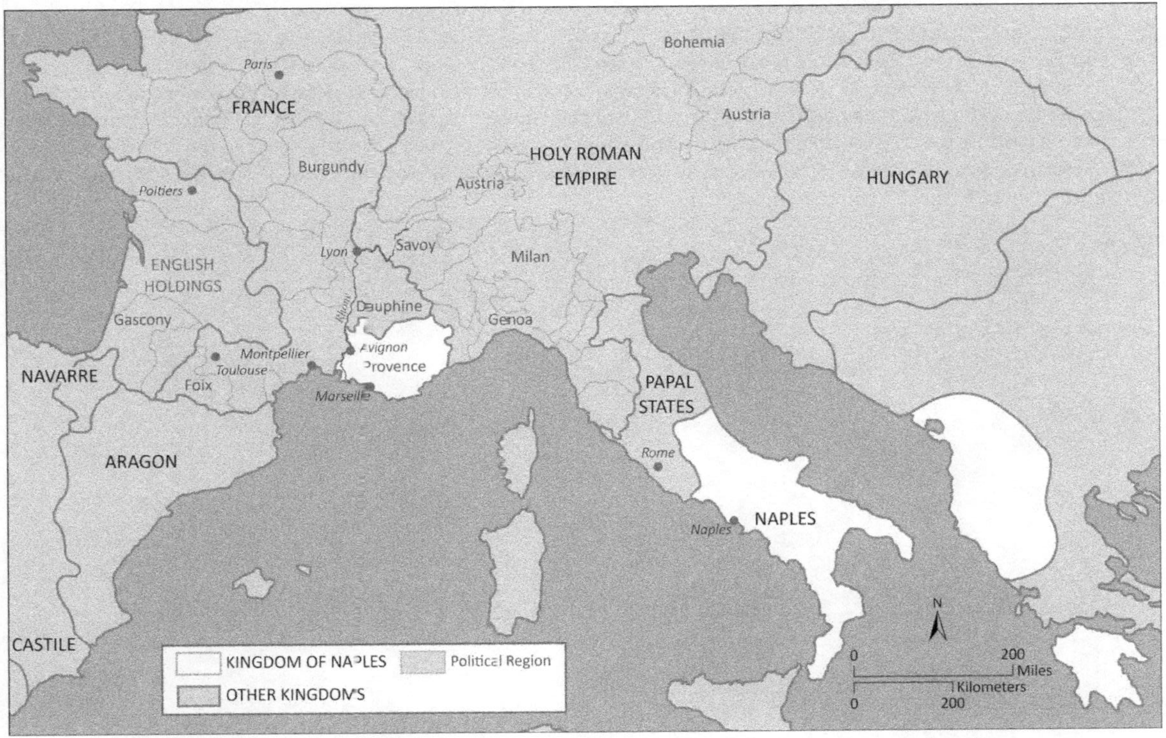

Map 1. The Kingdom of Naples and Approximate Political Boundaries in 1360. Created by Joshua Reyling, Geospatial Centroid, CSU, using ArcGIS® software by Esri. ArcGIS®, ArcMap™, and ArcGIS Pro™, which are the intellectual property of Esri and are used herein under license. Copyright © Esri. All rights reserved. For more information about Esri® software, please visit www.esri.com. Spatial Reference: Datum and Coordinate System—GCS European 1950; Projection—Europe Lambert Conformal Conic; Map Scale—1:11,500,000. Sources: Donald J. A. Matthew, *Atlas du Moyen Age* (Paris: Editions du Fanal, 1996); Léon Mirot and Albert Mirot, *Manuel de géographie historique de la France* (Paris: Picard, 1980); and Wikimedia Commons.

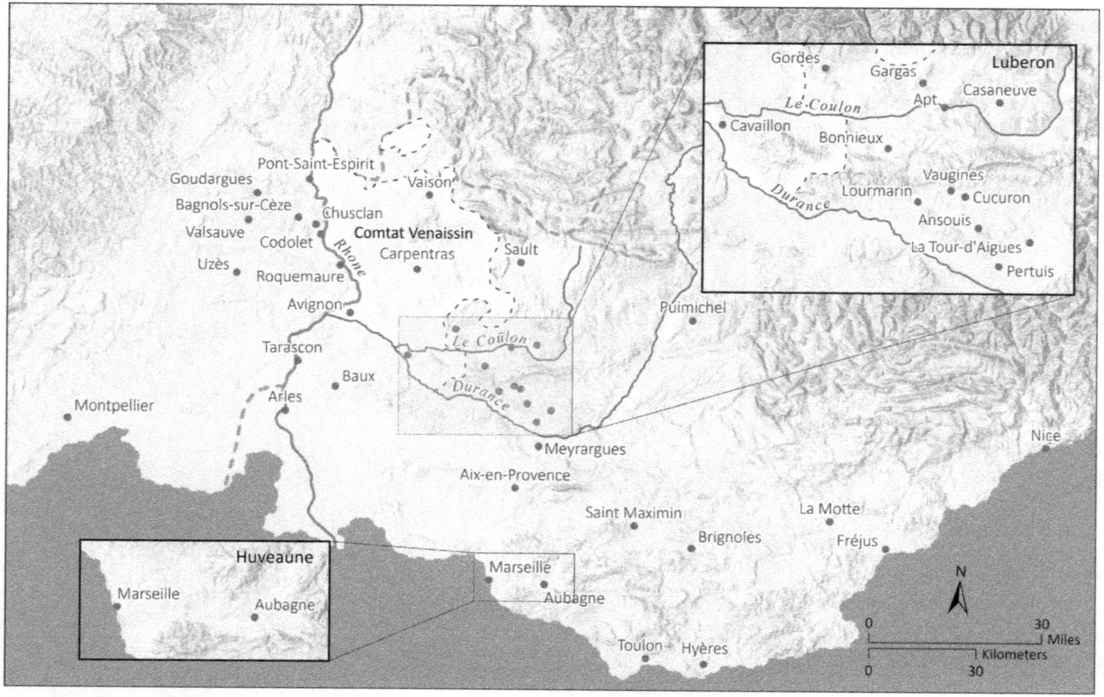

Map 2. Provence, the Luberon region, and the Huveaune valley. Created by Joshua Reyling, Geospatial Centroid, CSU, using ArcGIS® software by Esri. ArcGIS®, ArcMap™, and ArcGIS Pro™, which are the intellectual property of Esri and are used herein under license. Copyright © Esri. All rights reserved. For more information about Esri® software, please visit www.esri.com. Spatial Reference: Datum and Coordinate System—GCS European 1950; Projection—Europe Lambert Conformal Conic; Map Scale—1:1,500,000. Sources: Édouard Baratier, *Atlas historique: Provence, Comtat Venaissin, principauté d'Orange, comté de Nice, principauté de Monaco* (Paris: A. Colin, 1969); Wikimedia Commons; and Esri; Airbus DS; USGS; NGA; NASA; CGIAR; N. Robinson; NCEAS; NLS; OS; NMA; Geodatastyrelsen; Rijkswaterstaat; GSA; Geoland; FEMA; Intermap; and the GIS user community.

SOULS UNDER SIEGE

Introduction

Telling Stories of Danger in Fourteenth-Century Provence

In Provence, people spoke of a holy woman who healed sadness, grief, and anxiety during the late fourteenth century, when the Black Death killed a quarter of the population and the Hundred Years War threatened the rest. Her name was Countess Delphine de Puimichel. After she died in 1360, her family and community tried to get her canonized. The papacy held a legal inquest to decide if she should be a saint. This book is not about Countess Delphine, but is instead about the witnesses in her inquest, who told stories of plague, war, and confession in a swiftly changing world.

In the summer and fall of 1363, sixty-eight witnesses spoke in the canonization inquest for Countess Delphine. Most stood before two papally appointed commissioners—the archbishop of Aix-en-Provence and the bishop of Vaison—in the cathedral of St. Anne in Apt, Provence. A scattering of other witnesses testified from within convent walls or, in a private house in Avignon, and one special witness even testified from her own bed. For the majority of witnesses, two notaries, one local and one appointed by the papal court, wrote their testimonies down. Papal instructions ordered the notaries to stay as faithful as they could to witnesses' words even as they transformed testimonies from first person to third person and spoken Provençal into Latin.[1]

These witnesses had astounding stories to tell. Every one had survived the first wave of plague in 1348 and the second wave in 1361. They had survived the mercenary invasion of 1357–1358 and a much larger invasion of the Great

Companies in 1361, when mercenaries seized one of the main bridges over the Rhône River. They had all lived through the turbulent transfer of the throne of Naples from King Robert the Wise to his granddaughter, Queen Johanna I. Queen Johanna was just coming out of the shadow of her second husband, Louis of Taranto, as witnesses spoke to the papal commissioners in 1363. Witnesses told commissioners stories of war and plague and how their holy countess had saved them, their loved ones, or their colleagues. Through their stories, these sixty-eight witnesses show how they adapted to new pressures between 1343 and 1363. Because the canonization inquest happened when and where it did, the testimonies of these sixty-eight pious people can provide insight into the experience of the crises of the fourteenth century in Provence and perhaps in much of Europe.[2]

The witnesses included a range of people: servants and noble lords, local nuns and future cardinals, merchants and soldiers. They were linked to one another by their experiences with their holy woman and willingness to speak on her behalf. But the links often went deeper. Some had traveled together, worked together, or witnessed each other's miraculous healing. Some were extended family. Others shared relationships of vassalage. Many attended the same churches, heard the same sermons, read the same books, and visited the same confessors. And they all had political and social identities outside of the inquest. They were members of the papal court, the royal court of Naples, the Franciscan community, the merchant community, or local households. They lived in networks that shared stories of their holy countess's sanctity and miracles, at times across Provence and the kingdom of Naples, at other times across the street.[3]

How can we best use these stories about a local saint to understand the lived experience of crisis in mid-fourteenth-century Provence? While canonization inquest testimony has strengths and limitations as a historical source, which I will address in a moment, using these stories first requires scholars' awareness. We must avoid imposing modern assumptions about plague, war, and confession on people who had, in many ways, a very different worldview. And if we want to understand the witnesses' view, we must deeply contextualize their testimonies in order to understand how they perceived their experiences, the events and people they referred to, and the politics and culture that shaped their reactions.[4] We need to see the world that they shared with the papal commissioners who questioned them.[5] This was a world they did not feel that they had to explain, and which therefore can elude the modern reader who does not share it. At the same time, however, we do not want to lose sight of the broad picture of profound change during these decades. Nor do we want to lose voices that speak to surviving crisis across time and place. Therefore, the historian's bird's-eye view is also crucial, but should not obscure the view on the ground.

This process of combining deeply contextualized individual stories with the historian's broad view does not result in one clear statement about how medieval people handled these crises. But the diverse experiences and reactions of this specific group can give modern scholars insight.[6] Perhaps the most profound insight the stories reveal is that these crises were not separate for people living through them, as they can be for modern researchers far removed from them. Instead, each element of the crises became interwoven into a story. And witnesses used the language of sickness of body and soul to frame that story.[7] As people spoke to each other in the process of trying to understand and survive the many dangers they faced, they shared stories of remedies—for plague, political violence, and the difficulties of confession—to return themselves and their region to health.

Studying the Crises of the Fourteenth Century

When modern audiences consider the crises that afflicted western Europe in the fourteenth century, they tend to pick one or another to focus on, rather than considering them all at once. Plague is usually the one that first comes to mind, with good reason. The first wave of plague, what is now commonly referred to as the Black Death, lasted from 1347 to 1351 and killed an estimated 40 percent to 60 percent of the population.[8] Even at a time when epidemics could be annual events, this plague was different. Letters and descriptions spread before and during this plague. City governments improved public health measures and disseminated medical texts.[9] Several authors wrote of this plague as a punishment from God.[10] More wrote of it as a moment when social bonds broke down.[11] Notarial evidence shows that bishoprics and city governments struggled for months with the loss of life before they regained their footing.[12] The impact on inheritance challenged families, landowners, and renters.[13]

When the second wave moved through Europe in 1360–1362, however, the epidemic changed in people's minds. While still devastating, it was no longer a one-of-a-kind catastrophe. It became an illness with symptoms that doctors could identify and start to heal. It remained disruptive, but towns, cities, and kingdoms developed ways to respond.[14] By studying testimonies collected in 1363, this book captures this post–second wave understanding of the plague.

Individuals' stories from the time, however, reveal that plague was only *one* crisis that people faced. And for the community at the center of this book, it may not have been perceived as the worst one. At the same time that plague swept through, mercenary violence was destabilizing much of the European continent.[15] Mercenaries had always existed, but by the mid-fourteenth century constant warfare between city-states and kingdoms spurred the demand for hired soldiers until they became the main troops in Europe.[16] Thousands of fast-moving, battle-experienced companies were organized around successful leaders with little kingdom affiliation. When unemployed, especially during truces, many mercenary companies lived off the land, attacking towns and cities until they were hired again. Due to the growing number of mercenaries in the mid-fourteenth century, the experience of warfare changed for witnesses in this canonization inquest.[17] What had before felt like a dispute between lords that negotiation could often solve, by the mid-fourteenth century began to feel like a leaderless free-for-all.[18]

Surviving documents show that mercenary warfare was just as devastating as plague. Like the plague, it disrupted the physical and cultural structures of daily life.[19] For example, towns and cities reshaped their physical boundaries by abandoning or destroying structures outside city walls, including monasteries, grain storage buildings, and even whole suburbs.[20] Mercenary violence undermined pilgrimage, trade, and bureaucracy by making travel extremely dangerous. When mercenaries moved through a region they disrupted agricultural production and sanitation.[21] On a cultural level, mercenary violence undermined social and political expectations.[22] Local lords could no longer protect their communities or their own honor against these highly trained troops, many of whom were from a lower social status. Instead of fighting, local lords had to go into debt to hire more mercenaries to protect their communities.

Combining witness testimonies with the history of plague and war in Provence reveals that for people at the time, these crises were interconnected through the moral worldview of sin. Concern about sin formed the core of how this community understood and presented their own and others' behavior, whether those others were neighbors, violent mercenaries, or warring aristocratic lords. Sources show that the perceived sinfulness of political leaders, for example, increased the sense of widespread spiritual sickness.[23]

The language of health and healing was also the language of spiritual concern. The health of the body was linked to the health of the soul through words like *remedia* and *salus*, which were used simultaneously for physical and spiritual illness.[24] In this community, individuals described outward behavior—like violence against the Christian community and warfare—as sicknesses of the soul that caused people to sin continually, risking not just physical but also spiritual safety. In this way, groups like the mercenary companies were in constant spiritual danger. In contrast, peacefulness was a sign of spiritual and physical health.[25] In one plague treatise, for example, written for the people of Lerida in 1348, pestilence was both natural—a change in air—and moral—"a change in the spirit and in the thoughts of people, resulting in enmities and rancours, wars and robberies, destructions of places and deaths far beyond the ordinary."[26] This view is quite different from germ theory, which links a specific disease to a specific virus or a bacterium. Instead, pestilence was a change in the natural and spiritual (or moral) environment.

One important way that one healed spiritual illness was through the sacrament of penance. This idea had spread throughout the European Christian community in the thirteenth century through sermons, literature, and the increasing practice of the sacrament itself.[27] Confession—not just the face-to-face encounter with a priest, but all the elements of a complete confession—was necessary to heal spiritual sickness. In the mid-fourteenth century, waves of plague and war could increase the anxiety surrounding sin and make access to confession, especially the crucial deathbed confession, uncertain. At the same time, the desire for spiritual health during waves of plague and war made the sacrament of penance more attractive.

While a complete confession could heal spiritual illness, the elements of a complete confession were physically and spiritually demanding, and the results often less than desired. The pious people at the center of this book described their need for the sacrament of penance to be a fulfilling, transformative experience.[28] But according to their stories, that need was rarely met. They struggled to understand what they should confess and how they should perform penance. They struggled against their dying bodies to remember all of their sins and say them aloud. Many struggled with worldly demands at odds with the demands of the sacrament. They did not feel the consolation they expected. This quiet crisis of confession made healing the spiritual damage of war and plague difficult, if not impossible.

Souls under Siege brings all three crises together by exploring the testimonies of one group of diverse people in Provence, all of whom faced the dangers of plague, war, and confession just like others on the continent. The book focuses on twenty crucial years when fundamental changes occurred in Europe and people adapted to new problems, some of which are well known, like plague, and others harder to see, like the difficulties of confession.[29] The book deeply contextualizes these individuals' stories, showing how people at the time understood the different crises as symptoms of widespread spiritual sickness.

Testimony from 1363

Individuals' stories anchor *Souls under Siege* in fourteenth-century experience.[30] Witness testimonies reveal a community—a group of men and women of varying status surrounding Delphine, which we see in figure 0.1 in an anonymous painting of her vigil.[31] The community shared her values, though they practiced them at a much less exalted level, and they believed in her grace. While they did not all live in the same town or share the same social status, they shared a point of view shaped by their piety and their experiences in Provence. Their testimonies are this book's primary vantage point onto the transformative crises of the fourteenth century.

Like other research that uses canonization inquest testimony for social and cultural history, *Souls under Siege* turns the spotlight away from the saint and onto the inquest witnesses and organizers.[32] Although the stated goal of a canonization inquest was to collect information on the sanctity of a holy person, the questions and testimonies can end up revealing more about the goals and fears of the community surrounding the holy figure.[33] Witnesses in this inquest turned to Delphine in times of need because they saw her—like other saints—as someone with a special relationship to God who could therefore aid them at difficult moments.[34] Delphine could heal their illnesses, because nothing is beyond God, and she had God's ear. Between 1343 and 1363, when these witnesses started to face plague and mercenary invasions—new symptoms of widespread spiritual sickness—they turned to their holy woman for healing. When danger, physical weakness, or confusion disrupted their practice of the sacrament of penance, they also turned to Delphine. The inquest, therefore, provides fascinating insight into how people manipulated the "tools" they had, such as saints and the miracles that could occur through them. Through Delphine, the witnesses understood waves of plague and mercenary attack as symptoms of a sickness that she could heal if they were worthy of miracle. The anxiety they then felt for their souls shows they understood how miraculous healing worked and strove to be worthy of God's grace.[35]

In all of these witness narratives, we see people presenting their perspective of events to the commissioners. Their stories, whether or not they were "true," revealed the ways they had come to make sense of catastrophe.[36] They explained how they experienced waves of plague, the dangers of warfare, or the moment of confession. A key component of making sense was placing the events and behavior in a moral framework. As Elinor Ochs and Lisa Capps reveal about the modern world, "Everyday narratives of personal experience elaborately encode and perpetuate moral worldviews."[37] While these were not everyday or modern narratives, they did reflect witnesses' morality. This is not

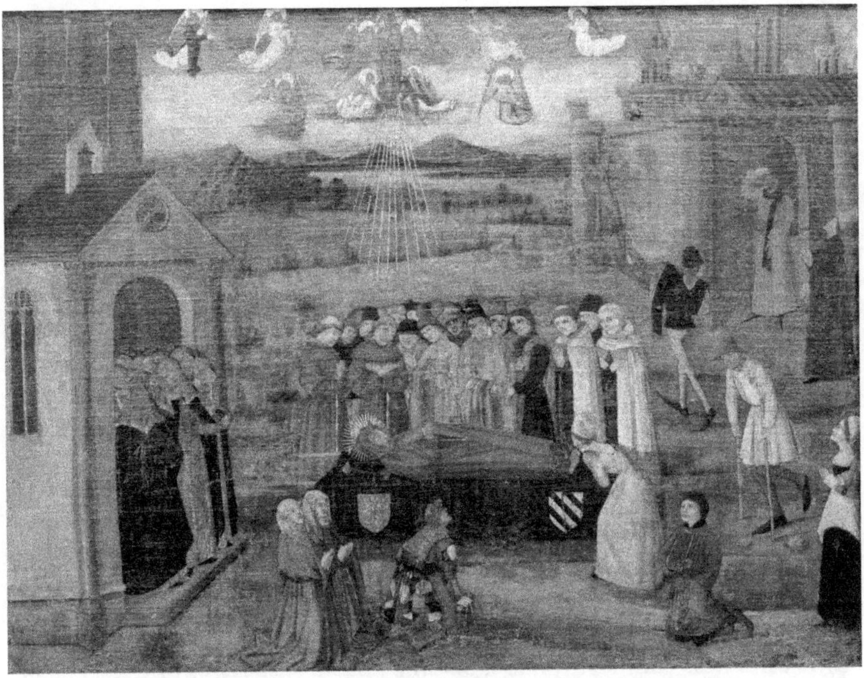

Figure 0.1. The Vigil for Delphine de Puimichel. Used with permission from Prof. Yann Codou

to say that witnesses believed they had survived because they were morally better than other people. Instead, their testimonies reveal how they wove events and people into a moral worldview that included crisis. The first wave of plague became the morally charged backdrop to the spiritual sickness of civil war. The anxiety surrounding confession revealed the struggle to be worthy of God's healing forgiveness. The struggle was embodied in narratives about giving up possessions and wearing humble clothing.

Witnesses used the language of health and sickness to speak of this moral framework.[38] Sinful behavior indicated spiritual sickness. Spiritual healing appeared publicly as reformed behavior. Again, this fit the local moral worldview of these witnesses. As Arthur Kleinman puts it, "Local cultural orientations (the patterned ways that we have learned to think about and act in our life worlds and that replicate the social structure of those worlds) organize our conventional common sense about how to understand and treat illness; thus we can say of illness experience that it is always culturally shaped."[39] The witnesses understood war, plague, and difficulties with the sacrament of penance as sickness and sought Delphine's voice and touch for a remedy.

Witnesses' language of morality and health in these narratives frequently included emotion words. As John Arnold reminds us, "Much of the vocabulary of emotion [in the West] is drawn from the language of sin, confession, and penance."[40] Witnesses described these life and soul threatening events as moments of transformation of their own and others internal states, therefore their testimonies can give us insight into their emotional world at this highly charged time.[41]

Some instances of emotion in Delphine's inquest fit clearly into studied patterns. For example, emotion words used in articles and testimonies mirrored legal, political, and medical expressions of hatred and love common at the time. Hatred expressed through warfare was a scandal and a sickness of the soul that could be healed with love and affection.[42] Witnesses also used emotion words to describe their reaction to extreme experiences.[43] Mercenaries, plague, and the complexities of confession inspired fear, confusion, and sadness.[44] Through protection, physical healing, and clear explanation, the witnesses perceived that Delphine transformed their internal, negative emotional states.

In medical understandings of emotion, negative emotional states could damage a person's health, while positive emotional states could improve it. Interestingly, several witnesses paired the experience of sorrow with particular physical states. They lost volition, became unable to speak or to walk, and became unable to experience positive internal states. These descriptions resonated with medical understandings of melancholy that had been in circulation for centuries, but were gaining new notice through increasing access to university trained medical practitioners and the growing popularity of regimens of health.[45]

Internal transformation was a key component of witness narratives about plague, war, and confession. It was crucial to healing, peacemaking, and problem solving. For this pious, educated community, which shared a belief in Countess Delphine de Puimichel as a holy woman who could channel God's grace, solutions to many problems started inside. Solutions did not start with microbiology or a peace treaty; they started with healing sin and repairing the soul's relationship to God.[46] Understanding this, what historians refer to as penitence, helps us see how confession was a moment of danger as much as any wave of plague or mercenary invasion.

Individuals Telling Stories

These statements of witnesses' internal selves are not timeless or pan-European. These sixty-eight witnesses spoke in a canonization inquest in 1363 in Provence. Time and place shaped the cultural options open to express their experience of war, plague, and confession. And the genre of canonization inquest shaped the statements that they could make.[47] Testimony reflects a specific moment in time as witnesses struggled to adapt to a devastating disease that they had only recently realized could recur. It was also a specific moment in the history of warfare as the dangerous impact of increasing use of mercenary troops played out in the Rhône valley. And testimony reveals an awareness of and a desire to reform the internal self increasingly possible in the later Middle Ages.[48]

The witnesses in Delphine's inquest lived in Provence—a key county of the kingdom of Naples, the residence of the papacy for much of the fourteenth century, and site of the major Mediterranean port of Marseille. And while they were not a random sampling of fourteenth-century Provençaux, they were still a relatively diverse group.[49] The group included roughly half men and half women. Many witnesses had traveled, were wealthy, and were educated. Many male witnesses were highly politically connected, and included a cardinal, the bishop of Avignon, the master of accounts of Provence, and a seneschal of Provence. Many female witnesses were from important families enmeshed in the political events of these twenty years of crisis.[50]

Many witnesses moved in the highest circles of Provençal power, and some of them influenced a broader political world. Because of who the witnesses were and because of who Delphine was, the witness testimonies were not spontaneous, neutral stories about life in Provence in the fourteenth century. They were constructed narratives influenced by the witnesses' status, political events, and the demands of a canonization inquest. In many ways, the things that appear to limit witness testimony make it even more revealing. For example, what witnesses do not talk about resonates in their stories as much as what they do mention. Or, when they talk about a significant crisis in an unexpected way, it sheds light on how they understood that crisis as part of their lives.

We find in their stories that the three crises were understood as affecting all of Europe but were simultaneously understood as extremely personal and local. Personal understandings and expressions of crisis were shaped by local and regional politics and events. It quickly becomes clear that local political figures and structures shaped how people understood and described plague, warfare, and sin and confession in their communities, even if they were active in much broader political spheres. In other words, for several witnesses, the perception of the queen of Naples, enmeshed in a scandal over the death of her first husband, shaped the Provençal experience of plague, war, and confession. But it shaped the perspectives of those who knew her more than those who did not. For those with a less extensive political network, things like food production needs, local rivalries, and faith in local saints shaped their experience more.

So when trying to understand the large crises of the fourteenth century, an in-depth local study reveals a different picture from a broadly comparative one. A local, contextualized study can bring these three crises together by showing how people found ways to understand and even confront the destabilizing experiences of war, plague, and confession in their lives. But testimony was embedded in its political and cultural landscape. When reading the testimonies of politically connected individuals, we have to dig deeply into political disputes at times to understand what witnesses reacted to and how. The contextualization is worth it to see how these people used their holy woman to address, and at times resolve, the dangers they perceived.

An important contextual step is to uncover witness perspectives of the holy person they spoke about. In this local study, witnesses spoke about Countess Delphine de Puimichel. Delphine was seventy-five years old when she died in 1360.[51] For most of the witnesses, who on average were between thirty and forty-five years old, she had been part of their whole lives. Witnesses had a lot to say about Delphine because they had known her and interacted with her, sometimes for decades. As an inhabitant of various towns in Provence, she had gone to mass, spoken at convents, and even begged in the streets. As a noblewoman of Provence, Delphine had been politically connected to its major families, the royal court, and the papal court.

In the fourteenth century, the county of Provence was part of the discontiguous kingdom of Naples held by the Angevins (see map 1).[52] The kings of Naples were the counts of Provence, and the Provençal aristocracy swore fealty, and paid taxes, to them.[53] Delphine's title, however, was the Countess of Ariano, which was a small region near Naples in the Italian peninsula. Her husband, Count Elzear de Sabran, received this title for his service to King Robert of Naples.

For witnesses, Delphine was their "holy countess."[54] The term encapsulates a paradoxical identity. Witnesses and organizers described her as extraordinarily pious, exemplified by the fact that they believed she had practiced lifelong virginity, vigils, fasts, and prayer. She was also the widow of a candidate for sainthood, a kind of living relic of her saintly husband. At the same time, she was part of the political world. With Elzear, she had developed a close relationship with King Robert and Queen Sanxia, living in their court for years at a time.[55] Delphine was also present, at Queen Sanxia's invitation, for King Robert's death and the transfer of political power to a council overseeing the minority of Johanna I in 1343. For many witnesses, their holy countess was in a unique position to influence the specific dangers they faced.

While a few witnesses were Delphine's social equals or held positions at the papal or royal courts, more were from the local Provençal aristocracy and their households. These were the aristocracy of cities rather than part of the royal court of Naples.[56] For these witnesses, their relationship with Delphine raised their status and linked them to the broader political sphere. Not all witnesses were aristocratic, however. Others were Franciscan friars, Augustinian and Benedictine nuns, and merchants. Delphine also gave these witnesses a voice in the broader political sphere that affected them on a daily basis, but over which they had little control. With different social status, ages, and gender, they did not experience the political events of the 1340s through the early 1360s in identical ways. Their testimonies give us the perspectives of leaders and servants, soldiers and clergy, and men and women.

Although witnesses spoke carefully in this official inquest, their stories about Delphine's sanctity were not politically neutral. Not only were witnesses involved in political events, but they spoke of a woman who had been involved in Provençal politics at the highest levels. Even the forum of a canonization inquest was deeply political.[57] No one involved could just tell a story. There were rules and expectations to their encounter in the inquest, and their words had an impact beyond just the moment of giving testimony.[58]

For the witnesses, both Delphine's and their own complex identities shaped every encounter. For example, Lord Giraud de Simiana, the lord of Apt and a future seneschal of Provence, described Delphine speaking in the papal court of Clement VI in support of her husband Elzear's canonization with wondrous clarity and influence. For Lord Giraud, she spoke not just as a holy woman but as his family member, Elzear's widow, and as a countess living an exemplary life of poverty and piety. He, in turn, told the story to the papal commissioners as a member of the upper aristocracy of Provence. Who he was, who Delphine was, and the rules of the canonization inquest encounter shaped everything he said. This shaping was not active suppression or censorship imposed by a nefarious entity—"the Church," for example—but instead the shaping force of self and audience that we all experience as we tell a story.[59]

Witnesses in Provence could not separate Delphine's friendships from the political sphere, not at a time when friendship was a political status.[60] These witnesses never forgot that Delphine and her husband, Elzear, had been the close associates—friends—of King Robert and Queen Sanxia of Naples. And the witnesses did not forget that Delphine had known but had *not* been a friend of Queen Johanna and King Louis of Taranto, who ruled Naples after Robert died. During her life, Delphine had spoken as a noblewoman, a countess, and a holy woman whenever she spoke. For these witnesses, when they spoke of Delphine's life, therefore, they were speaking of political events and spiritual relationships that they were still navigating even after her death.[61]

The identities of the witnesses were as diverse as that of the holy woman they spoke of.[62] When Lord Guilhem Enric spoke of Delphine's life and miracles, for example, he spoke as a pious Christian who believed that Delphine's sanctity had saved Ansouis from mercenary attack. But he did not stop being a legal professional in the royal court of Provence. When Cardinal Philippe Cabassole testified, he did not stop being the titular patriarch of Jerusalem. Even Delphine's maid, Bertranda Bertomieua, spoke with awareness of the broader political sphere she inhabited because of her relationship to Delphine.

This complex of identities was true for every witness, not just politically connected ones. For witnesses who saw her locally, for example, she may have cleaned the kitchen in the hermitage of Cabrières, but she had at one time been the *domina* of the region, living in the nearby castle in Ansouis. None of the witnesses nor those conducting the inquest forgot this. Some witnesses even described themselves as her vassals, even though Delphine tried to give up her titles and sell all of her property in her search for humility.[63] These multiple identities in each testimony help us see the diverse, flexible ways that people encountered plague, war, and confession and how they tried to make sense of their experiences.

The Inquest as an Event

If what the witnesses did and did not say was shaped by the canonization inquest that brought them together, it is useful to understand this kind of inquest. By the fourteenth century, canonization inquests were large-scale legal procedures sanctioned and run by the papacy that explored the life events and reputation of candidates for canonization.[64] They were not overly standardized, however. For example, while all canonization inquests had witnesses, the number, social status, and sex distribution could vary widely.[65] And while all inquests included descriptions of life events and miracles for the holy person, these materials could be written and organized in very different ways.[66]

Countess Delphine's inquest included sixty-eight witnesses, roughly half men and half women, from a range of social and political backgrounds. They were all given the opportunity to answer almost one hundred questions about their holy woman. Their testimonies survive in the notarial record of the hearings, rather than in a summary format or preliminary sketch.[67] Witness testimony in this record was not sorted by miracle or life event, but instead by the order in which witnesses testified.[68] This means that witnesses to the same miracle or life event could appear in very different places in the inquest. While this can be a bit confusing for isolating specific events or miracles, it does keep each witness's testimony intact. In this way a modern scholar can see more clearly how witnesses moved from one idea to another as they testified and may have created associations between events for their audience.

Delphine's official inquest began May 14, 1363, roughly three years after the holy woman died.[69] Like other official canonization inquests, Delphine's opened with the reading of the papal letters at the Franciscan house in Apt, describing the tasks and goals of the commissioners and proctor.[70] The last witness was questioned on October 18 of the same year.

A brief look at the day-to-day proceedings of Delphine's inquest gives a sense of what witnesses would have experienced and how the commissioners collected information. From mid-May to the beginning of July, one or more people were interviewed per day before the commissioners, the main notaries, and sometimes others. Most questioning occurred in the church of Apt, most likely the cathedral of St. Anne, though some took place elsewhere.[71] For example, the commissioners and notaries went to the convents of St. Catherine and the Holy Cross to question the nuns and other women who lived in the convents. They also went to the bedside of Delphine's maid, Bertranda Bertomieua, because she was too ill to walk.[72] And, after a two-month hiatus, five more witnesses were questioned in the city of Avignon between October 6 and 18.

During the inquiry, the proctor, Master Nicolau Laurens, a notary in Apt, was responsible for the witnesses and the questioning procedure.[73] He gathered the witnesses ahead of time, assured that they would arrive at a set day and time, and took an oath before the commissioners attesting to the truthfulness of the witnesses. Laurens had been associated with Delphine since he had conducted the canonization inquest for her husband in 1351.[74] Delphine's inquest reveals that he had been collecting material and witnesses for her canonization for almost a decade.[75]

Most importantly, Laurens also wrote the ninety-eight articles of interrogation that summarized Delphine's life events, characteristics, living miracles, and posthumous miracles. These articles captured witnesses' views and experiences of Delphine, since they were constructed from the stories that witnesses told Laurens as he gathered information for Delphine's inquest.[76] If we want to understand witnesses' testimonies, it is important to understand the articles they spoke in response to.

In all fourteenth-century canonization inquests, witnesses were read a series of articles of interrogation.[77] In some inquests, witnesses testifying to articles about the life of the holy person were mostly separate from witnesses for the miracles. We see this clearly in the inquest for St. Louis of Anjou, for example. Of the 207 witnesses in that inquest, 32 testified to the events of his life and 175 testified to his miracles. Only two witnesses who testified to his life events crossed over into the second group.[78]

This did not happen in Delphine's inquest. Every witness was given the opportunity to speak to all ninety-eight articles. Commissioners for Delphine's inquest had the articles read to the witnesses in Latin or their *lingua materna*, and witnesses responded in the language they knew.[79] After each article, the witnesses could either choose to speak about it or pass on. Witnesses spoke to whatever articles they had information for and passed over articles about which they claimed to know nothing. Alternatively, some witnesses opted not to hear all the articles and instead only spoke about one or two. In these cases, only those articles were read to the witness.[80]

As witnesses in Delphine's inquest spoke in response to the articles of interrogation, they did not stick to the articles like a script. They told the commissioners what they had seen and heard, even if it differed from the article of interrogation. They reinterpreted or redirected the articles in order to talk about different events or people than those mentioned. And they presented their understanding of important events, which could differ significantly from the article and other witnesses' versions.[81]

Perhaps the most revealing articles of Delphine's inquest for modern scholars, however, are two open-ended articles that all witnesses were given the opportunity to speak to. Article 1, the first article of interrogation, invited witnesses to tell the commissioners everything they knew about Delphine's life, living miracles, and posthumous miracles. Twenty-four witnesses chose to speak to this article, and many told personal, detailed stories unstructured by the language of the official articles of the same event. In some instances they described events and miracles that appear nowhere else in the inquest. The second open-ended article, Article 35, asked witnesses about any internal transformations—from sinful to pious or from anxious to assured—that they experienced, saw, or heard about. Twenty witnesses responded with stories of their own and others' sin and confession experiences, many of which included significant language of emotion. While this procedure would not have been ideal for evidence collection in a fourteenth-century legal procedure, these responses are fascinating for modern scholars looking at how people tell stories.[82]

The importance of these rare, open-ended articles cannot be overemphasized. While many articles highlighted what was important to the organizers and the papacy—like Delphine's virginity and poverty—the open-ended articles let witnesses speak about what was important to them.[83] These stories reveal the witnesses' needs, fears, actions, expectations, and reactions during crises of plague, warfare, and confession. For example, there were no articles of interrogation that asked about plague. Everything witnesses said about the first and second waves of plague appeared in answer to Article 1. In this way, testimonies tell us much more about the members of this community than they do about Delphine. They shed light on the perceived dangers these witnesses faced in mid-fourteenth-century Provence and their strategies for articulating those dangers.

After the witness spoke about an article, the papal commissioners asked questions about the testimony. The most common questions included those found in many legal inquiries in the fourteenth century, such as "When did this happen?" "Where did it happen?," "Who was there?"[84] The commissioners also prompted witnesses to speak more fully by asking if the witness remembered anything else.[85] A letter read when the inquest opened included these questions and urged that the words of the witnesses be faithfully recorded in writing.[86]

A testimony like that of Delphine's confessor and medical doctor, Master Durand Andree, who spoke about almost fifty articles, could have taken hours, while witnesses who spoke to only a few articles likely went through the process more quickly. Thirty witnesses, a little less than half of the entire number, chose to speak only about one article.[87]

Although it is not stated who was present at questioning every day, a few exemplary moments allow us to see the kinds of people who might be present. For example, in some instances a young person who experienced a miraculous healing, but was too young to testify, was brought in to be examined by the commissioners. On the day when the son of Savaric Bot was brought in, for example, the people in attendance included the commissioners, the primary notaries, Master Durand Andree, and Master Johan de Taffris of the Limoges diocese.[88] When Louis, the object of Article 87, was brought in for examination, the list included the commissioners, the primary notaries, Aycard Bot, Master Henri of Diepenheim, and Master Michael Engelberti.[89] From these two exceptional moments, we have some evidence that the commissioners and primary notaries were present each day, but other people, perhaps experts such as physicians, might be brought in as needed.

Overall, there does not seem to have been an order in which witnesses were interviewed. On the same day, men and women, noble and common, religious and lay were interviewed in the church of Apt or other locations. There also does not seem to have been a clear hierarchy of testimony based on social class. Servants and merchants often testified at greater length about Delphine's life and her miracles than high nobility.

June 8 is an interesting example of this mix of witnesses and the varying length of testimonies. On this day, commissioners saw five witnesses in succession: Ayscelena, wife of Peire Pelliceri of Apt; Louis Manenti, identified as a burgher and *syndicus* of Apt; noble lady Francisca, widow of noble lord Raymon Bot of Apt; noble lady Ysoarda, wife of noble lord Laugier de Gorda of Apt; and Alazays Mesellano, the widow of Johan Mesellano, a draper of Apt.

Both Ayscelena Pelliceri and Louis Manenti testified at various lengths to one posthumous miracle each.[90] Both noble ladies Francisca Bot and Ysoarda Laugier addressed Article 1—the open-ended article that asked witnesses to discuss everything they knew about Delphine. Francisca testified at length and included not just information about Delphine's life, but also information about how Delphine cured her of a fever. Ysoarda primarily supported Francisca's story about the fever.[91] The last witness of the day, the draper's widow Alazays Mesellano, spoke by far the longest. She gave a detailed testimony to Article 1, discussing both Delphine's life and her miracles. Her testimony revealed a perceived close relationship between herself and Delphine. Alazays also addressed Article 25 concerning Delphine's charity to the poor, Article 35 concerning the spiritual transformations Delphine caused in people, and Article 69 concerning Alazays herself being cured of a rupture caused by a fall.[92] This sample day shows the variety of testimony that the commissioners saw.

During the inquest, commissioners did more than just hear witnesses. They also visited sites of popular devotion. One of the commissioners' more interesting outings occurred on July 2, the feast of the Visitation of the Virgin Mary, when the commissioners examined Delphine's *publica fama*.[93] On this important feast day, when they could be sure a large number of people would come to mass, the commissioners and a large group of dignitaries attended mass at the church of Apt.[94] Lord Raymon, the bishop of Apt, led the mass for all assembled.[95] During the proceedings, the papal commissioner from Aix-en-Provence spoke in a clear and intelligible voice in the common tongue to everyone gathered there. He asked people to recall whatever they could about Delphine, so that the commissioners could perfect what they knew before going to the pope with the information.[96] He particularly asked them about Delphine's virginity, her donations to the poor, and miracles (both *in vita* and *post mortem*). At this point, the bishop of Apt went out to the congregation to explain what the commissioners wanted and ask people what they knew. The people swore that they knew about Delphine's holy life by raising their hands toward the altar.

After gathering information, the bishop returned to the commissioners and told them what he found out. The congregation was again asked to swear to what they said by raising their hands to the altar. Not all the people present took part in this pledge, but "a greater part raised their hands and extended them against the altar of the church."[97] The two main notaries repeated twice that they were asked to and did write down the proceedings. They listed all the regions where attendees were from and the names of people who were officially asked to witness the event. This ceremony likely had multiple purposes. On the one hand, it showed the papacy that Delphine had popular support. On the other, it gave organizers a chance to gather further information about Delphine and her miracles. This would prove useful if her first bid for canonization were rejected. Information gathered at this event could supplement the next inquest.

After the last witness deposition, there are two statements that conclude Delphine's inquest. The primary notaries—Iacob Octaviani de Guaschis from the papal court and Peire Thamiseri from Apt—stated that they worked together to collect all their materials, rewrite them into a clean draft, and create one book.[98] This text was presented to the commissioners and ultimately sent to the papal court of Urban V.[99]

Goals and Structure of the Book

Souls under Siege focuses on a group of individuals involved in a specific event—the canonization inquest for Countess Delphine. But instead of focusing on the inquest itself or the daily lives of individual participants, the book contextualizes their stories in the broader political and cultural world of mid-fourteenth-century Provence. The book uses witness stories of war, plague, and confession to reflect on larger events from the witnesses' perspective. For example, the serving woman Bertranda Bertomieua told several stories of the court of King Robert of Naples in 1342. This book tries to uncover the political context of her stories in order to reveal her response to King Robert's death and the political actions of his heir, Queen Johanna. This format allows us to explore the resonances of witness testimony for the history of this transformative moment.

Souls under Siege touches on broad topics—the Angevins, the Avignon Papacy, mercenaries, plague, and confession—all of which have a vast ecosystem of scholarship surrounding them. I have worked to ground the book in this scholarship, but many readers will have a far more nuanced understanding of each topic than I can cover here. It is important to point out, however, that the focus of the book is not any of these larger topics. Instead this is a book about how the witnesses in Delphine's inquest *spoke about* those subjects.

Therefore, the witnesses and the audiences of the canonization inquest are the focus of the book.

This book embraces testimony as crafted narrative shaped by the inquest format, audience, and purpose. Witnesses spoke carefully about every issue, and often their silences were as meaningful as their words. Each chapter highlights a specific witness or inquest organizer to explore the pressures of political identity that shaped every aspect of Delphine's canonization inquest. These pressures, too, give insight into the politics and culture of this region.

To analyze these crafted narratives, *Souls under Siege* owes a debt to Sharon Farmer's *Surviving Poverty* and Didier Lett's *Un procès de canonisation au Moyen Âge*, but also uses approaches adapted from linguistic anthropology. In discourse analysis, witness testimonies like these fall on a spectrum between living (or spontaneous) and practiced narratives.[100] The inquest documents show that Delphine's witnesses told some of their stories of miraculous survival again and again to multiple audiences over a span of time. But even though these were relatively practiced narratives, they were vivid for both teller and audiences. As in "danger of death" narratives in modern Western societies, the tellers likely partially relived the emotions of the moment each time they told the familiar story.[101] Other witnesses recall hearing these stories, even years later.

These miracle stories were also survival stories that served as problem-solving narratives, providing information about spiritual choices at dangerous moments. Witnesses described their own choices, but also saw the spiritual choices that others made, when they remarked on changes in clothing or behavior.[102] Finally, these testimonies functioned as moral narratives that reflected the ways the community gradually made sense of the crises and found different ways to adapt and respond.[103]

Because the goal of *Souls Under Siege* is to highlight the stories of people living through crises, I worked to avoid imposing my assumptions about those crises on them. What I discovered is that, while I and many other modern scholars were interested in their bodies and their physical world—what diseases they had, how many died of plague, the conduct and impact of warfare—the witnesses were equally, or more, interested in their souls and the spiritual world. They wanted to know the state of their own and others' souls and paid attention to what people wore, ate, and said as indicators of spiritual health. This is partly the result of the source. It *is* a canonization inquest, after all. But the stories they told revealed frequent, long-term consideration of both body and soul. Their concerns about the sacrament of penance and mercenary invasion were not separate concerns. For them, violence was too often a sin with as strong a spiritual impact as a physical one. Their stories revealed how they understood the multiple crises they faced as spiritual *and* physical crises.

To uncover the witnesses' perspective, and to limit imposing my own assumptions, I paid attention to moments when at least five witnesses spoke about one event as particularly perilous or about one moment in time as having many dangers. In this way, I uncovered two types of what I refer to as "moments of danger" from the witnesses' perspective. The first type was chronological. These were moments when war, plague, or both destabilized Provence. The second type was sacramental. Each witness would have experienced the sacrament of penance, but not at exactly the same time. It is clear many found it to be a moment of danger for their soul. These two types of "moments of danger" structure the book.[104]

Chapters 1–4 look at four main chronological moments of danger when witnesses turned to their holy woman for aid. Chapter 1 explores a destabilizing moment of change that underlays the chronological moments of danger in witness testimony. This was the death of King Robert of Naples in 1343. Sources outside the inquest present this as a moment of political transition for Provence and Mediterranean kingdoms. One witness who knew Delphine longer than anyone used his death as a time marker for several of Delphine's healing and protection miracles, framing this as a moment of missed opportunity for healthy peace. The first chronological moment of danger that witnesses described stemmed from political turmoil after 1343. In 1348–1349, witnesses experienced a narrowly averted war among Provençal lords as the first wave of plague, what they called "the first mortality," killed up to half of the population. Witnesses and their associates saw these events as symptoms of spiritual sickness that they used their holy countess to heal.

In the second and third chronological moments of danger, witnesses struggled to understand and speak about changes in warfare and violence. Witnesses described their experiences during a mercenary invasion in 1357–1358 and told the papal commissioners about transformation and protection miracles they experienced and heard about. Finally, in the third moment of danger, witnesses described their needs and experiences in 1361 during a second wave of plague simultaneous to a massive mercenary incursion during a truce in the Hundred Years War. These three chronological moments of danger reveal the swiftly changing experience of plague, warfare, and sin in the mid-fourteenth century.

Chapters 5 and 6 look at a sacramental, rather than chronological, moment of danger when witnesses could not complete the sacrament of penance or were not sure of the internal state of their souls. Over half the witnesses in the inquest testified to experiencing some kind of difficulty with one or more element of a complete confession, including memory loss, inability to speak, and anxiety-inducing confusion about penance. Witnesses also described a profound need to be assured about the state of their souls—a feeling they expected, but did not often experience, as part of the sacrament of penance. They found wondrous clarity and assurance in Delphine's voice and touch. Many experienced internal transformation and in turn changed their outward, sinful behavior.

In all of the moments of danger, the witnesses presented behavior as a reflection of the internal self. For the witnesses, sinful behavior, which included spiritually damaging violence as well as vanity and pride, indicated a soul at odds with God. This moment of danger could be a personal moment, when someone could not complete confession. Or it could be a public moment, when violence between noble lords threatened the souls and bodies of many in Provence. In all of these moments, the witnesses described how Delphine's words and actions provided a remedy for spiritual sickness. Their conception of sin as sickness shaped their understanding of events and gave them a solution through their local holy woman.

In their testimonies, witnesses appeared to be seeking control and consolation in situations rapidly moving beyond the scope of their political and spiritual leaders. Rather than whip themselves in the street—like the flagellants that so many histories of the time mention—these educated, pious, influential individuals found ways to use their holy woman for protection, healing, and internal transformation.[105] Through their narratives about her sanctity, they critiqued the institutions that had failed them. And through her voice and touch they took control of dangerous situations for themselves. Often control meant internal transformation for oneself or others. Healing the spiritual sicknesses caused by war, plague, and confession meant transforming political hatred into love, sorrow into consolation, or doubt into certainty. The witnesses used their holy woman to accomplish these transformations and survive twenty years of intense political, environmental, and social change.

Chapter 1

Bertranda Bertomieua and the Death of King Robert of Naples, 1343

The death of King Robert of Naples, the Count of Provence, was a precarious moment. His sons were dead, and a host of powerful lords had claims to the throne. Despite the strategies set out in King Robert's will, decades of violent political machinations emerged from this moment. For many witnesses in Delphine's canonization inquest, King Robert's death was the root of the first two chronological moments of danger: the narrowly averted civil war in Provence and the first mercenary invasion.[1]

The witness who provided the most insight into the death of King Robert in 1343 and the immediate transfer of political power was not a cardinal or a nobleman. Instead it was Delphine's maid, Bertranda Bertomieua. As Delphine's companion for almost fifty years, Bertranda lived with Delphine in Naples in 1342 and 1343 when Delphine was a guest of Queen Sanxia. Bertranda experienced the events in Naples neither from a political insider's view nor from the bird's-eye view of the historian. She brought instead the personal perspective of a member of Delphine's household.

Bertranda's testimony is a useful reminder that each witness in the inquest not only brought his or her own perspective to events, but they also saw different events. A witness like Bertranda saw what happened where she lived and to the people she knew. And through her individual background, her testimony gives us access to a specific political, social, and cultural moment. Members of the papal or royal courts, for example, would have presented events differently than she did. They had different experiences and information to draw on. Bertranda, as our closest vantage point in the inquest to King Robert's death, had a perspective shaped by her respect for Delphine's sanctity and her concern for Delphine's safety and reputation. She valued those who imitated and respected Delphine and critiqued those who did not, even if this meant subtly critiquing Robert's heir, Queen Johanna of Naples. We can use her testimony to understand the roots of two chronological moments of danger that witnesses faced. At the same time, we can also use her testimony as an introduction to what it meant to testify in this canonization inquest.

Bertranda Bertomieua as a Witness

Unlike the majority of witnesses—who were significantly younger than Delphine and had only known the holy woman for fifteen to twenty years—Bertranda had been Delphine's companion for almost five decades. She had entered Delphine's household shortly before Delphine's husband Elzear died in 1323 and lived with Delphine afterward. Bertranda slept in the same room as Delphine, ate with her, and traveled with her. From Bertranda's testimony, we learn about Delphine's private moments away from the eyes of various courts and convents. Bertranda gives an intimate view of Delphine as a wife. She described how Delphine and Elzear had practiced an intimate chasteness—lying in bed together as a married couple should, but remaining clothed. She even described how Delphine washed and cut Elzear's hair.[2]

Bertranda was an observant person, who, through Delphine, had spent years attached to the royal household in Naples and Provence. She saw how Elzear and Delphine had been close to the royal couple. King Robert had made Elzear Count of Ariano—a region close to the city of Naples—and depended on him as a political adviser who could handle difficult tasks with fairness. Elzear brought Delphine from Provence to live in Robert and Sanxia's court in Naples in the early 1300s. Delphine and Elzear were considered a pious couple and critiqued by some for having a court more like a monastery, in which they discouraged displays of wealth and activities such as dancing or gossiping.[3]

Most importantly for this study, Bertranda was present in Naples when King Robert died in 1343. Within Bertranda's poignant description of Countess Delphine as a caring, pious, and defiant woman, we also see a world of political instability. Her testimony about events in Delphine's life in 1343 reveals her impression of Naples and the royal court. Bertranda described how Delphine was insulted and threatened in the streets of Naples. But she also described how Delphine was welcomed into Sanxia's court and solved problems even King Robert could not solve.

We must keep in mind, however, that the stories Bertranda told as an inquest witness in 1363 were shaped by the twenty complicated years that had passed since King Robert's death. The ugly political infighting that followed his death had cast a dark and violent shadow over political relations with Provence. To understand her reaction to King Robert's death and her understanding of its implications, we have to listen closely. We ought to consider the stories that Bertranda chose to share not as random memories, but as selected stories from a woman who saw and heard a great deal as a member of Delphine's household.

What we know about Bertranda as a person comes from the inquest and from inference. At the time of Delphine's inquest, Bertranda was in her sixties, somewhat younger than Delphine, but still of a similar generation. Although her own testimony does not indicate where she was from, another witness referred to her as Lady Bertranda, and still others indicated that she was a member of the lower aristocracy from Puimichel, where Delphine's family had lived.[4] This makes sense for fourteenth-century Provence, where women from the lower aristocracy would serve in the households of powerful women.[5] Just as Countess Delphine and other aristocratic women of Provence waited on Queen Sanxia, Bertranda waited on Delphine. We also know from inquest testimony that Bertranda shared Delphine's commitment to avoiding a worldly lifestyle. Perhaps the strongest indication of this is that Bertranda never married. Instead she moved with Delphine from court to hermitage to convent.

At the time of the inquest, Bertranda was living in the Holy Cross convent in Apt, Provence, where Delphine had had her own room. Bertranda was very ill and could not get out of bed. But she was such an important witness that the papal commissioners, the proctor, and the notaries relocated to her room in order to hear her testimony. Not surprisingly, Bertranda has one of the longest testimonies in Delphine's inquest. She spoke to forty-eight articles of interrogation, and as she testified, we see a household member's perspective of this moment of political transition. Even when she was not present for important events, people of diverse social levels spoke to Bertranda, including King Robert of Naples, noblewomen of Provence, and other household servants.

Bertranda was a significant source of information about other people. In her testimony, Bertranda referred to over seventy-five people, all but a handful of whom she claimed to have spoken to directly or seen in person. Only about a third of these people were other witnesses in Delphine's inquest in

1363. So Bertranda's testimony brought many perspectives into the inquest. When the papal commissioners asked questions such as "Who told you this?" or "Who was there?," Bertranda's answer brought another person into the inquest. And by doing so, she shared their stories of the dangers they faced and how Delphine had helped them.

Twenty people that Bertranda mentioned were people she spoke to in Naples. Although this was a troubled time, Bertranda's stories of living in Naples with Delphine were not overly negative. She focused on what she had seen, which was mostly Queen Sanxia's household, including miraculous healings and the impact of Delphine's divinely inspired prayer. There is no sense in her testimony that she was circumscribed by the articles of questioning or limited to formulaic or uniformly positive statements.[6] Nor was this like a heresy inquest where a witness like Bertranda might have to speak carefully because people's lives and property were at stake. Bertranda had relative freedom to speak. If there was censorship of content, it was likely self-imposed.

The political and social events of 1363 shaped how Bertranda talked about 1343. Bertranda spoke at a transition point—a possible end to the troubled relations between Naples and Provence. In 1363, Queen Johanna of Naples was in a new position of political strength. Her second husband, Louis of Taranto, had died, and she was able to act on her own. This was a moment when Queen Johanna could be a powerful support for Delphine's canonization. And this was not an unlikely idea. Historian Gábor Klaniczay describes Queen Johanna, as part of the Angevin monarchy, as an active supporter of saints, especially those like Delphine's husband, Elzear de Sabran, who were connected to the Crown.[7] Historian Elizabeth Casteen also presents Queen Johanna as supportive of saints, particularly Birgitta of Sweden.[8] So overt criticism, while not forbidden to a witness like Bertranda, was not a savvy option for Delphine's canonization.

But a critique of Queen Johanna gradually emerged, especially in Bertranda's answers to the papal commissioners' questions.[9] The stories she chose to tell about 1343 brought events from Johanna's early reign to mind. Perhaps the strongest critique emerged in what Bertranda did not say. As Bertranda answered commissioners' questions about who had told her about events or whom she had seen interacting with Delphine, she never named Queen Johanna. Bertranda obviously thought it important to include names. She named seventy-five different people. So her silence is powerful. Bertranda left Queen Johanna out of Delphine's experience of Naples. As we will see below, this was not an oversight, but a conscious choice.

A more subtle critique of Queen Johanna emerged in how Bertranda spoke about time. The commissioners frequently asked her when an event happened.

This is a common question in all types of inquest, but people answered it in different ways.[10] Like many medieval witnesses, Bertranda rarely recalled specific years or months. Instead, she dated events in relation to significant events she recalled. In Bertranda's case, these events were most often deaths. She organized Delphine's life events and miracles as coming before, after, or at the same time as significant deaths. The death of Delphine in 1360 was, of course, a fixed point in Bertranda's testimony. For example, if she were talking about Delphine's saintly characteristics, she described them as lasting from when she met Delphine until the time of Delphine's death. If she described an illness Delphine suffered, she described it as afflicting Delphine until her death. Another important moment of death was the "first mortality"—the *prima mortalitas*. This is the phrase that many witnesses used to describe the first wave of plague in 1348. It was a fixed point in Bertranda's understanding of the past. Bertranda used this phrase five times in her testimony to date other events.[11]

Both of these significant moments of death—Delphine's death and the *prima mortalitas*—in turn shaped the events that Bertranda described by giving them a positive or negative impression. By placing a miraculous healing before Delphine's death, for example, she infused Delphine's life with God's grace and the miraculous healing with Delphine's sanctity. In other words, God's grace and the person being healed were linked by Bertranda's testimony in the minds of the papal commissioners and anyone who read her testimony. At the same time, the healed person and the event of their healing became infused with God's grace. In contrast, by placing an event in the same year as the first mortality or even several years before or after, Bertranda brought the plague to listeners' minds and permanently linked the first mortality in the recorded testimony to the event she described.[12]

Bertranda's expression of time also emphasized for her audiences—from the papal commissioners to the readers of this book—that she was linking her past and present. She might be speaking about 1343 or 1348, but all the events of the intervening years shaped how she described those times in the testimony she gave in 1363. All the moments of danger that emerged in witness testimony weighed on her answers to commissioners' questions. This is an important point to revisit. While the first part of this book builds a chronological narrative, we must remain aware that witnesses' perceptions of the past and the ways they described the past were shaped by later events. For Bertranda, who was so very ill in 1363, perhaps death seemed the appropriate way to mark time. But the deaths she spoke of reflected on more than just her own situation. They reflected on the personal and political events she described.

A third significant death, which bears directly on Bertranda's presentation of Queen Johanna, appears as a time marker in Bertranda's testimony. She used the death of King Robert of Naples to date two events. Both of them, according to Bertranda, occurred shortly before his death. First, Bertranda recalled that Delphine's voice and touch miraculously healed a noble woman, Lady Johanna de Meleto, in the royal court.[13] Second, Bertranda described how Delphine was ridiculed for her humble clothing near the chapel of the Duke of Calabria in Naples.[14] Both events seem minor to modern audiences because we have little context for them. But for the papal commissioners listening to Bertranda's testimony, as well as any in the papal court who read it, both events evoked the political upheaval of the 1340s.

To understand why Bertranda's stories dated by King Robert's death would have resonated with her audience we need context—the historian's bird's-eye view—from which to view this healing miracle and life event. We need to take a step back from Bertranda's personal stories and trace the political landscape of Naples from shortly before the death of King Robert in 1343 to the eve of the first mortality in 1348. For Provence, this was a time of significant change.[15] Bertranda's testimony about personal events brought names and places to her audience's minds that would immediately recall the scandal, assassination, and remarriage that pushed a wedge between Provence and Naples for decades and caused several of the moments of danger that witnesses spoke of in their testimonies. Bertranda managed to recall this moment without directly mentioning or criticizing Queen Johanna of Naples. But she evoked Johanna, and the young woman's actions after the death of her grandfather, King Robert, just the same.

From the Death of King Robert to the Eve of the First Mortality

The death of a king was a dangerous political moment. The dying ruler tried to transfer authority to an heir in a way that retained (or regained) the loyalty of subjects and staved off outside claims to the throne. Higher nobility saw this transfer as a moment to renegotiate their status and responsibilities. They could enter the new ruler's confidence, often by displacing others. Those with ties to the dynastic line had the chance to enter royal favor or even the ruling family through marriage alliances. It could be a moment of violent instability as rivals fought for political dominance.[16]

So although no witnesses, even Bertranda, directly marked the death of King Robert as a moment of danger per se, in many ways it was the root of several dangers they all faced.[17] Robert's efforts to secure the throne of Naples for his granddaughter, Johanna, set in motion rebellions among his heirs that made Provence a battleground for decades. The assassinations and invasions directly after Robert's death colored perceptions of the first wave of plague and the increasingly difficult relations between Provençal lords and their counts.[18]

The reasons King Robert's death was particularly disruptive require us to immerse ourselves in the minutiae of inheritance practices in the kingdom of Naples. King Robert's position was particularly difficult since both of his sons predeceased him. Robert knew it was a problem that he had no clear male heir. As soon as his son Charles died, Robert began looking for another heir. But Robert was navigating a broken inheritance system that had far too many possible heirs.

This break in the inheritance system happened before King Robert came to the throne. When Charles II (Robert's father) died, his oldest son, Carobert, should have inherited the throne. At that time, however, Carobert was in the process of consolidating his hold on the kingdom of Hungary, so he was not a good choice. Ideally, Carobert's son would have inherited the throne, but Carobert's son was too young. Instead of having a very young king with a regent, Charles II instead chose another of his own sons, Louis of Anjou, as heir. Louis abdicated the throne in order to become a Franciscan friar, however, so Charles II chose his son Robert. This process of choosing an heir from his own younger sons, rather than following the line of primogeniture, created the precedent that younger sons of Charles II could inherit the throne of Naples.

In most royal families at the time, this would have been tricky. But for the Angevin royal family in Naples at this moment, it was a catastrophe. Charles II had had twelve children, many of whom survived to adulthood and had children of their own.[19] Robert, therefore, had far too many options and faced intense in-family striving when choosing a new heir. At the risk of oversimplifying a complex dynastic battle, the main contenders in 1343 included Carobert's sons, Louis and Andrew of Hungary. Louis was already King of Hungary, however, so Andrew was the more obvious choice. The contenders also included Robert's granddaughters, Johanna and Maria, who were the oldest children of his own sons. Further strong contenders included Robert's nephews, Robert and Louis of Taranto and Charles of Durazzo.[20] All of the contenders had valid claims to the throne and the means to pursue those claims. Their pursuit ultimately created some of the most dangerous moments that Delphine's witnesses faced.

In 1333, King Robert chose one of his own granddaughters—Johanna, the eldest surviving child of his eldest son—instead of the son of one of his brothers.[21] Knowing that he had just created perhaps the most desirable heiress in western Europe, King Robert also chose her husband. In 1333, Johanna was promised in marriage to Andrew of Hungary, younger brother to the powerful Louis of Hungary, who was now king of that region. Johanna was seven and Andrew was six. They were both raised in Naples.

Johanna's marriage to Andrew of Hungary was an attempt to resolve decades of political uneasiness between the Neapolitan and Hungarian lines of the Angevin family. By arranging a marriage between Johanna and Andrew of Hungary, King Robert might end the primogeniture debate and remove the very real threat to Johanna that the King of Hungary posed.[22]

King Robert's last will of 1343 suggests his ideal political transition. In it, he planned for Johanna to remain a minor until she was twenty-five. He established a council to act as regent, with Queen Sanxia as its leader. For supporters of King Robert, Johanna's long minority under a council of his choice would create political continuity and associate Johanna with Robert's court, which many chroniclers portrayed as wise, just, and pious.[23] It would also associate Johanna with the lords of Provence, since the council had a strong Provençal presence. As we know from several witnesses, Delphine was present in Naples at this time at Queen Sanxia's request, though she was not a member of the council. The council did include Bishop Philippe Cabassole of Cavaillon, one of Delphine's witnesses. Cabassole was a prominent figure in Provençal politics and an increasingly important figure in the papal court in Avignon.[24]

King Robert's will also used a variety of methods to oppose other claims. For example, Robert made Johanna sole ruler of Naples. Her husband, Andrew, was given the title Duke of Calabria, but he would never be king. He would only have the title of consort. If she should die before Andrew and if they did not have a child, the throne would pass to Johanna's younger sister Maria. The will limited Maria's marriage options to members of the French Valois family or the Hungarian Angevins.[25] By tying all authority of the throne to Johanna, however, Robert left the now sixteen-year-old Andrew in the dangerous position of having little authority, being far from his family's support, and being in the way of several ambitious families. The chronicler Domenico de Gravina called him "a little lamb among wolves."[26]

Almost immediately after Robert's death in 1343, the will was broken, starting a trail of violence and instability that lasted for decades. Pope Clement VI broke it first. He disregarded the council set up in Robert's will, and acted as regent for Johanna himself. He sent a legate to Naples as his representative to report back on political events. The will was broken again in early 1344 by Agnes of Périgord, the wife of John of Gravina and sister of the famous Cardinal Talleyrand of Périgord.[27] She negotiated a political coup by marrying her son, Charles of Durazzo, to Johanna's younger sister, Maria.[28] This put her son in line to inherit the throne of Naples if anything happened to Johanna and Andrew.

In a little over a year, therefore, the political situation turned from one that favored Provençal, French, and Hungarian interests to one that favored the families of Robert's younger brothers. For almost two years, the court of Naples was a political storm navigated by mothers of rival suitors. Agnes of Périgord, now Maria's mother-in-law, installed herself in Naples. Elizabeth of Hungary, Andrew's mother, also came to Naples, perhaps to protect her sixteen-year-old son.[29] Catherine of Valois was already a powerful figure in the court of Naples.[30] She was the influential wife of Philip I of Taranto and mother to the potential inheritors, Robert and Louis of Taranto. Meanwhile, Queen Sanxia's political clout waned. Sanxia was not Johanna's grandmother, so she did not have direct familial ties that might have translated into political influence. With the council of Johanna's minority disbanded, she had little influence.[31]

By late spring of 1345 the courtly landscape had shifted in favor of Catherine of Valois and Louis of Taranto. Agnes of Périgord had died (possibly from poison). The papal legate had been removed, and Elizabeth of Hungary had departed. King Robert's widow, Sanxia, had entered a Clarissan convent that she had founded and which housed her late husband's tomb.[32] This left Catherine of Valois and her son, Louis of Taranto, as the main influences on the young royal couple.

Much of what we know about these tense years after King Robert's death comes from chronicles. Like today's newspapers, however, late medieval Italian chronicles usually supported a political faction, shaping their accounts of events to favor one side and vilify another. Other sources, such as royal records, for example, are sometimes difficult to come by after the bombing of Naples in World War II, so historians often work with the stories chroniclers told.[33] Even more than witness testimony, however, chroniclers' accounts are constructed narratives. These chroniclers were not sworn to tell the truth and testify to papal commissioners. So while we use chronicles to learn about events, chroniclers were embedded in political events and working with different political leaders. When building a narrative of Neapolitan politics in 1343–1347, therefore, every historian navigates many politically influenced versions of events.[34]

For most chroniclers, the transition to Johanna's reign took a violent turn on the night of September 18, 1345, when two men called Johanna's husband, Andrew of Hungary, out from his sleeping apartment and strangled him.

Multiple accounts of the assassination survive. One chronicle described Andrew as a helpless victim, lured out, dragged down from a second-story gallery into a small garden, beaten, cut, and finally strangled by someone wearing an iron gauntlet.[35] An official letter that circulated after the crime, however, had a different tone. It claimed that Andrew was a reckless boy accustomed to going out at suspicious hours of the night. He had refused a guard and shut the door of his apartments behind him.[36] The official account of this event, which would shape the perception of Queen Johanna's reign in Provence, appeared self-serving and cold. For many chroniclers it increased the perception of her guilt.[37]

Some historical analyses, however, suggest that Queen Johanna had little to gain from Andrew's assassination and much to lose.[38] The powerful Hungarian branch of the Angevin family, led by Andrew's brother Louis of Hungary, could and did use the event as a reason to invade the Italian peninsula and unify their Angevin holdings. Charles of Durazzo, married to Johanna's younger sister, could accuse Johanna of murder and depose her. Finally, Catherine of Valois and her son, Louis of Taranto, could use Andrew's death as an opportunity to gain the throne of Naples through marriage to the newly widowed Johanna.[39]

A local inquest quickly found the assassin, but few were satisfied with this initial investigation.[40] The results seemed too easy and self-serving for those at the court of Naples. King Louis of Hungary and his family rejected the investigation and accused Johanna and everyone near her of complicity in Andrew's murder. Riots and rebellion erupted in Naples, and leaders of other Italian city-states prepared attacks. Louis of Hungary began preparing to invade the Italian peninsula.[41]

The reaction from Provence was skeptical as well. Pope Clement VI immediately sent diplomats to the Hungarian and Neapolitan courts to negotiate peace. Among other dignitaries, Clement sent the Provençal lords Uguo and Bertran de Baux to Naples to learn what they could and to tell him what was happening there. Like Count Elzear, Delphine's husband, Lord Uguo de Baux had been a strong supporter of King Robert, who had made him seneschal of Provence and Count of Avelino. Their presence reflects the importance of Provençal lords under King Robert and their continued importance to the Avignon popes. Count Uguo de Baux, present at this precarious transfer of political power, would ultimately play a complex role in witnesses' testimonies in Delphine's inquest.

Soon after sending the Baux cousins, Clement declared his own official investigation into the murder, couched in the language of pastoral care. He instigated the investigation "for the health of the souls of those he cared for," meaning not just Andrew, but also anyone who might have been involved in the assassination.[42] Lordly violence was a serious sin and could lead to damnation if the guilty parties did not confess and repent. Pope Clement put Count Uguo de Baux in charge of opening the investigation in Naples.[43]

The ongoing papal investigation of Andrew's murder sought to question Johanna and members of the other two branches of the Angevin family in contention for the throne. In this way, Pope Clement VI hoped to assuage the anger of the Hungarian branch of the Angevin family and stave off an invasion. Clement supported Johanna's queenship. But his efforts at peaceful transition were at odds with her refusal to participate in the investigation into Andrew's murder.[44]

Pope Clement VI's efforts for peace were undermined by Johanna's choice for a second husband as well. Johanna chose Louis of Taranto, a man who had been close to her through her marriage to Andrew and the political fallout of his assassination.[45] But he was also a suspect in Andrew's assassination. This choice went so directly against her grandfather's will and against so many interests of the various branches of the Angevin family, however, that Johanna and Louis needed the blessing of the pope to make it official. But it was difficult for Clement VI to condone this marriage because Louis of Taranto also refused to participate in the papal inquest.[46] Papal resistance did not stall Johanna and Louis long, however. By mid-August 1347, Louis of Taranto secretly married Johanna in Naples. By September, Johanna relinquished some of the sole authority given her by her grandfather by naming Louis vicar-general of the kingdom.[47]

In the four years after King Robert's death, every part of his will, which had been designed for a peaceful transition, had been dismantled. Fissures that had always unsettled the kingdom of Naples had opened into rifts. The fissures between powerful families that had claims to the throne, especially the Hungarians, the Taranto, and the Durazzo, would continue to widen with constant efforts to seize control. King Robert's will and Johanna's choices had not transferred authority to Johanna in a way that retained the loyalty of her subjects. They had also not managed to stave off outside claims to the throne. Higher nobility throughout the kingdom saw this transfer as a chance to renegotiate their status, displace others, and perhaps even become part of the ruling family. As we shall see, this included the Provençal noble Lord Uguo de Baux, who tried to marry his son to Johanna's younger sister, Maria, with disastrous results.

Death and Silence in Bertranda Bertomieua's Testimony

Bertranda did not talk about any of these political machinations in her testimony. But this broad political picture, at least part of which she saw first hand, gives us insight into the two events that she associated with the death of King Robert and insight into her silence about Queen Johanna. Her experience testifying in Delphine's inquest can help us see how she could express subtle critiques.

In 1363 Bertranda was lying in her bed, giving testimony about a holy woman she had known and served for most of her life. Bertranda was sworn in on June 2, twenty difficult years after the events she mentioned in conjunction with King Robert's death. Although a pre-inquest does not survive, there is evidence that she had been questioned by the inquest proctor, Master Nicolau Laurens, long before this moment. Laurens wrote the roughly one hundred articles of interrogation used for Delphine's inquest. Several of the articles reflect information only Bertranda could have known, so it is likely he based those articles on his conversations with her. Bertranda mentioned him five times in her testimony as someone she spoke to or saw present at important events in Delphine's life.

Bertranda's testimony begins with her swearing in. She "pledged on the holy Gospel of God to speak purely, directly, and fully and to testify truthfully about that which was written in the articles of interrogation."[48] The inquest was recorded in Latin, but this was not a language she spoke. Before her testimony to Article 1 begins, the inquest states that the articles were read to her in her mother tongue (*lingua materna*), which was likely Provençal.[49] She would have responded in the same language, and the notaries recorded her testimony in Latin for the convenience of the polyglot papal court. They also transformed her testimony from first person (I) to third person (she), likely also for the convenience of the readers in the papal court.

The importance of having two notaries, one local to Apt and one from the papal court, becomes clear at this point. With members from all over Europe, the papal court functioned in Latin. All clergy in the papal court were familiar with this language and could read and speak it. Bertranda's testimony had to be translated. But many of the phrases that someone like Bertranda used would have been unfamiliar to an outsider and hard to capture or translate. By involving a local notary, the papal court did not lose the local voice that was so important for the success of a canonization inquest.[50]

After being sworn in, Bertranda immediately began to address the open-ended Article 1, which asked her to tell the commissioners everything she knew about Delphine's life events, living miracles, and posthumous miracles. The papal commissioners knew that Bertranda had lived with Delphine for decades, so they prompted her to tell them how she knew about Delphine's reputation for sanctity.[51] In response, Bertranda began to speak about Delphine's life.

Bertranda's testimony gives us insight into the ways witnesses told stories. These were seldom fully elaborated stories, like those found in saints' lives. Saints' lives, often written for a didactic purpose, usually had a story line—a beginning, middle, and end—that would highlight a specific aspect of the holy person's sanctity and conform to contemporary readers' expectations.[52] Most importantly, the stories revolved around the saint, often leaving other people in the story in the background.

Instead, witness narratives like Bertranda's are more of a hybrid, similar to both those found in miracle collections and those found in other kinds of inquests. Miracle collections included stories often gathered at shrines when people who had received miraculous aid came to complete their vows. The stories showed the efficacy of the saint and could help sustain the shrine.[53] Witness statements in Delphine's inquest also bear a resemblance to testimonies in criminal, civil, or heresy trials, since a canonization inquest included many of the same components.[54] The stakes were very different for witnesses in these different kinds of inquests, but the procedures that elicited testimony were often similar.[55] Because of the nature of an inquest, stories could take many different shapes. Some of Bertranda's stories were very concise, little more than "I heard" or "I saw" and a few details. Some narratives emerged almost exclusively through the commissioners' questioning.[56] Others had significant detail and a beginning, middle, and end. Overall, witness narratives recounted the past and had a roughly linear structure, but their stories could take many shapes.

Most importantly, however, the stories often revolved around the witness, including what the witness saw and heard. The witness in canonization inquest testimony often becomes the "main character," with the saint appearing only at the end of the story. In this way, we get the witness's vantage point on events, rather than the hagiographer's.

In response to Article 1, Bertranda explained Delphine's reputation for sanctity, especially holy speech and humility, which caused many people to seek her out while she lived. In King Robert's court, Bertranda described Delphine praying with Sanxia's courtiers with spectacular results. She also told a story about how Delphine healed a woman who was also receiving medicine made by King Robert. In her stories, she wove Delphine into the lives of King Robert and Queen Sanxia, showing how they respected and supported each other at important moments.[57]

Bertranda dated two of the events that happened in Naples as occurring shortly before King Robert's death in 1343, thereby evoking this difficult political moment when she recounted them to the papal commissioners and to readers in the papal curia. According to Bertranda, Lady Johanna de Meleto, a member of Queen Sanxia's household, became gravely ill with a protracted fever. The doctors consulted had no hope that she would live. Delphine visited Lady Johanna and touched her. According to a certain woman named Almodia, who had been present at Delphine's visit to Lady Johanna, Lady Johanna's fever diminished during the night after Delphine's visit, and in three days she was well enough to visit Queen Sanxia's palace.[58]

After Bertranda described this event, the two papal commissioners asked Bertranda a series of questions. Several of Bertranda's answers to these questions—as well as the short miracle story itself—would have recalled the political tensions of 1343–1348 to the minds of the commissioners and future readers. For example, the commissioners asked Bertranda to more fully identify Lady Johanna. Bertranda said that Lady Johanna "was from Meleto [also known as Mileto de Porto Salvo] under the Duke of Calabria."[59] In 1343, the Duke of Calabria was Andrew of Hungary. This was a title King Robert gave him as his granddaughter's consort. Bertranda's testimony therefore linked Lady Johanna to the assassinated Andrew of Hungary.

The commissioners also asked who was present when Delphine visited Johanna during her illness. According to Bertranda, in addition to Almodia, Johanna's daughter, Maria, was present. Including young Maria in Johanna's sickroom may have reminded the commissioners of Queen Johanna and her younger sister Maria, who were the focus of so much political scheming between 1343 and 1348.

Finally, the commissioners asked how long Bertranda saw Lady Johanna healthy after Delphine's touch healed her. This was a common question in canonization inquests meant to show if someone had been truly healed or had only recovered briefly. Bertranda said that she saw Lady Johanna healthy for about half a year, but did not see her after that because she and Delphine returned to Provence. This statement indicated to the commissioners that Delphine did not stay long in Naples after the death of King Robert. We can only speculate why Delphine left so quickly, but she, as a guest of Queen Sanxia, may not have been welcome after the council that was supposed to oversee Queen Johanna's minority was dissolved. Between 1343 and 1345, Catherine of Valois and her son Louis of Taranto rose in power in Naples at the expense of other claimants to the throne. By the time Andrew was assassinated, the widowed Queen Sanxia was no longer in the palace.

At the very least, this short miracle story brought the names of Johanna, Maria, and the Duke of Calabria to the minds of the papal commissioners in 1363. While it may have been a coincidence, it also reminded them of the dangerous political events of 1343–1345 by describing Delphine leaving Naples soon after King Robert's death. To go a bit further, the healing miracle also offered an alternative history of events. In Bertranda's story, *this* Johanna was transformed from sick to healthy by speaking with Delphine. *This* Johanna worked with the medicine offered by King Robert and associated herself with Queen Sanxia. *This* Johanna was healthy in body and soul. All of these details would have highlighted what *Queen* Johanna had not done.

Bertranda used the death of King Robert as a time marker for one other event, which also evokes the danger of the city of Naples, especially at this transition point of 1343. In response to Article 25, which asked witnesses about examples of Delphine's profound humility, Bertranda recalled several instances when Delphine embraced the ridicule of her peers for her choice of humble clothing and for her practice of begging in the street. Bertranda's example from Naples was subtle, but ugly. While walking down the street, Bertranda saw and heard certain youths in the chapel of the Duke of Calabria make derogatory comments about Delphine, whom they knew was a countess. One pointed at her and asked, "Who is this *bizoca*?"[60] There are multiple definitions for the term *bizoca*, including beggar-woman. Delphine accepted this humbly, however, as befitted a proto-saint. When the commissioners asked when this happened, Bertranda replied that she "saw it twenty years ago, before the death of King Robert."[61]

This event may not seem particularly shocking to a modern reader, but for Delphine an accusation like this one could have had serious repercussions. In the fourteenth century, a person's reputation, or *fama*, was part of the basis of their standing in society. It could affect everything from their access to legal courts to their standing among their neighbors and peers.[62] Although writing about twelfth-century Tuscany, Chris Wickham captures this well. As he states, "What the public environment accepted as true was, indeed, valid in law as well."[63] This value of reputation was certainly important in Delphine's inquest. Every witness was asked not just about what they knew of Delphine, but what they had heard about her. The commissioners wanted to know Delphine's common reputation and what was publicly said about her in Naples, Provence, and Avignon.[64]

So these youths who accused Delphine of being a beggar living in doorways because of what she wore were attacking her status in Naples society through her public *fama*.[65] Bertranda defended Delphine's *fama* by explaining that her humble clothing was a sign of extreme virtue rather than destitution. So on one level, the youths' crudeness allowed Delphine's humility to shine brighter. But on another level, the youths' public speech reveals something about Bertranda's perception of the event. As she testified in 1363, the Naples that she recalled was in transition from one ruler to another. In Bertranda's memory, Delphine had interacted in pious ways with King Robert and had "great familiarity [with] the most serene lady Sanxia, Queen of Jerusalem and Sicily."[66] In Bertranda's remembered Naples at this moment of transition, Delphine was a *bizoca* to the followers of the new generation of leaders.

In contrast to Queen Sanxia and King Robert, Bertranda did not mention Johanna of Naples. There is every likelihood that Delphine knew and interacted with King Robert's granddaughter during her minority and after she became queen. Bertranda's testimony shows that Delphine was in Naples in 1342–1343, from shortly before King Robert's death through when the council first took authority during Johanna's minority. Delphine was there at the request of Queen Sanxia, so she was moving in the same circles that Johanna would have moved in. Delphine, and by extension Bertranda, would have known about, and perhaps interacted with, the council named in King Robert's will. For example, Bishop Philippe Cabassole recalled meeting Delphine in Naples at this time and being impressed with her piety.[67] He was an increasingly influential figure in the Avignon Papacy during Delphine's life and a man who would become one of the strongest supporters of her canonization. Cabassole certainly interacted with Johanna while in Naples and later in Provence and would have been a likely point of contact. Even after Delphine left Naples, Queen Johanna visited Avignon and surrounding towns when Delphine lived in Cabrières. Regardless of evidence that they likely crossed paths, however, Bertranda did not mention any meeting between these two women.

Bertranda's silence was not an oversight or a coincidence. In other canonization inquests from fourteenth-century Provence, organizers and witnesses worked to associate the potential saint with politically powerful people.[68] This strategy could move the canonization process through the papal bureaucracy much faster. In 1363, Queen Johanna of Naples—the Countess of Provence—was one of the most politically powerful figures in the region. For a witness like Bertranda not to mention even a limited relationship—a discussion or a visit between the two women—was significant. Instead, Bertranda worked to associate Delphine with King Robert and Queen Sanxia. In this way, Bertranda's silence separated Delphine from Queen Johanna.

1343: The Root of Many Dangers

Bertranda Bertomieua gives us an insider's view of Delphine's life in Naples. Hers was a close but narrow vantage point on the events surrounding the transfer of power from King Robert to his granddaughter, Johanna, and the various family members battling for political power. Bertranda's access to the aristocracy came from her proximity to Delphine. She was present for events because she accompanied the holy countess. She spoke to people from many levels of society because she was in Delphine's retinue. Noble women told her stories. Lower-status women asked for favors.

Bertranda's depiction of Delphine in Naples and her strong relationship with King Robert and Queen Sanxia gave the commissioners a picture of two couples who respected each other and shared the same values. While Sanxia and Robert did not have a chaste marriage like Delphine and Elzear, they were both devout people.

Bertranda's silence about Johanna, therefore, placed Delphine in opposition to Johanna. In a spiritual sense, Bertranda described Delphine as a humble woman turning her back on luxury and worldly power just as Johanna was accused of murder in order to expand her own. In a political sense, Bertranda aligned Delphine with King Robert and Queen Sanxia, who had brought the aristocracy of Provence into their government at the moment when Johanna and her new husband, Louis of Taranto, broke King Robert's will and started to draw away from Provençal lords as political allies.

But Bertranda did not openly speak against Queen Johanna in her testimony. Instead she offered an alternative Johanna, one who was healed by Delphine's miraculous touch. While there is no evidence that Bertranda was involved in Provençal politics of 1363, she did not appear to be unaware of the political impact of her canonization inquest testimony. This comes as no surprise for one who spoke to and was mentioned by some of the most politically powerful witnesses in the inquest.

Bertranda's testimony opened a small window on a dangerous moment. Combining the historian's bird's-eye view with Bertranda's perspective has helped us see that moment better. While witnesses did not describe Robert's death as a moment of danger like the others, it was in many ways the birthplace of those dangers. The rival claimants for the throne of Naples hired mercenary troops to attack Provence after this point. The rise of Louis of Taranto and Niccola Acciaiuoli, who valued Provence less and Sicily more, occurred here. Witnesses' experiences from 1343 to 1363 were shaped by King Robert's death.

Chapter 2

Bishop Philippe Cabassole and the "War of the Seneschals," 1347–1349

The first moment of danger—the first event that five or more witnesses with diverse backgrounds described—was what several historians of Provence refer to as the "war of the seneschals."[1] The "war" centered on the removal of Lord Raymon d'Agoult as seneschal of Provence by Queen Johanna, who tried to replace him with her trusted ally, Lord Giovanni Barrili. This act, among others, split the lords of Provence. Some supported Queen Johanna, like Lord Uguo de Baux and the lords of Marseille. Others opposed this action, like Lord Raymon and other lords of the Estates, based in Aix-en-Provence.[2] This inspired a feud between Lord Uguo and Lord Raymon, in which they and their supporters cut off trade and armed their cities for war.

The quotation marks around phrase "war of the senenschals" remind us that this is a modern term for the event. The witnesses used multiple words to describe it. And even their use of a word like *guerra* had complex aspects of feud and rebellion that modern audiences may not bring to a word like war. The quotation marks around the word war can help the reader remember that this was a local event and a local feud that was dangerous for witnesses in Delphine's inquest, but perhaps not a fully erupted civil war.

Several witnesses were involved in the "war," but none of the witnesses described the political background in detail. Because this was an inquest into Delphine's sanctity, witnesses focused their testimony on how they saw

Delphine care for others and endure physical suffering in order to bring peace to the feuding lords. Six very different witnesses told the papal commissioners about how Delphine changed the hearts of Lord Uguo de Baux and Lord Raymon d'Agoult. She helped them move from a dangerous state of hatred and violence to exchange the kiss of peace. One witness, the focus witness of this chapter, Bishop Philippe Cabassole, helped put the event in perspective. Cabassole was the papacy's chief negotiator between these lords, and he understood this as a moment of crisis for Provence. As Cabassole put it, "If [peace] had not been made, there would have been, as he believes, a great division in Provence and great scandal and war."[3]

The witnesses' circumspection reflects the demands of speaking in a canonization inquest. The members of the Agoult and Baux families and the servants of the Crown and papacy who testified in Delphine's inquest had to navigate political relations in 1363 as they made sense of events happening fifteen years earlier. The witnesses who spoke chose to emphasize the moment of peace, in which Delphine was directly involved.

At least one witness, however, chose silence. Master Guilhem Enric, was directly involved in the war of the seneschals.[4] But he was also an important figure in the royal law court in Provence. From 1331, he held the title doctor of law and was a proctor and advocate of the king. He was named *juge mage* in 1348 and was a judge of first appeals in 1361.[5] Enric did not mention the "war" in his lengthy testimony even though he was an associate of Bishop Philippe Cabassole and other witnesses who did speak. We cannot know why he remained silent, but his silence is a powerful reminder of the choices witnesses had as they testified.

As historians, however, we can step back and put the "war" in the context of the time. This allows us to better see how witnesses shaped a politically difficult story. They wanted to tell this story because it revealed the grace and sanctity of Delphine. But for them, it was very much part of several larger, more uncomfortable stories, that captured the danger they perceived. Witnesses knew that the "war" had its roots in the death of King Robert in 1343, Andrew of Hungary's assassination in 1345, Louis of Taranto's quest for the throne of Naples, and Louis of Hungary's invasion of Naples in 1347.[6] Some saw the violent politics in Naples as dangerous for Provence.

But political transition was just one part of the story of this moment of danger. For the witnesses, describing these political events evoked the larger moment when those events occurred. This included the first wave of plague in 1348. As we saw in chapter 1, Bertranda Bertomieua used the phrase "*prima mortalitas*" five times as a time marker for other events. And each time she did so, it placed that event in the experiences, one could say in the shadow, of the

Black Death. Bertranda was one of the witnesses to this "war," and she used the first mortality as a time marker for it.

Bertranda's use of the time marker helps us remember that war and plague were not separate stories in the experience of these witnesses. Plague and violence were part of the same epidemic. Epidemic death, violence, and the destructive internal states of despair and anger affected the physical and spiritual health of the region.

Witnesses did not have to explain the impact of plague to the papal commissioners, who had lived through it as well. It is useful for modern audiences, however, to consider how people experienced this moment. Literary sources give us a sense of the danger of this moment. Economic sources, wills, and letters help us reconstruct some of the witnesses' shared experience. For these sources we move outside the inquest to Bishop Philippe Cabassole's other duties and his larger social circle. Cabassole's fiscal work for the papal court gives us a vantage point from which to see the effects of this moment. And Cabassole's friends, especially Francis Petrarch and Louis Heyligen, were involved in the "war of the seneshcals," lived through the plague, and wrote in moving detail of their experiences.

Bishop Philippe Cabassole in the Political World of Provence

Bishop Philippe Cabassole could act as a papal negotiator attempting to avert this "war" in Provence because he was a pivotal figure in the court of Naples, in the papal court, and among the lords of Provence. He does not provide the intimate view that Bertranda Bertomieua did on Delphine's life. Instead his role in these negotiations, his network of friends and associates, and his writings give a modern reader the scope to understand the many layers that made up this complex moment of danger.

Cabassole was roughly sixty years old when he testified and, like Bertranda Bertomieua, had known Delphine for decades.[7] The opening of Cabassole's testimony identified him not as the bishop of Cavaillon, but as the patriarch of Jerusalem. This prestigious title might explain why he did not testify in Apt, like most other witnesses. Instead, he was read the articles of interrogation and gave his answers in Avignon at the dwelling of Bishop Nicolau of Toulouse, a member of the College of Cardinals.[8] In this last stage of the inquest, the papal commissioners were staying with Bishop Nicolau. The proctor of the inquest, Master Nicolau Laurens, the notary from Apt, was also present.

On October 9, 1363, Cabassole was sworn in and asked to tell the truth as he had seen and heard it. He was given an opportunity to hear and respond to all of the articles of interrogation. He chose to address twelve of them. He started his testimony with the open-ended Article 1 and began immediately to describe his impressions of Delphine in Naples and Avignon. Although he kept his testimony focused on Delphine's sanctity, it is clear that he moved in the highest circles of Neapolitan aristocracy. Despite his lofty titles, Philippe Cabassole was not from the high nobility of Provence. His family members were legal professionals and well-connected diplomats. Cabassole's uncle, Isnard, was the *viguier*, the royal representative and one of the highest authorities, of Arles in 1315 and the *viguier* of Avignon in 1356.[9] Cabassole's father, Johan, over the course of a long career was a *juge mage* of Provence and a proctor in the court of King Robert of Naples, and was involved in the canonization inquest of King Robert's brother, Louis of Anjou.[10] He was a trusted official in Naples and Provence.

Philippe Cabassole continued and expanded this service to King Robert and also served several Avignon popes. In 1334, he became the bishop of Cavaillon, an important city in the Comtat Venaissin—the papal territory within Provence.[11] In 1343–1344, he was vice chancellor of Naples and, as we saw in chapter 1, he was part of the short-lived council that King Robert had appointed to act as regent for Johanna before she became queen.[12] In the years before and after Delphine's inquest, Philippe Cabassole became more influential. In 1360, Cabassole received the title patriarch of Jerusalem. This was a nominal title, since the Crown of Naples had no direct claim on the holy city. But it was a politically meaningful title nonetheless, since ruler of Jerusalem was included in the official titles of the king and queen of Naples. In 1362, the year before Delphine's inquest, Cabassole became the rector of the Comtat Venaissin.[13] He oversaw much of the work to repair this region after the waves of plague and mercenary invasion.

But Philippe Cabassole's titles tell only part of his story. His active life in Avignon brought him into contact with the humanist poet Francis Petrarch.[14] The two visited frequently and wrote letters when they lived in different cities. Petrarch dedicated his *De vita solitaria* to Cabassole, whom he described as a great admirer of his writing.[15] Like Cabassole, Petrarch was deeply involved in the "war of the seneschals."

Their circle of friends included the well-connected diplomat Cardinal Talleyrand of Pèrigord, whose sister Agnes died in the court of Naples during Johanna's brief minority. It also included the chanter Louis Heyligen (Petrarch's "Socrates"), who wrote an account of the 1348 plague in Avignon.[16] Both of these men were well aware of, and involved in, the political events of the Crown of Naples. Philippe Cabassole's view of the "war of the seneschals" and the meanings of the first wave of plague were influenced by these men.

Philippe Cabassole was not just the friend of writers. He also wrote an intriguing work of his own. After King Charles II of Naples discovered Mary Magdalene's relics in the church of St. Maximin in Provence, Cabassole wrote the *Libellus hystorialis Marie beatissime Magdalene*.[17] This book, one of several histories of the discovery of the Magdalene's relics, was the only one to tell the complete story of the relics' survival and discovery. The book was one of only two based on personal experience.[18] This book showed Cabassole's support for the Angevin dynasty and his support for a holy woman with powerful speaking abilities.[19]

Diplomat, bishop, patron of poets, and recorder of female sanctity—Bishop Philippe Cabassole brings many vantage points to our view of 1347–1349. While his testimony was relatively circumspect, he was involved in all of the events surrounding the first moment of danger that witnesses described in Delphine's inquest. We can use his diverse roles and connections to understand this "war" in the midst of the Black Death. What appears in witness testimony to be a simple story of seigneurial warfare was, as Philippe Cabassole knew, the tip of the iceberg in a broader story of rebellion as members of the ruling family of Naples warred against each other and forced their vassals to choose sides. And all of it took place as the worst epidemic in centuries killed tens of thousands of people in Provence and millions throughout Europe.

Article 38 and the Framing of the "War of the Seneschals"

Like the other five witnesses who testified about the averted civil war, Cabassole spoke about it in reference to Article 38. To better understand Cabassole's and other witnesses' testimonies about the "war of the seneschals," it is useful to have a clear sense of the article they responded to. Even if they did not repeat its words, they heard it before they spoke. It shaped how they thought about the moment and presented a frame of reference for this dangerous moment.

Article 38, like many of the articles of interrogation that the inquest proctor, Master Nicolau Laurens, wrote, allowed witnesses to speak about different events and saintly characteristics of their holy woman. It includes details from witnesses' stories about this "war," but none of the names of those involved. It opened up several ways for witnesses to describe Delphine's regard for peace and her ability to bring peace to those around her. It also valued love and affection while criticizing the violent as offending God. Witnesses such as Bishop Philippe Cabassole who chose to address this article had a flexible framework within which to speak of the first moment of danger. Article 38 reads:

> Moreover, in common speech, common belief, and common assertion, it was and is public voice and *fama*, in parts of Provence and other places that Lady Delphine, while she continued in her human life, was filled with great fervor of love and affection for God and her neighbor, and she greatly rejoiced and desired that the souls of men be made healthy; therefore she was not afraid to sustain great worries and great care. And because, when she heard of the conflicts and disagreements of others, on behalf of the harmony of these, she worked most affectionately and she even carried herself to remote places where she hoped to settle the scandals even though she could neither ride a horse nor walk on account of the impediments of her age and weakness. And on account of this, she had herself carried by men in a cheap and humble litter with great strain and harm to her body. And because this same woman, whenever she heard of grave sin which seriously offended God, by the companies or unfaithful Christians and others of low state, that same lady poured out great tears and afflicted her body, to such a degree that frequently on account of her weakness fever grew strong in her.[20]

The article has three main parts. The first part is a general statement about Delphine's love and affection. The second describes her reaction to violence. And the third was her reaction to sin, particularly those sins done by the violent. To better understand how this article allowed witnesses to address the "war of the seneschals" in 1349, as well as other moments of danger, as we will see in chapters 3 and 4, we have to put the article in its fourteenth-century cultural and political context.

The first part described Delphine's love and affection for those around her and how she expressed it. According to the article, Delphine's emotional state mirrored the spiritual health of the people around her. Delphine felt joy when people's souls were healthy. Her desire for the health of the souls around her was so strong, however, that she did not fear to take on great worries and care to help them.

The emphasis on emotion, especially love, is a strong indication that this article is not just about the love of God, but also about political relationships. For centuries, lords at political odds with one another were described as existing in a state of hatred.[21] By the fourteenth century, hatred had become a conventional term of "medieval secular jurisprudence used to describe an enduring public relationship between two adversaries."[22] By describing Delphine as full of love and affection, the article placed Delphine in the opposite state. When she encountered discord, however, she suffered pain and anxiety. In other words, Delphine did not feel hatred. She did not take a side in the earthly dispute. Instead, she interceded in the discord by feeling worry and anxiety, which, in some cases, could have a positive effect on the souls of others and ideally change discord into peace and hatred into love. In this way, the souls of those around her could be healthy.

The second part of Article 38 continued to describe Delphine's response to political discord. When she heard about conflict, she worked to bring harmony. This work entailed physical suffering as she traveled to visit those in conflict. Two implications emerge here. First, Delphine's physical suffering, not just her emotional suffering, could have an impact on the relationships of people in conflict. Experiencing the pain of being carried in a humble litter could influence the souls of those she was traveling to visit. On the most basic level, this reflects the common theme of the holy person suffering for the sins of others.[23] The second implication is that, since Delphine was traveling for the purpose of visiting the lords, her presence after her arrival (not just her difficulty traveling) would help settle the discord. In other words, the physical proximity—the presence—of the holy woman was an important space. She was well known for the power of her voice to change those around her, as we will see in later chapters, so this article could allow witnesses to speak of that as well.

The third part of the article discussed Delphine's reaction to other grave sins and offenses to God and the subjugation of Christians. In this situation, Delphine wept and afflicted her own body, causing herself fever. There is no indication, however, that her suffering could have an impact on those offending God in this case. Instead, her weeping and self-affliction reveal her sensitivity to the suffering of others and the affront to God.[24]

Overall, Article 38 made several revealing statements about conflict and violence. It grouped conflict and discord with the activities of the unfaithful. Discord was wrong and potentially sinful, whether perpetrated by Christians or non-Christians. The main difference was that Delphine could bring peace among Christians, but she could not bring peace to non-Christians, though she could suffer for those oppressed by them.

The article also described discord as sickness of the soul, putting discord in the framework of health. This was a common view in the fourteenth century. The state of hatred underlying political discord was linked to anger, one of the passions or accidents of the soul.[25] Both medical doctors and spiritual doctors (i.e., those administering pastoral care) would have put the passions into the category of nonnaturals—those things (like air and food) that influenced the body but were not of it (like blood or internal organs).[26] So hatred was not just a political status. The anger that hatred produced was also a physiological experience that had an impact on body and soul. It was particularly linked with disrupting the reasoning ability of the brain.[27]

By putting Delphine in the role of *healer* of discord through her love and affection, the article evoked the familiar language of healing both through opposites and through pastoral care. The two appeared commonly together in metaphor. The priest, bishop, or confessor cared for the health of the soul just as a medical doctor cared for the health of the body.[28] A healthy anger that got the blood flowing could cross over into the deadly sin of wrath. A fourteenth-century confessor would have been aware of this for those people under his pastoral care.

The three parts of Article 38 provided the frame that Master Laurens chose for this event, and it resonated with witnesses, not just for the averted "war" but with other violent episodes at the time. Delphine's ability to heal the souls of warring men by transforming discord into harmony would appear in many ways in witness testimony.

Rebellion and "War" in Provence, 1347–1349

As Bishop Philippe Cabassole heard the language of Article 38, it would have reminded him of the complexity and potential danger of this moment for Provence and Naples. A highly educated witness like Cabassole, with theological training and on-the-ground knowledge of political issues, would have been aware of all of the spiritual and political nuances in Article 38. He also knew the people involved, some quite well. He had seen this "war" build from the death of King Robert onward. He interacted with Provençal lords involved in the dispute, with the papal court, and with Queen Johanna. Bishop Philippe Cabassole gives us the different vantage points to understand this as a moment of danger for both body and soul.

The first thing that becomes clear is that Delphine's witnesses tell only the end of a long story. For witnesses, Delphine averted a "war" in 1349, so this is what they described. The roots of that "war" started much earlier, and the larger story was what made this moment crucial for six very different witnesses. The political details are not simple, but they are worth delving into in order to understand why witnesses saw the "war" as the main danger of this time period and how the lived experience of the Black Death was woven into that "war."

The two lords involved—Lord Raymon d'Agoult, lord of Sault, Count of Agunto, and Lord Uguo de Baux, Count of Avellino—represented two of the most powerful families in Provence. They had both served as seneschal of Provence and had both been servants of King Robert of Naples and were now servants of Queen Johanna of Naples.[29] Both lords held titles in Provence and southern Italy. While both lords had ties to royal, papal, and local courts, their dispute reveals regional fissures in the county of Provence exacerbated after the death of King Robert.

The spark that threatened to ignite this "war" occurred in 1349, when Lord Raymon, acting as seneschal of Provence, seized property from Lord Uguo. But the tinder for this conflagration had been building for years. A chronology of events, necessarily limited but useful nonetheless, will help modern readers see the context of the witnesses' stories of Delphine bringing peace to warring lords in 1349.

As we saw in chapter 1, in late 1347, Queen Johanna married Louis of Taranto, a man many thought to be responsible for Andrew of Hungary's death. Louis of Taranto's desire for the Crown of Naples was not a secret. By 1347, Johanna had already named him vicar-general of the kingdom of Naples, and he worked inexorably to make himself king, rather than just consort.[30] King Louis of Hungary, the son of Carobert, saw this as a direct political attack. By Andrew's death, he had lost influence over the Crown of Naples, which by right of primogeniture he should have had.[31] In response to the assassination of his brother, Andrew of Hungary, and the refusal of Queen Johanna and Louis of Taranto to take part in the papal investigation, King Louis of Hungary invaded Naples.[32]

Rather than bring his own troops, he moved down the Italian peninsula with only two thousand mounted soldiers, negotiating safe passage and gathering more soldiers as he traveled. This tactic allayed fears that he was planning to invade the whole peninsula. His plan was to bring small numbers of men from Hungary and hire mercenary soldiers already in southern Italy.[33]

When King Louis of Hungary closed in on Naples at the beginning of 1348, Johanna fled to Provence, making an official visit as countess of Provence. At the same time that Johanna arrived in early January, however, the first wave of plague was spreading from Marseille to Aix-en-Provence and Avignon.[34] Queen Johanna did not bring the plague to Provence. It had broken out in Marseille in November 1347.[35] But her arrival and travel coincided with its spread, merging the two in the minds of some of the Provençaux.

Johanna's initial welcome in Marseille was positive, influenced largely by Lord Uguo de Baux and the powerful families of the city.[36] But many lords of Provence had grievances against the new rulers of Naples, including the extraordinary rounds of taxes for the marriage of Johanna's sister Maria to Charles of Durazzo. More importantly, the lords of Provence were unsure of their standing in the relatively new court under Queen Johanna and Louis. They had had a relatively strong presence in the Angevin court.[37] As with any change in political leadership, they feared losing influence.[38]

When Johanna and her retinue left Marseille to attend a meeting of the Estates in Aix-en-Provence, Lord Raymon d'Agoult, one of the coleaders of the Estates, had Johanna's retinue arrested on suspicion of Andrew of Hungary's murder.[39] Lord Uguo de Baux, who was also coleader of the Estates, did not take part, however, putting him at odds with Lord Raymon.

Several historians understand this action as the lords of Provence asserting their independence within the kingdom of Naples, rather than rebelling against it.[40] They were making a bid to change the treatment of Provence by the new queen when she was in a moment of weakness and need. The Hungarian invasion and Johanna's continued refusal to participate in the papal inquest into Andrew's death made her vulnerable to such power plays. By arresting Johanna's retinue without the support of Lord Uguo, however, Lord Raymon also set into motion the political maneuvering that underlay the "war of the seneschals" that Delphine helped avert.

Lord Raymon's bid for more independence succeeded, at least temporarily. On February 17, Johanna vowed that high officers of Provence, like seneschals, should be Provençal, not Italian. To demonstrate her sincerity, she made Lord Raymon seneschal, replacing Filippo di Sangineto.[41] She also conceded that the various regions of the county of Provence could not be sold individually, a worry that many lords of Provence shared.[42] In return, Lord Raymon released Queen Johanna's retinue and, on February 19, when Johanna made a speech to the Estates, they swore fealty to her.

After her tumultuous visit to Aix-en-Provence, Johanna wished to travel to Avignon. This was also politically complicated. On the one hand, Pope Clement VI had close ties to Johanna, for whom he had acted as a regent during the brief time she remained a minor.[43] He also had close ties to the rulers of Naples for territorial reasons.[44] On the other hand, representatives of the King of Hungary were also in Avignon demanding justice for Andrew's assassination. To solve the difficulty, Clement VI had Queen Johanna stay outside the city. By the middle of March 1348, as the plague outbreak continued and the King of Hungary's invasion of Naples wore on, Louis of Taranto also made his way to Provence, staying in Villeneuve Avignon, just across the Rhône from the pope's court.[45]

Between March and June, Johanna and Louis's fortune changed. Even though they continued to disregard Clement VI's citation to testify in the official inquest into Andrew's death, Clement invited them into Avignon on March 14 and 15 and recognized their marriage soon after.[46] Also, by the middle of May 1348, the battle in the kingdom of Naples had turned against King Louis of Hungary. He had lost the popular support of the people of the kingdom of Naples. His severe punishments for the death of his brother Andrew, especially the beheading of Charles of Durazzo (son of Agnes of Pèrigord and husband of Johanna's younger sister Maria), led to riots and uprisings against him and his troops. In addition, the month of May marked the height of the plague outbreak in the city of Naples.[47] This likely diminished the available troops in the region and may have also had an impact on his popularity. Louis of Hungary was forced to leave the Italian peninsula, which allowed Johanna and Louis of Taranto to leave Avignon in July and return to Naples.[48]

Queen Johanna and Louis of Taranto's visit to Provence was not the peaceful visit King Robert and Queen Sanxia had enjoyed in the region in the 1320s. Violence, distrust, and plague overshadowed the new royal couple's entire visit, but they could not leave. Only when King Louis of Hungary's invasion of Naples failed was Queen Johanna free to return to the peninsula. Before leaving Avignon, however, she did two things. First, she sold Avignon and the Comtat Venaissin to Clement VI for 80,000 gold florins.[49] The sale likely made it easier for the pope to recognize her marriage and to continue to overlook her refusal to testify in the inquest.[50] It also gave the royal couple needed funds for the military effort to remove Louis of Hungary's remaining supporters.[51] Second, Johanna conferred on her second husband the title of Count of Provence. This gave Louis equal authority to Johanna throughout Provence, allowing him to make political decisions that would eventually complicate the "war of the seneschals" even further.

Soon after their return to Naples, Queen Johanna and Louis of Taranto confirmed the privileges of the nobles and cities of Provence, ratifying their obligation to choose officers, such as seneschals, from the native population of Provence, and reinstituting the jurisdiction of the judges of Provence.[52]

Some privileges proved short-lived. When Lord Raymon seized lands from Lord Uguo de Baux in early 1349 and refused to return them, Queen Johanna, in her capacity of Countess of Provence, removed Lord Raymon as seneschal and replaced him with Lord Giovanni Barrili.[53] This was an opportunity to get rid of a lord who had openly defied her and put someone in his place that she trusted.[54]

Queen Johanna trusted Lord Barrili after his help during her complicated minority. But many lords of Provence saw Barrili as a foreign lord being imposed on them only a few months after Queen Johanna promised she would do no such thing.[55] Lord Barrili's appointment caused a rift among the lords of Provence that threatened open rebellion and civil war.[56] The witnesses to Article 38 focused on Lord Raymon and Lord Uguo, but their feud happened in this broader moment of danger.

The cities of Provence, especially Aix-en-Provence, which was the seat of the Estates court, refused to hear Lord Barrili's oath of office and continued to support Lord Raymon as seneschal. By March 1349, only Marseille had officially accepted Barrili. Messengers sent to Aix were mistreated and incarcerated. In response, Lord Barrili and the Marseille council officially cut off trade ties with the supporters of Lord Raymon d'Agoult and reinforced Marseille's walls. They removed or incarcerated any members of their governing council faithful to Raymon and replaced them with men from Florence, further turning this dispute into a perceived struggle between the people of Provence and outsiders.[57]

Nobles and city representatives from around Provence supported Lord Raymon or at least withdrew their support for Barrili. For these men, Raymon was not an upstart lord rebelling against Queen Johanna, but a defender of Provence standing against an oath-breaking overlord. Although Lords Giovanni Barrili and Uguo de Baux were skilled diplomats and not seen as enemies of Provence, Queen Johanna's letters and tactics did not put them in a good light.

By the end of March 1349, Pope Clement VI was involved in the dispute. He supported a truce until May 12 and invited both parties to come to Avignon to negotiate resuming trade and ending hostilities. Pope Clement highlighted the importance of safeguarding the peace, though by this time Provençal lords had already attacked and seized lands of several lords of Marseille, refusing to return the property until Marseille renounced support for Barrili as seneschal. In response the lords of Marseille armed themselves further, including recruiting cavalry and placing arbalests near the walls.[58] They also sought support from lords in cities west of the Rhône, like Arles and Tarascon, where many had strong ties to the lords of Baux and Marseille. Several of these cities retracted their active support of Lord Raymon d'Agoult and the Estates, though they hesitated to fully support Barrili, creating even more dissension in Provence. This is the great division, scandal, and war that Bishop Philippe Cabassole had seen.

In mid-April 1349, Clement entrusted peace negotiations to Bishop Philippe Cabassole. For many reasons, Cabassole was a perfect choice. He had been a longtime supporter of the Angevins of Naples. He had acted as a royal officer under King Robert and Queen Sanxia and traveled frequently to Naples. Finally, like Lord Barrili, he was a friend of Petrarch, so he could bring a sense of shared friendship to these difficult meetings.[59]

But these negotiations between the two seneschals never happened. In an awkward turn of events at the end of April 1349, Queen Johanna renounced her support for Lord Giovanni Barrili.[60] Letters sent by Johanna and Louis of Taranto stated their desire to maintain the peace of Provence by recalling Barrili. Some scholars, however, see this as Louis exercising his authority as Count of Provence by forcing Johanna to remove Barrili, who was chosen without Louis's consent.[61]

While this maneuver removed the problem of having two seneschals, it did not restore good relations between Lords Raymon d'Agoult and Uguo de Baux. Louis and Johanna's abrupt turnaround placed the lords of Marseille and Uguo's other supporters in the awkward position of having as seneschal a lord they had openly defied and with whom Uguo had an ongoing land dispute.

In early May, before the end of the official truce, Pope Clement VI asked Bishop Philippe Cabassole to negotiate with Lord Uguo de Baux, Uguo's Marseille supporters, and Raymon d'Agoult.[62] Cabassole convinced these lords to come to Cavaillon, where he negotiated a successful peace.[63] As part of the negotiation, he called upon Delphine to speak with the lords. It was at this point that, for the witnesses to Article 38, she averted the "war." In the words of Article 38, she healed the discord between Lords Uguo and Raymon by creating harmony between them. Cabassole did not explain the background of this moment—Delphine's inquest was not the appropriate place—but he knew the complexity of the moment, as would many of the readers of the inquest documents in the papal court. The political details help a modern audience, however, see the connotations shared by many audiences of this wondrous moment.

Bishop Philippe Cabassole's choice to invite Delphine to the negotiations reflected the cultural view of the emotions associated with lordly violence. The emotion language of Article 38 showed how Delphine could diffuse political discord with affection and heal the sickness caused by lordly violence with her own suffering. By bringing in Delphine, Cabassole was caring for the souls of men and offering them a kind of sacred space in which to transform their discord into peace. This solution resonated with Pope Clement VI's language in his official inquest into Andrew's death as care for the souls under his charge. It was not simply religious hyperbole or affectation. It was a way of understanding and negotiating violence.

A letter from Petrarch to his friend Giovanni Barrili, the man who was briefly seneschal of Provence, gives further insight into this sense of emotion and political negotiation. Petrarch wrote the letter to calm Barrili, who was having a significant disagreement with the royal seneschal of Naples, Nicola Acciaiuoli. In one section, Petrarch wrote:

> Having thus directly located anger in the breast and lust in the region of the heart, he [Plato in his three-part understanding of the soul] placed reason in the head as in a fortress, so that its very location would reveal it as the controller and mistress of the passions. . . . I believe you should be briefly reminded about what every learned person knows, namely, that where passions dwell, there too reside the hideous clouds and dreadful darkness of the soul, and to put it clearly, the total eclipse of reason . . . if we wish to be happy with that happiness which may be enjoyed in this mortal life—although through it we aspire to another—it is necessary, I say, for it to partake significantly of the divine mind so that, as is said about Olympus's loftiest peak, no mists of passion may touch it.[64]

In this letter we see the same link of emotion and political relationships. Petrarch's language goes beyond that used in Article 38. He evokes and conflates ideas expressed in theological and medical texts about the way anger affected the body.[65] Anger was believed to heat the blood and cause it to rush from the heart to the extremities. While a small amount of anger was good to get the blood flowing, continuous anger overheated (literally burned) the blood, which could then become black bile and rise as a mist to the brain. This obscured the rational faculties.[66]

Petrarch's letter, however, also incorporates the spiritual effects of anger, namely, that the mist of passions also obscures the rational mind's ability to seek earthly and spiritual happiness. The eclipse of reason precludes men from spiritually healthy friendship and causes them to continue in irrational, angry actions. Actions governed by anger separated a person from God.

The language of Cabassole's friend, Petrarch, suggests what witnesses believed that Delphine accomplished politically, physically, and spiritually when she calmed the anger between these lords. She healed the sickness of violence caused by anger that the political disruptions of 1347–1349 had caused. The context of plague, invasion, and political division reveals this moment as more than just another skirmish among the lords of Provence. This was a moment of danger for the people of Provence, and Cabassole's choice to use Delphine as a negotiator reflects how he and others understood that danger in the interplay of emotion, political relationships, and spiritual health.

Witness Testimony to Article 38

While Delphine's inquest was not a place to directly air political grievances, it was the place to describe moments when Delphine had protected the faithful from harm. And the political events of 1347–1349 had harmed the people of Provence. Witnesses navigated this situation by emphasizing the making of peace, emphasizing Delphine's suffering, and attesting to the *fama* (in this case, the public awareness) of the event, if not the political backstory.

Bishop Philippe Cabassole's testimony shows how a witness could make his political views clear without making direct statements. When Cabassole spoke to the open-ended Article 1, his first statements about Delphine concerned her actions and reputation in Naples. His framing of the "war" in Provence in 1349 started here.

His framing is clearest in the list of people he spoke to in Naples about Delphine. He stated that he heard about Delphine from King Robert, Queen Sanxia, and Duchess Agnes of Pèrigord.[67] He also mentions hearing about Delphine from his own family members and Lord Raymon d'Agoult. He did not mention Queen Johanna, though as a member of the council appointed for her minority he would have interacted with her. This list of people who spoke to him of Delphine puts him on a side in the political dispute of 1347–1349. Not only did he associate with Lord Raymon and *not* Lord Uguo, but he aligned himself with Cardinal Talleyrand. For Cabassole, mentioning Lady Agnes of Pèrigord, Talleyrand's sister, and not Queen Johanna was a choice. It was not a direct attack, but it was a statement. Although decades had passed, he had not forgotten that Louis of Taranto and Louis's mother, Catherine of Valois, were implicated in Agnes's death. Queen Johanna was now associated with them.

Philippe Cabassole's testimony emphasized the danger of the political discord and put it obliquely in the larger picture of royal politics in Provence. He started his testimony to Article 38 with a restatement of Delphine's love and fervor for God. He then put the event in the larger context of the death of King Robert by telling the papal commissioners about Delphine traveling to Naples to console Queen Sanxia, who was ill.[68] He used this as an example of Delphine's love and good will, but because of the political overtones of Article 38, it also spoke to the dangerous political atmosphere in Naples in 1343. In other words, Cabassole put Delphine in Naples to console and support a sick friend, but she was also in a position to heal political discord there. In addition, this brief statement, coming directly before the story of the civil war, created a link for the inquest commissioners between the transfer of the Crown of Naples from King Robert to Queen Johanna and the civil war in Provence. Cabassole did not directly state the link. He did not mention Queen Johanna. He did not have to.

After mentioning Queen Sanxia, Cabassole related a brief version of the story of Delphine coming to Cavaillon in order to settle the discord between two great men of Provence. He made no mention of Delphine's suffering, which appeared in Article 38. Instead he focused on the resolution. He stated that she settled their discord and returned them to peace and concord. Although he organized this negotiation and could have included a personal narrative, he chose not to. Cabassole still had to tread lightly in a politically difficult time. Even though Clement was no longer the pope in 1363 and both Lord Raymon and Lord Uguo had died, Queen Johanna was still in power and at the beginning of a new stage in her reign. For Cabassole, peace was the important detail here. His worry that if Delphine had not brought peace there would have been a great scandal and war made him the most directly critical of the political discord of all six witnesses.[69]

Along with Philippe Cabassole, there were five other witnesses—Bertranda Bertomieua, Lady Catherine de Pui, Friar Bertran Jusbert, Friar Giraud Raybaud and Master Durand Andree.[70] If we think of the six witnesses to this article as a representative sample of people who told the story, they were a surprisingly diverse group. They represented diverse social statuses, included both men and women, and included both religious and lay people. Through simple narrative construction (he saw / he heard), witnesses remembered and presented the event. They included none of the details of political discord, which would not have been appropriate in Delphine's inquest and, as we have seen, were potentially harmful to the success of her canonization.

Each witness emphasized a different element of the event. I have chosen three stories that provide three different perspectives. Friar Bertran Jusbert described the act of making peace in the most detail, and his testimony gives us a way to think about how witnesses understood the peacemaking process. Friar Giraud Raybaud revealed that the story of Delphine bringing peace to warring Provençal lords had been shared for years among many groups of people. Finally, Bertranda Bertomieua emphasized the timing of the event, placing it in relation to the "first mortality."

Like Cabassole, Friar Bertran Jusbert also assessed the danger of the discord, and emphasized the making of peace. Friar Bertran was the *guardianus* of the Franciscan house in Apt. He had become one of Delphine's confessors in 1348. Though he did not see the negotiations, he had heard about them from the inquest proctor, Master Nicolau Laurens, who Friar Bertran claimed had witnessed them. Friar Bertran named the lords involved and offered judgment by describing their controversy and dissensions as dangerous.[71]

Friar Bertran used formal language to describe the peacemaking process. He specified that after Delphine made peace and concord between Lords Uguo and Raymon, the lords exchanged "the kiss of peace," and thus withdrew in friendship.[72] By using this language, Friar Bertran linked Delphine's negotiation to the long tradition of curbing constant warfare among lords by transforming hatred into love. The kiss of peace became a politically binding event during the Peace and Truce of God movements that emerged in the tenth and eleventh centuries.[73] In these movements, not only did local lords and bishops attempt to limit warfare through law, but they also held large, at times ecstatic, meetings in the presence of relics that brought combatants together in a spiritually charged moment where they could make peace without loss of honor.[74] For bishops and lords responsible for the health and souls of those in their care, this was a way to protect monastic and ecclesiastical property, defuse feuds, and reintegrate those who had engaged in violent conflict into the broader Christian community.

The "war of the seneschals" in 1349 has some similarities to the violence that the Peace of God events tried to control. For example, there was a growing feud between these lords that would result in danger to local people and likely destruction of Church property. As in the earlier Peace of God events, there was also low institutional control at this moment. The people of Provence could not expect Queen Johanna to solve this problem.

Inviting Delphine to speak to these warring lords was a solution similar to the use of relics in the Peace of God movement. For the witnesses, the living Delphine was like a relic. Miracles had already started happening around Delphine in the early 1340s, revealing her sanctity. These included miraculous healings in the court of Naples that Bertranda Bertomieua described, healings on the steps of St. Louis of Anjou's church in Marseille, and a holy light that had appeared in her room starting in 1348.[75] For the inquest witnesses, these miracles had proved her special relationship to God and the potential for her to be a liaison between God and the people of Provence.[76] Her difficult and painful travel and her physical presence at the negotiation also functioned in a similar way to relics in the earlier Peace of God movement, which were carried to the place where feuding lords met.

These elements made up the drama of peace and the careful staging that went into these events.[77] In both ways her presence as a source of God's grace created a sacred space for the lords to meet and allowed them to show each other mercy without losing status.[78] This "war" was not identical to the Peace of God movement, and certainly Friar Bertran Jusbert did not consciously evoke it here. But in his testimony and even in Article 38 we see negotiators using a living holy person like a relic in order to solve a political dispute similar to those encountered in earlier centuries.

Delphine as a relic is just one way to see how witnesses understood her ability to bring peace, however. For both the witnesses and the audience of these testimonies, Delphine made sense as someone who could intercede. Even without any special sanctity, noblewomen were often seen as being able to influence warring relatives.[79] Delphine was related to one of the men involved in the "war"—Lord Raymon d'Agoult—and had lived in a convent with two of his daughters.[80] Lord Raymon and several of his supporters had great respect for Delphine. In addition, she called to people's minds her late husband, Lord Elzear de Sabran, Count of Ariano, who had been remarkable for his fair dealings with lords under his rule and was the subject of a canonization inquest in 1351.[81] As historian Florian Mazel explained, "The grace of these two saints [Elzear and Delphine] permitted them to limit the violence around them and contribute to the reestablishment of peace in their noble group."[82] Together and separately, they had embodied an ideal of Christian behavior that others could use to transform anger and violence between lords into love and peace.[83]

In combination with her status, Delphine's sanctity—based on her poverty, virginity, and humility—also gave her influence over nobles in dispute.[84] For witnesses, Delphine was a noblewoman who had renounced great wealth to work alongside residents of a hermitage outside Ansouis and nuns in the Holy Cross convent. She was a virgin who inspired others to that sacred state and had a successful chaste marriage.[85] Delphine's extraordinary piety made her suffering special. Her suffering created a way for them to stop sinning. For the witnesses, Delphine's presence helped the lords overcome their discord and return to a relationship of peace. In light of Article 38, she not only suffered for their sins, but created a way for them to stop sinning.

Another witness, Friar Giraud Raybaud, gives insight into public opinion of the event, revealing that people outside Delphine's immediate circle knew about the danger and Delphine's role in healing it.[86] Friar Giraud, at age seventy, was one of the oldest witnesses in Delphine's inquest, nearly as old as Delphine had been when she died. He had been an important witness in the inquest for Delphine's husband, Elzear, in 1351, making him an associate of the holy couple for a long time. His full testimony not only described his experience of Delphine in Naples, but showed him to be a significant social networker in Naples, Nice, and Provence.[87]

Through Friar Giraud's testimony we see the apparatus of *fama* at work. He claimed to have heard in 1350 about Delphine's exhausting travel in the humble litter "to a place where she hoped to bestow concord on those experiencing discord."[88] He knew the names and titles of the lords, and where the negotiation had taken place. When asked by the commissioners where and from whom he had heard about it, he stated that he had heard in Avignon from Peire Raoli and Malosaguine of Monteus. When these two men described the event, there were others present, including Friar Peire Polli and Friar Peire

Reversati. These names, which never appeared again in Delphine's inquest, provide a glimpse of the story of averted civil war passing among various social levels and social groups in Provence. When the commissioners asked Friar Giraud if his statement represented common belief and statements in Avignon and Apt, his "yes" implied a regional awareness of a dangerous moment and a way of understanding that moment.[89]

Like other witnesses, Bertranda Bertomieua described Delphine's difficult travel and named the lords involved in the dispute. But she also located these events as occurring after the first mortality. As we saw in chapter 1, Bertranda framed several events by placing them in relation to important deaths. The first mortality was a very important moment for Bertranda. She used it five times in her testimony as a reference date for Delphine leaving Naples and the worldly life, returning to Provence, and living humbly. The last time she used it was in reference to Article 38. When asked by the commissioners when the event happened, "she said that [it was] after the first mortality."[90]

She was not alone. Friar Bertran Jusbert also used the plague as a time marker for this "war."[91] By linking the discord of Lords Uguo and Raymon to the first mortality, Bertranda and Friar Bertran remembered plague and political discord together and brought them together for the commissioners and later readers of these documents. They added the psychological weight of the first mortality to the political discord caused by Queen Johanna and Louis of Taranto. And in contrast to either of these political leaders, Delphine brought peace and health for men's souls.

Bishop Philippe Cabassole and the First Mortality in Provence

The "war of the seneschals" was inseparable from the shared knowledge and experience of the first mortality. In Delphine's inquest thirteen witnesses and two articles of interrogation used the phrase "at the time of the first mortality" as a time marker. This is the second most common time marker in the inquest, after Delphine's death. Witnesses did not describe the general events of that time, however. They were not asked and did not describe their general experiences of plague. They could assume that the papal commissioners and everyone who read these documents would know what they meant by the phrase because those people had lived through it too.

Modern readers, however, can never fully understand the psychological weight of the phrase "the first mortality." Over six hundred years later, we can only try to get a sense of what they might have experienced, how they made sense of those experiences, and how they tried to solve the problems that emerged from this devastating epidemic. Again, Bishop Philippe Cabassole and his broader social circle provide vantage points from which to understand the physical and psychological impacts of the first wave of plague, which so shaped witnesses' perception of the "war of the seneschals."

One of the things we understand immediately from the phrase "the first mortality" is that there had been more than one wave of plague. By the time they testified in 1363, all the witnesses in Delphine's inquest had lived through two waves of epidemic. Their perspective is different, therefore, from sources that were written directly after the first wave.[92] (One wishes that the canonization inquest testimony for Delphine's husband, Elzear, had survived. Testimony from 1351 might provide an interesting contrast for these testimonies from 1363.)

Generations of historians have used tax records to see the physical impact of plague on Provence. Edouard Baratier's demographic study of medieval Provence includes basic taxation data on many cities and towns. Apt, where the inquest took place and where almost half of the witnesses lived, was among the second-tier cities in terms of population.[93] In the early fourteenth century Apt had roughly six hundred hearths and its *bailie* had three thousand hearths.[94] A larger city, like Aix-en-Provence, had roughly fifteen hundred hearths, and Provence as a whole had roughly fourteen thousand hearths.[95]

Many cities and towns of Provence experienced gradual population decline before the first wave of plague.[96] However, after waves of epidemic in 1348, 1361, and 1399, the number of hearths dropped significantly and stayed low.[97] For example, by 1400, only 250 hearths paid the *droit d'albergue* levied against all the hearths in Apt.[98] Claude Faure, in his study of the finances of the Comtat Venaissin, found that tax income for the Apostolic Chamber dropped from roughly six thousand florins in 1343 to twelve hundred florins in 1349.[99]

Daniel Lord Smail has tracked the impact of plague in Marseille from another angle by looking at the sale of property in the city's records. He found that property changed hands quickly at this time as people inherited land and houses from dying relatives. But inheritors could not always pay the taxes, so they often sold the property, abandoned it, or in some cases married someone who could help them pay for it.[100]

Other kinds of economic records can reveal the impact of plague.[101] An economic inquest conducted in 1358 by the royal court in Aix-en-Provence shows the changes in food availability and prices at this time. The goal of the inquest was to understand changes in prices from 1346 to 1358. Master Raymon Ysoard, who was a notary as well as the *clavaire* (a type of financial official) for the court, was sent to five grain-producing towns in eastern Provence. There he interviewed people involved in producing and selling grain, recorded the measures used in each town, and read documents produced in this thirteen-year span. These records reveal that in 1347 and 1348, wheat prices went up to seven or eight times as much as usual.[102] This was particularly true for spring prices, which were traditionally higher because communities relied more heavily at this time of year on stored grain. Prior to the appearance of plague, two poor growing seasons had already reduced the availability of grain and increased prices. As historian Louis Stouff points out, the plague arrived in an area that had been suffering from a serious supply crisis for many months.[103]

Taxation records and other economic sources can show the drop in population and changing economic choices after the plague, but these records do not help modern audiences understand the lived experience of the plague. Survivors had to make sense of this moment for themselves. Historians have studied both short- and long-term reactions. Francine Michaud, for example, looked at the success of pilgrimage in the years after the first wave, especially travelers in Marseille for the jubilee year of 1350.[104] Jacques Chiffoleau, in his broad study of Avignon in the second half of the fourteenth century, looked at the preambles of wills, as well as funerary art, to see how people reacted to the plague. He argued that we can understand the lived experience of plague by exploring how people prepared for death, such as using their wills to micromanage their funeral processions and paying for thousands of masses to be said after they died.[105] Chiffoleau sees this process as interacting with the long-term issues of urbanization and movement to the city, because people were no longer as worried about their ancestors in the long term (being buried in the family plot and being part of a long family history). Instead they were worried about themselves. This appeared in their desire for grand funerals even if they were not noble or wealthy, their desire for many masses, and their desire to be buried somewhere important, such as in a tomb or a religious institution rather than a cemetery.[106] Bishop Philippe Cabassole's relatively grand tomb with a marble effigy reflected some of these changes.[107]

Recent studies of funeral practice during the first waves of plague reveal that mourners and families showed great care for the dead, even when burying them in mass graves. Bodies were carefully placed, individuals had shrouds, and some of the dead even had ornaments, suggesting that the family took care to prepare their loved one.[108] One miraculous healing from the first wave of plague gives us a glimpse of the attempt to maintain funeral practices, even at a time when so many were dying. Lady Maria d'Evenos, of the upper aristocracy of Provence, related a story that her husband had told her of his experience of the fever and buboes of the illness of the first mortality.[109] According to Lady Maria, Lord Giraud was near death, his sister had already died, and their family had already prepared the candles and gold cloth at the sepulcher. He was far too sick to travel to the location of the sepulcher, however, so his doctor and friends cared for him at the Holy Cross convent in Apt. Delphine was not present, but the people caring for him laid him in the pious woman's bed, "hoping for his recovery."[110] According to Lady Maria, Lord Giraud knew this was happening and did not consider himself worthy. But in Delphine's bed he was able to rest and sleep, and eventually he regained the ability to eat. When his doctors later came to question him, they found the fever gone, though he was still weak.[111]

Lord Giraud was a member of one of the powerful Provençal families, so his experience does not reflect that of the average person. But it does show how one family experienced the death of multiple members and still prepared the candles and cloths expected at a funeral for someone of high status.[112] As with archeological evidence from fourteenth-century burials, we see that his family did not abandon him, as some literary texts suggest, but instead provided him with medical care and prepared an elaborate funeral for him and his sister.

Lady Maria's story about her husband shows that we must be cautious with literary depictions of the first wave of plague.[113] But while literary sources may include hyperbolic language or exaggeration, they can reveal the psychological impact of plague on Provence. Although no letters survive from Bishop Philippe Cabassole or others in the inquest about this moment of plague, Cabassole's friends Francis Petrarch and Louis Heyligen of Beeringen did write accounts.[114] They took very different approaches to this catastrophe, which allow modern audiences to see a range of reactions.[115] Their letters give insight into what the witnesses meant when they used the phrase "the first mortality."

During the first ravages of the plague in Provence, Petrarch left Avignon for his solitary retreat on the banks of the Sorgue. Both Bishop Philippe Cabassole and Louis Heyligen visited him there. During his time near the Sorgue, Petrarch wrote his *Vita Solitaria*, which he dedicated to Cabassole, but he also wrote a series of letters to Heyligen.[116] In these letters, Petrarch described 1348 as a time "which not only robbed us of our friends but the entire world of peoples. If anyone remained, the coming year gathers those survivors, so that whoever survived that storm is being pursued by death's sickle. . . . When was anything similar ever seen or heard? In what chronicles did anyone ever read that dwellings were emptied, cities abandoned, countrysides barren, fields laden with bodies, and a dreadful and vast solitude covered the earth?"[117]

Petrarch especially struggled with the sudden loss of friends. He described meeting a new friend after returning to Italy only to sit at the man's deathbed a few months later. The letters have hyperbolic language describing death on a massive scale, and evidence that people still cared for the dying and dead, as we saw in the miracle concerning Lord Giraud.

Throughout the series of letters, Petrarch struggled to understand the cause of the plague. Many works written at the time searched for the underlying cause, not just the immediate, terrestrial cause. Understanding the underlying cause could help people understand how to fix the "real" problem so that they could bring an end to the epidemic. Petrarch believed the plague had to come from God rather than the workings of nature, because if it did not, then that meant God did not care about mankind. But he could not see why his age was being punished more than others. As he wrote to Louis Heyligen, "Therefore either we are really the worst of all, something which I would like to but dare not deny, or else we are being saved through these present evils by becoming more experienced and more pure for future blessings, or else there is something involved which we are simply unable to fathom."[118]

Petrarch ultimately left God's purpose an open-ended question and focused instead on his response as a man guided by reason.[119] He mourned, but he tried not to mourn too much. He used this moment, instead, to emphasize the idea that what many men considered life was actually a dreaming sleep. When people woke from sleep (i.e., died) they would feel none of the sorrow of their fleeting dreams.

The recipient of Petrarch's letters, Louis Heyligen, also wrote about the first wave of plague, but in a very different way. Heyligen was a chanter in the household of Cardinal Colonna in Avignon. In a letter Louis sent to his colleagues in Bruges, he described the first wave of plague in Avignon.[120] Like Petrarch, he too struggled to understand why the plague happened. And even more directly than any of the witnesses, he linked the violent political instability of Queen Johanna's early reign to the epidemic of 1348.

Louis Heyligen's letter brings together the medical, political, and spiritual meanings of the first wave of plague for an educated cleric in mid-fourteenth-century Provence. Although I do not claim that everyone in this social group thought the same way, Heyligen's letter can give us insight into how a witness like Bishop Philippe Cabassole understood the implications of the 1348 wave of plague.

The letter began with a common contemporary medical description of plague and its spread.[121] Heyligen reported reading a letter about rains of frogs, snakes, and scorpions in India followed by lightning storms that caused uncontrollable fires. The two combined to send large amounts of poison into the air, which reached the western Mediterranean through wind. He also included the story of the plague ships, packed with irresistible silks and spices, which went from port to port, including Marseille, moving the plague via trade goods and greed.[122]

Heyligen then described the impact of the plague on the Rhône valley, and especially Avignon. He claimed to have seen over seven thousand houses empty and alms going unused because so few of the poor survived.[123] Outside sources also indicate the toll the plague took on the Comtat Venaissin, including the deaths of the *clavaires* of Cairanne, Sorgue, Bollène, Cavaillon, Mornas, and Malaucène. In several of these towns the position could not be filled for years.[124]

According to Heyligen, Pope Clement VI led processions and bought and consecrated new fields to use as cemeteries. Other sources show that Clement VI remained in Avignon for the seven months of the plague and paid for doctors for the sick, carters, and gravediggers. In the field that he bought outside the city, a long, deep trench was dug for the thousands of bodies that overwhelmed the city's cemeteries. Clement had a church built there, dedicated to the Virgin Mary, and developed a mass for the plague.[125] The pope's actions show the continued care for bodies and souls even when preparing mass graves.

In Avignon, Heyligen also saw fear. In general, even amongst the clergy, epidemics were thought to come from widespread corruption of the air that then corrupted other elements, such as water.[126] Even if the ultimate source of an epidemic was God's anger, the distribution method of an epidemic was terrestrial—hence the rains of poisonous creatures that then caught fire. This process corrupted the air on a scale massive enough to explain an epidemic of this size. Heyligen observed that large groups of people feared to drink the city water or eat fish. And he saw many people so afraid of poison that poor men carrying powders, which might poison water, were burned.[127]

Although he did not specify that Jews were targeted in these attacks, they were frequently accused of poisoning wells at this time. The danger for Jews became so great that in July 1348, Pope Clement VI reissued the bull *Sicut Judeis*, which reminded Christians that the Jews were under the protection of the Church and ordered Christians not to harm Jews physically or financially.[128] The danger continued, however, and Clement supplemented the bull in September with a letter to clergy urging them to actively protect Jews in their communities. He sent a long letter in October, urging bishops to suppress the flagellants and their supporters who were targeting Jews.[129] Although Louis Heyligen did not mention it, we know that the Jewish community in Apt was attacked in 1348. In 1349, Lord Raymon d'Agoult ordered the offending lords to pay a fine for harming the Jewish community.[130]

Like Petrarch and other writers at the time, Heyligen considered the underlying cause of the plague and, through that, the way to heal it. Petrarch had offered multiple ideas about God's motives; the one he chose for himself was the idea that the plague was purifying. In this scenario, people could not do anything to stop the plague, but they could endure it and in the process become better prepared for eternal life. Heyligen posited that the plague was a punishment for sinful behavior, and therefore people could purify themselves by changing their behavior and then asking God for forgiveness. Many at the time took this view, which led to what some historians refer to as "moral sanitation." Different people considered various causes of God's displeasure, which in part led to persecution of the Jews and the removal of people seen as morally corrupt, as well as ill, from cities.[131]

Heyligen described efforts in Avignon to heal moral corruption. Pope Clement VI lead large processions in Avignon, including up to two thousand people—some in hair shirts, some barefoot, and some whipping themselves. For modern audiences, these processions can seem bizarre. But they were ultimately trying to solve the underlying problem of plague by recognizing God's punishment and expressing the contrition and sorrow that would repair the relationship with God. If they could repair this relationship, they could potentially stop the epidemic. There are many accounts of cities praying to saints for intercession and holding processions. For them, it was a valid solution to the problem.

Concerning the cause of God's punishment, Heyligen hinted at contemporary political violence. He stated, "What beginning or what end, God knows; certain people still fear that for the death of King Andrew, who was slaughtered, God scourges the world by these evils."[132] This was a clear reference to the 1345 assassination of Andrew of Hungary, Queen Johanna's first husband. It is also an oblique reference to the papal inquiry into Andrew's death, in which Queen Johanna and Louis of Taranto never participated.

The fact that Heyligen, and the "certain people" he mentions, considered the death of King Andrew as the cause of the plague is a powerful criticism of Louis of Taranto and Queen Johanna. He suggested that Andrew's assassination was a serious enough sin that it made God punish the world. We cannot know if Heyligen's friend Petrarch was one of these "certain people," but we do know that Petrarch was not a strong supporter of the new administration in Naples and that he wrote scathing letters against them.[133] And we have seen that the Bishop Philippe Cabassole mentioned Queen Sanxia and Agnes of Pèrigord in his testimony, but not Queen Johanna.

The first wave of plague, what witnesses called the first mortality, was traumatic for those who lived through it. Delphine's witnesses and their friends and colleagues had different reactions to the great numbers of dead. As we saw in Petrarch's and Louis Heyligen's letters, people navigated the fear of "death's sickle," the loss of loved ones, and the feeling of guilt and bewilderment that their sins, or their leaders' sins, had caused God to send this punishment.

Political disaster and epidemic were linked in the minds of many in Provence. The plague began to ravage Provençal cities and towns just as Queen Johanna fled to Provence to escape the invasion of Andrew's brother, Louis of Hungary. This conjunction of events—plague, rebellion, and civil war—could not be separate in people's memories. It shaped how people in Provence perceived Queen Johanna and the plague. That several witnesses used the phrase *prima mortalitas* as a time marker for the 1349 "war of the seneschals," for example, linked the overwhelming death and sorrow of plague to this moment of political danger.

Conclusions and Codas

Bishop Philippe Cabassole testified to Article 38 in 1363 as a trusted servant of Pope Urban V. Cabassole was rector of the Comtat Venaissin by this time, and continued to travel on diplomatic missions for the papal court.[134] But remembering what he called the "great division," "scandal," and "war" that an earlier pope had asked him to help avert would have brought the political and spiritual complexity of that moment back to his mind.[135] The effects of Andrew of Hungary's assassination, the effects of the plague, and the political turmoil of Louis of Taranto's efforts to become King of Naples rather than just Johanna's consort were part of the story of "the war of the seneschals" that he could not share with the papal commissioners questioning him, but he did not forget. Starting his testimony with the names of King Robert, Queen Sanxia, and Agnes of Pèrigord and including Queen Sanxia in his testimony to Article 38 give the modern reader clues to his perception of events and the story he was trying to tell.

Article 38 and witness testimonies about the lords' discord emphasized peacemaking and concern for the sickness that violence caused for the soul. Political discord angered God and threatened everyone involved. Cabassole's friend, Louis Heyligen, wove Andrew of Hungary's assassination into the story of plague in Avignon and the world. Delphine's care for the health of men's souls and her closeness to God gave her the ability to heal discord through her suffering and holy presence. She transformed lords on the brink of war from enemies to friends who could exchange the kiss of peace. Witnesses like

Philippe Cabassole perceived that Queen Johanna and Louis of Taranto had, in contrast, inspired violence and war.

Two codas to the peace negotiations between Lords Uguo and Raymon give further insight into the spiritual and political impact of 1348. The first coda comes from Delphine's inquest. Articles 42 and 43 reveal Delphine's continued concern for the soul of Lord Raymon d'Agoult. In Article 42, Delphine was wondrously aware of Raymon's death at the moment it occurred in 1356. She wept for him and said an office of the dead.[136] Article 43 described Raymon's daughters, Tiburga and Rossolina, who lived at the Holy Cross convent, questioning Delphine about the state of Raymon's soul at death. Delphine revealed that his soul had been healthy, which consoled them.[137] For the papal commissioners and everyone who read these testimonies, these articles reveal the moral framework in which this story existed. According to the inquest articles, this lord, who was close to Delphine and changed his behavior because of her, had healed his soul and achieved eternal life.

The second coda reveals that the other figure in the "war," Lord Uguo de Baux, remained engaged in the destructive political maneuvering for the throne of Naples. This information did not appear in Delphine's inquest, but Bishop Philippe Cabassole and others would have known the end of his story. In 1350, Lord Uguo de Baux, with the support of Pope Clement VI, aided Queen Johanna and Louis of Taranto when the King of Hungary invaded for a second time. Uguo arrived in Naples's port with six Marseillaise galleys and tipped the balance of the fighting against the King of Hungary. After negotiations concluded, Uguo agreed to meet with Johanna and Louis, who were in Gaeta. Before doing so, however, Uguo took on board Johanna's younger sister Maria, who had been a widow since the King of Hungary's first invasion. Uguo oversaw the marriage of Maria to his son.[138] This was a significant bid to enter the royal family of Naples, since Maria was in line to inherit the throne.[139]

When Lord Uguo de Baux arrived in Gaeta, however, Louis of Taranto accused Uguo of treason and soon after stripped him of his titles.[140] Louis arrested Uguo's sons and brought Maria back under his own control. This, and other acts, allowed Louis of Taranto to defeat other claimants to the throne and gain the title and powers of King of Naples, which he did in 1352.[141] Several Baux family members rebelled in 1357–1358, in what emerges from witness testimony as the second moment of danger, which we will explore in chapter 3.

These codas give a sense of how people understood the interconnectedness of political violence in the midst of plague. Bishop Philippe Cabassole tried to limit that violence through his association with the holy woman

Delphine and through his personal relationships with the lords of Provence and Naples. In his and other witnesses' testimony, Delphine brought peace to warring lords through her presence, her words, and her own suffering at the time of the first mortality. The story of the averted "war" between Lord Uguo and Lord Raymon brought order and a sense of control to a time when thousands died of a mysterious illness while political leaders fought each other for worldly power.

Chapter 3

Master Nicolau Laurens and the Mercenary Invasion of 1357–1358

The second chronological moment of danger that emerged from witness testimony occurred in 1357–1358. Over the course of this year, roughly four thousand mercenaries entered Provence, captured towns, and laid siege to Marseille and Aix-en-Provence.[1] The mercenaries were the first wave of the companies mentioned in Article 38, who offended God with their violence and for whom Delphine wept. Although there would be larger invasions later, this was one of the first significant mercenary invasions of Provence, and it stayed in witnesses' memories.

From the bird's-eye view of the historian, we can see that this moment was a continuation of political wrangling for the Crown of Naples and the strained relationship of Queen Johanna and (now) King Louis with the lords of Provence.[2] In this flare-up of violence, potential heirs from the Durazzo branch of the Angevin royal family joined forces with the disgruntled lords of Baux in an attempt to seize the county of Provence and weaken Queen Johanna and King Louis.[3]

From the historian's perspective, we can also see this moment as a turning point in the nature of violence at this time. As historian Justine Firnhaber-Baker, writes, "From the mid-1350s, violence that was not directly inflicted at English or French command also became a growing problem as mercenaries, left unemployed during truces, formed companies and took up arms on their own behalf."[4] The people of Provence were drawn into the fringes of the Hundred Years War, not by direct attack from the English or French, but by the increasing availability of mercenary soldiers to fight local battles.[5]

But Delphine's witnesses did not take this bird's-eye view. For them, this was not only a moment of danger; it was a moment of confusion. Although many witnesses spoke about the dangers of this time, and some likely understood the political maneuvering, the large-scale mercenary presence was different. Witnesses did not even have a consistent way to refer to the new kind of warfare. This was not "war" between local lords, as they had seen in 1349. Nor was it any other kind of war they were familiar with.[6] This was something else. Their struggle to name this violence so that they could describe it to papal commissioners reflects the changing nature of warfare and the difficulty that people who were living through the change had in coming to terms with it.[7] So, while witnesses may not have had a modern historian's perspective, putting their testimonies into a broader context helps us better understand what they experienced and how they spoke about it.

Several witnesses referred to this moment as "the war with the Gascons." While this invasion was led by the Gascon mercenary leader Arnau de Cervole, Provence was not at war with Gascony in the mid-fourteenth century, and the witnesses knew this. Cervole did not represent the duke of Gascony or anyone else, for that matter. More likely, these witnesses meant that there was general fighting with mercenaries, who were sometimes referred to as Gascons and in this case were led by a Gascon. Cervole and his troops usually fought for the king of France, but in 1357–1358 they were being paid by the Durazzo and Baux and were available because of a truce in the Hundred Years War.

But the phrase "war with the Gascons" helps us understand how witnesses tried to put a new kind of violence into a familiar frame of reference. Some witnesses tried to understand it as war, even though they knew it did not conform to the same rules and could not be ended using past methods, like the kiss of peace we saw in chapter 2. Witnesses also struggled to protect themselves during mercenary invasions. The lords of Provence—caught between warring sides of the Angevin royal family—could not depend on their count and countess for military aid. They ultimately had to put aside their differences to protect themselves. Local lords, far less experienced and trained than the mercenaries, had to lead town militias in an effort to protect their people from attack. Even people who were ideally considered noncombatants, like women and clergy, had to find ways to protect themselves and their towns. By combining the broad context of the Hundred Years War and the local warfare in Provence with witness testimonies, we gain insight into how people understood this violence as both physical and spiritual, opening the way for spiritual solutions.

Master Nicolau Laurens as the Shaper of Testimony

A useful way to explore the lived experience of the second moment of danger is through a participant in Delphine's inquest who had a bird's-eye view of all the inquest testimony. A witness is not the best choice, since even the most politically connected witness would have a limited view of the many different ways witnesses spoke about this moment of danger. Instead, the proctor of the inquest, Master Nicolau Laurens, is a better guide through this moment. Laurens was the person who collected evidence of Delphine's sanctity for over a decade, was part of Delphine's entourage during the events, chose and gathered most of the witnesses for the inquest, and wrote the articles of interrogation used for questioning witnesses.[8]

Master Nicolau appears to have been part of Delphine's household.[9] We learn much about him through witness testimonies. Witnesses give him different titles, including *magister, notarius, familiarus* of Delphine, and *servitore* to Delphine. In their stories we see him as a witness of Delphine's life and miracles, starting in the early 1340s when she returned to Provence from Naples. He was present for several important events, including the negotiations between Lords Raymon and Uguo in 1349, and, according to witnesses, he spoke about these events frequently. Friar Bertran Jusbert, for example, recalled hearing about the "war of the seneschals" from Master Nicolau. Witness testimony also reveals that Master Nicolau was not a distant or impartial observer of Delphine's saintly behavior. For example, he was actively part of a group who tried to hide her books about saints when her efforts to imitate their behavior harmed her health.[10]

Another way to understand Master Nicolau is by considering the role of proctor in an inquest. Historian James Brundage describes proctors as "useful all-purpose agents" who appeared in every level of legal courts and performed many tasks.[11] They were usually trained as notaries, sometimes had training as advocates, and were the workhorses of any inquest. They gathered evidence and witnesses, wrote and collected necessary paperwork, and understood the procedure of a large formal inquest.[12] As the proctor of Delphine's inquest, therefore, Master Nicolau had a profound influence on the stories collected in the inquest documents. He chose almost all of the sixty-eight witnesses, so he influenced who spoke about Delphine to the papal commissioners. He also wrote the articles of interrogation. As the articles were read to witnesses, they influenced what witnesses said about events.[13] As we saw in Article 38, Master Nicolau's articles were flexible enough to allow witnesses to speak to several events, but they also included enough specific information that he had gathered in advance so that the articles elicited specific stories rather than generalized statements.

Inquest testimony and documents show that Laurens understood the events of 1357–1358 to be a crucial moment for Delphine's sanctity. Many different people turned to her during this time, and she aided individuals and whole towns. As proctor of the inquest, Laurens included four articles of interrogation about this moment. The articles described Delphine's protection of combatants and noncombatants and the transformation of a mercenary into a penitent. He constructed these articles partly from his own experience and partly from speaking with many of the witnesses for years before Delphine died.[14] Witnesses also used the open-ended Article 1, which Master Nicolau wrote, to describe events at this time.

Master Nicolau went to great lengths to collect and include testimonies about these events. Overall, a large, diverse group of people testified to dangers they faced in this year. At least thirteen official witnesses described events in 1357–1358. As we will see below, Master Nicolau also included three testimonies that he heard and wrote down shortly after the events occurred.[15] Men and women, clergy and lay people, soldiers and serving women all told different stories. Master Nicolau brought those stories together. We can see his vantage point—his bird's-eye view of Delphine's life and sanctity—in the many articles of interrogation and witness testimonies he collected about this moment.

The stories that emerge in articles and testimony show that he understood why the moment mattered to political and spiritual leaders like the pope in Avignon and the lords of Provence. He used inquest procedure to frame the moment around Delphine's ability to heal discord and inspire peace. She protected those who avoided violence and transformed those who had committed violence if they were truly penitent. For Master Nicolau and the witnesses, the spiritual and political were deeply intertwined in this moment of dangerous warfare. Master Nicolau's framing of events in the articles of interrogation dovetailed with papal efforts to control mercenary violence through pastoral care at a time when there was a Europe-wide dependence on mercenary soldiers.

But the way witnesses described the violence and how they turned to Delphine for help were subtly different than in the "war" a decade earlier. While there were no lords for Delphine to visit and heal, Master Nicolau and the witnesses still emphasized Delphine's ability to bring peace. The mechanisms of peace in 1357 and afterward were much more complicated, however, and not within the witnesses' control.[16] As the articles of interrogation and witness testimony reveal, the mechanisms of peace were not fully within leaders' control either. Turning to God through Delphine's sanctity was a way witnesses had to heal the violence they lived through.

While historians have studied this lack of protection of local communities in 1357–1358 as a political and economic problem—the damage of military attack and the failure to raise funds for local armies to fight against mercenaries—Delphine's witnesses and inquest organizers raised complex issues of fear and the spiritual damage of violence.[17] The actions of the mercenaries under Arnau de Cervole made Delphine weep for the sickness of men's souls. Mercenaries risked eternal damnation by committing grave sins, and, according to Master Nicolau's articles, Delphine wanted to help them.

Through these testimonies a tension emerged between the ideals of healthy peace and the expectations of witnesses' social milieu. While local lords felt they had to fight to defend their communities, Delphine strove to protect their souls and contain the spiritual sickness of violence. In some inquest testimony, defenders were even subtly criticized for using violent methods. By focusing on spiritual dangers of violence, Master Nicolau's articles and the witness testimonies to them frame the spiritual sickness of violence and reveal the profound ambivalence about these mercenaries. For example, while killing was presented in articles and testimonies as always wrong, the mercenaries were not a faceless, monolithic evil. Master Nicolau allowed witnesses to criticize the mercenaries, but he also allowed mercenary testimony to inform the inquest. In particular, he also highlighted how mercenaries could be brought back into the Christian community. And he, in fact, brought them back into the community by allowing them to testify.

As we saw above, Master Nicolau did not just write the articles and collect testimony. He also actively spread stories of Delphine's sanctity. Like Bertranda Bertomieua, witnesses frequently mentioned speaking to Master Nicolau. Twenty witnesses—twelve men and eight women—mentioned Master Nicolau as a person who told them a story about Delphine. He was mentioned in conjunction with twenty-four different articles of interrogation. As we saw with Friar Giraud Raybaud in chapter 2, the information witnesses provided about where they heard about the miracles and who told them shows how certain individuals, Master Nicolau included, acted as contact points between courts, cities, and social groups. In this way, Delphine's inquest reveals that there were many links between social groups outside of known institutions and that people of all social levels shared stories whenever and wherever they met. Some of those stories—especially about how their holy woman protected them from violent attack and transformed the heart of a mercenary—spread across communities. For them, Delphine was a pious leader providing a solution to the problem of mercenaries, partly by addressing the problem as a spiritual one rather than a political or economic one. This wasn't unique to Delphine or the community around her, but this canonization inquest gives insight into how and why people might turn to their saints.

Master Nicolau's articles give us a sense of the problems that mercenary companies introduced. His view appeared in Articles 54–57. Each article emphasized a different event during this year of violence. Article 54 emphasized Delphine's ability to protect the bodies and souls of both noncombatants and combatants. This article described the miraculous appearance of guards around the town of Ansouis when mercenaries planned a night attack. Through testimonies from some of the highest-ranking witnesses in the inquest who had spoken to captured mercenaries, we see how mercenaries attacked vulnerable towns. More importantly, we see the excitement that a thwarted attack could generate among a group of people living in fear.

Article 55 describes a defender's response to the mercenaries. The *domicellus* of Cucuron, Lord Ferrier, described how Delphine protected him from death in an ambush. Through the article and his testimony, we see the dangers local lords faced as they took up arms against professional mercenaries; specifically, we see his fear of the shame he would face if he did not fight. Ferrier believed that Delphine's intercession saved him from death, shame, and spiritual harm. His testimony even subtly questioned the use of violence to retake conquered towns.

Articles 56 and 57 concern the miraculous rehabilitation of a mercenary, Durand Arnau de Rupa Ayneria, who was captured by the men of Ansouis. Prior to what should have been his execution, he devoted his heart to Delphine. As a result, he miraculously survived execution. He then visited Delphine and became a penitent. The popularity of this miracle among aristocratic men testifying in Delphine's inquest reveals how they navigated their ambivalent attitudes toward the invaders. The way the internal transformation of a mercenary in this miracle resonated with papal efforts to describe and control the mercenaries reveals how Master Laurens shaped the inquest to address many contemporary attitudes toward these events.

Mercenary Companies and Warfare in the Mid-Fourteenth Century

Before exploring these articles and the testimonies they generated, it is useful to take a step back in order to place this moment of local danger in larger events. For the witnesses and organizers of Delphine's inquest, the thing that was different between the "war of the seneschals" in 1349 and the "war with the Gascons" in 1357 was the presence of mercenary troops under a mercenary leader. The invading mercenaries were in large part a by-product of the Hundred Years War, but also of changes in warfare that had happened much earlier. Changes in the conduct of war during the thirteenth and early fourteenth centuries—an outgrowth of the long-term trend of replacing feudal service with money payments—had led to the emergence of professional soldiers.[18] Contemporaries and historians give them a variety of names, including *routiers*, Gascons, brigands, stipendiaries, mercenaries, and heretics. Petrarch called them "raging dogs," among other, less flattering things.[19] Their many names highlight how difficult it was and still is to categorize these men in the military world of the late Middle Ages. This world traditionally included military categories that could look a lot like mercenaries, but were not, such as conscripts, men-at-arms, or individual noblemen called upon for defense or a particular fighting season.[20]

The fighting between England and France would change how war was conducted from the mid-fourteenth century onward. The mercenaries increasingly functioned in groups that people at the time called companies, as we saw in Article 38. These were established groups of twenty to several hundred men who followed a specific leader and did not permanently disband after each battle or fighting season. Mercenary companies sometimes had their own treasurers, secretaries, and counselors.[21] The number of companies exploded during the Hundred Years War.

In a letter Pope Innocent VI wrote in 1357 begging the king of France for aid against Arnau de Cervole and his troops, Innocent described the depredations of the mercenaries and the reaction of local communities. He wrote: "Each day we hear that the children of the Church are disturbed, robbed, oppressed, tortured, decapitated, and killed with various punishments. The men corrupt virgins, seize women, violate widows, and hold in their sacrilegious hands virgins consecrated to God. People fleeing no longer find safety within the walls of sacred places. To escape so many evils, fathers and mothers run away, abandoning their children to the enemy and children flee, abandoning their parents."[22] For Pope Innocent, the mercenaries did not conduct war in an ideal Christian manner. They disregarded the safety of churchmen and noncombatants and had no respect for Christian places or persons. By evoking the hyperbole used so often for disasters like the plague—that family members abandoned each other—Pope Innocent captured the magnitude of mercenaries' devastation and the suffering and fear it caused.

But they were at the same time indispensable to great lords throughout Europe, including Pope Innocent. Historian William Caferro's study of soldiers in Florence in 1348–1350 explores the complex place of these soldiers in an urban community and its finances.[23] City governments needed them, but also frequently paid them to go away. Overall, without national armies or nation-states, it was unclear who the mercenaries were and where they fit in Christian society. The historian Jonathan Sumption, generating a picture from a variety of contemporary chronicles, describes the mercenaries as "unemployed foot soldiers and archers; professional criminals from the towns; penniless gentry; and a handful of knights."[24] Many of these men and their leaders came from southwestern France, especially Gascony, hence the title Gascons even for diverse groups made up of men from Germany, Spain, Italy, France, England, and elsewhere.

Their leaders were at times lower nobility or younger sons—men with military skill but few inheritance prospects. They used the Hundred Years War and ongoing warfare in the Italian and Iberian peninsulas and elsewhere to expand their wealth, status, and lands.[25] Particularly skillful leaders, like Arnau de Cervole, could become kings' allies or dangerous enemies.

Not surprisingly, these groups often did not follow the laws of war as they were understood in the fourteenth century.[26] The mercenaries were not primarily inspired by a sense of loyalty to their land, their king, their local lord, or a religious leader like the pope. These professional soldiers did not share quite the same ethos of honor and shame as those with official ties and titles, like *miles* or *scutifer*. And their leaders' reputations as defenders of the Christian faith were not at stake in the battles they fought. This meant that the mercenary companies were very difficult to make peace with in any of the standard ways that relied on the political emotions of hatred and love.[27] And since these men functioned in relatively autonomous units, even if their employers negotiated peace, it was no guarantee that the mercenary troops would leave the area. This is not to say the mercenaries could not be influenced by spiritual or honorable means, but like mercenaries in any time period, they responded best to money.

Protection offered by regional lords and royal houses was increasingly ineffective against these mercenaries. Semi-autonomous mercenary bands with their own leaders could leave the main group of an army and threaten towns far from the main fighting areas. The process of gathering taxes to raise an army or sending out a call for individual lords and men-at-arms to gather and then organize a defense was often too slow against these fast-moving, always-ready groups.[28]

Individual towns, cities, and counties, especially in the frequently threatened region of Languedoc, had found ways to defend themselves, however. Effective defenses included repairing the walls of a major town or city, hiring soldiers, stocking major cities and towns with surplus supplies, and preparing the local populace to run to the city when the mercenaries appeared.[29] Towns might preemptively destroy large churches or religious houses that were outside the city walls so that they could not be held as strongholds by invading mercenaries, a process that the nineteenth-century Dominican historian Henri Denifle called "self mutilation."[30]

Cities also tried to hire their own mercenaries or negotiate with invaders. Problems occurred, however, when contracts ended. If they received a better offer, hired men might leave to fight *for* the army they had just been fighting *against*.[31] Negotiation was also affected by money. While a city might successfully negotiate with the mercenary leaders and pay them to go elsewhere, this was no guarantee that those same mercenaries would not come back and attack again.

The upper nobility had ambivalent attitudes toward these mercenaries. They feared the mercenary leaders and their professional troops who caused significant damage to property and morale. Local militias could rarely stand against them, and the mercenaries fought better than most other troops. But this meant that the nobility needed these professional soldiers. When a truce during the Hundred Years War ended, these men would rejoin the armies of the kings of England and France and their regional leaders. But as Justine Firnhaber-Baker shows, kings and higher nobility had a diminishing ability to control these companies, even when they tried to create legal limits to private violence.[32]

The pope in particular had a fraught relationship with these professional soldiers. In the first half of the fourteenth century, popes John XXII and Boniface VIII had repeatedly hired professional troops to retake and protect territory in the Papal States.[33] Later popes wanted to send the mercenaries on crusades to fight non-Christians on the borders of Hungary and Spain. At the same time, however, when mercenaries turned on religious houses, the popes condemned and excommunicated them.[34]

Excommunication did not mean that the pope no longer cared for the souls of these men, however. Continued violence against Christian communities posed a danger to the mercenaries' souls that the pope and other religious leaders had to address. The pope and the clergy had to protect the souls of everyone in their care. Excommunication had two uses in this situation, therefore.[35] It severed ties between these men and faithful Christians who might be in legal or feudal relationships with them. It also revealed the strained ties between these men and God. This process was meant to push these men to reform their behavior and re-enter the Christian community in order save their souls.[36] In a way it functioned as an extreme form of pastoral care.

Arnau de Cervole and His Troops

The mercenaries became an immediate problem for Avignon and Provence after the truce of Bordeaux in 1357. The Hundred Years War between Edward III, king of England, and Jean II, the king of France, had been simmering since roughly 1328, but fighting had mostly taken place in northern, central, and western France. The Rhône valley, which marked the southeastern boundary of French lands, was relatively far from the contested region. Provence, as a county under the control of the king and queen of Naples and ultimately held by the Holy Roman Emperors, had not been a target.

The devastating battle of Poitiers in 1356, however, had led to the capture of King Jean, his youngest son, and many of his closest advisers. In a position of political stability, King Edward III negotiated a truce that was supposed to last from 1357 to 1359.[37] A truce meant that these companies of professional soldiers and their energetic leaders were not employed by either the king of France or the king of England and could join local warfare like that in Provence.

Arnau de Cervole, who led the mercenary attack on Provence, was one such energetic leader.[38] De Cervole's shifting political loyalties and constant engagement in warfare as a profession reveal the shift from local fighting to professional violence.[39] De Cervole was best known in chronicles as the Archpriest of Vélines. Although he accrued other titles and significant property in the region of Berry in northern France, chroniclers continued to call him the Archpriest. Several of Delphine's witnesses used this title as well, suggesting that a broad audience remained aware that Arnau de Cervole was not of the upper nobility by birth (even though he was very definitely a noble of the sword) and had used violence to increase his fortune and status. By leading his soldiers to Provence, we see de Cervole's continued engagement with mercenary warfare, even as his status in relation to the king of France changed and even as King Jean wrote laws criminalizing such activity.[40] After the battle of Poitiers, the Treaty of Bordeaux in 1357 released many mercenary leaders, like de Cervole, who chose to fight in local warfare.

Mercenaries in Provence in 1357–1358

Mercenary companies came to Provence as part of a local effort by the Durazzo and Baux to capture Marseille and Aix-en-Provence and weaken Queen Johanna and King Louis. Provence was a strategically savvy region to attack. In cultural terms, it had been the first foothold in the Mediterranean for the

Angevins. It was the step from which they reached out for Naples, Sicily, Achaea, and other Mediterranean regions. By the 1350s, Provence was a relatively stable source of tax money for the Crown of Naples. And Marseille, the major port city of Provence, provided naval support to Naples. Johanna and Louis depended on the stability of Provence to further their political goals in other areas. For example, by the end of 1356, Louis of Taranto and his highly effective grand seneschal, Nicola Acciaiuoli, had almost all of their military might invested in an attempt to regain Sicily—a lucrative source of grain and taxes.[41] Limiting the financial support Provence provided would undermine the Crown of Naples at a moment when it was extending itself.[42]

The Durazzo branch of the family had lost significant influence since King Robert's death in 1343. Both Agnes of Périgord and Charles of Durazzo had died. And King Louis of Naples directed more positions of power to his own family members. For example, his brother Philippe of Taranto was now vicar-general of the Crown of Naples in Provence.[43]

Several lords of Baux in Provence shared the Durazzo family's frustrations with King Louis of Naples. As we saw in the previous chapter, Louis and Johanna removed Lord Uguo de Baux's titles in 1350 after Uguo had his own son, Robert, married to Johanna's sister, Maria. Louis may have rid himself of Uguo, but the marriage to Robert was valid. In response, Louis of Taranto held Robert and his younger brother Raymon in prison. Robert de Baux died in prison in 1353.[44] In response, several members of the Baux family joined the Durazzo in almost continuous rebellion against the Taranto branch of the Angevins.[45]

The leadership of the 1357–1358 attack on Provence included Lords Raymon, Amiel, and Bertran de Baux.[46] It may also have included the support of a group of cardinals aligned with Cardinal Talleyrand. Although it is not directly clear how Arnau de Cervole came to be involved, some historians who explore this event suspect that Cardinal Talleyrand, with his family ties in Périgord, may have known Arnau de Cervole and influenced him to come to Provence.[47]

Because of the truce of Bordeaux, the Archpriest was able to lead his forces to Provence. King Jean and his son, the dauphin Charles, who acted as leader while his father was imprisoned, may even have supported de Cervole's efforts.[48] King Jean and Charles had quarreled with Queen Johanna and King Louis, especially resenting the sale of Avignon to Pope Clement VI in 1348.[49]

This assault on Provence built slowly over months.[50] But even though defenders in the region were aware of what was happening, they found it difficult to stop. The Durazzo and Baux began massing their own troops around Provence in the winter of 1356 and early spring of 1357. West of Provence, Raymon de Baux's forces threatened Arles and Orange. North of Provence they gathered near Valence. Arnau de Cervole left Paris on March 27 and gathered more men as he moved south, including his brother, Pierre de Cervole. By the time they reached Valence, he had at least four thousand men. They claimed that their goal was to march against their enemy, Philippe of Taranto, and make war on the lands and men of King Louis of Naples.[51]

Before Arnau de Cervole's troops arrived, other lords took advantage of the looming threat to Provence. Lord Jean, the count of Armagnac, decided to use the military threat of approaching mercenaries to press his claim to his father's rights over several Provençal towns. He threatened to attack Provence as well if not given his father's property. Or if his father's rights were returned, he offered to support Provence with mercenary troops and harass the Archpriest's men passing through his regions.[52]

At the same time, within Provence, Marseille found itself again torn between conflicting loyalties. The lords of Marseille had recently supported the kingdom of Naples, especially Queen Johanna. As we saw in the previous chapter, they had accepted Lord Giovanni Barrili as seneschal when many others in the Estates of Provence had not. An attack that harmed the king and queen of Naples would harm Marseille. Marseille was also strongly supportive of the Baux, however, who were some of the main instigators of the invasion. Many associates of the Baux held influential positions in the city. For example, Lord Raymon de Baux's brother, Lord Antoine de Baux, was the *prévot* of Marseille.[53] The various factions fought for control of this key Provençal city and its surrounding regions.[54]

In February and March, before the main body of the invasion force could arrive, Pope Innocent VI began an intense letter-writing campaign to head off Arnau's troops and negotiate support against the invaders.[55] Innocent's letters to Charles, the Dauphin of France, were unsuccessful. Charles claimed to oppose the rebellion, but his reply to Pope Innocent claimed that he could offer little help in the aftermath of the battle of Poitiers.[56]

Pope Innocent also wrote to the king of Hungary for support, perhaps expecting a positive response after helping in the successful negotiations that ended the war between Naples and Hungary. But Philippe of Taranto's presence in Avignon as vicar-general undermined Pope Innocent's credibility with the king of Hungary, and he received no support.[57] Innocent even wrote to Arnau de Cervole, a move that reveals the ambiguous position of mercenary leaders in mid-fourteenth-century politics. Arnau assured the pope that he would not attack Church lands, but this was thin reassurance from a man at the head of mercenary troops that often followed their own agenda.[58]

None of Pope Innocent's letters brought promises of military support for the county of Provence and the Comtat Venaissin, so the pope funded other defenses. As Arnau de Cervole's mercenary army continued to prepare for their attack, Innocent worked to repair Avignon's defenses.[59] But attempts to organize the defense of the Comtat Venaissin were hindered by the fact that Juan-Ferdinand de Hérédia, captain of the troops of the Comtat Venaissin, had also been taken prisoner by the English in the battle of Poitiers and was in the process of ransoming himself.[60]

Arnau de Cervole and his troops crossed the Rhône north of Valence in mid-July 1357 and moved steadily south.[61] Philippe of Taranto, the vicar-general, stood against them at Orgon on the Durance, but he had too few men to stop the invaders.[62]

From the end of July until October, the Durazzo and Baux, with their mercenary forces, gained the upper hand in Provence. Lord Antoine de Baux held Aubagne (roughly twenty kilometers from Marseille) and the whole Huveaune valley between Aubagne and Marseille. This was a strategic blow, since that valley was a major corridor through the mountains to Marseille and the Mediterranean (see map 2). It allowed Arnau de Cervole's troops to attack Marseille from two sides.[63] Arnau's troops also crossed the Durance and burned the town of Draguinan.[64] They captured Brignoles, the castle of Eguilles, and the city of Saint Maximin. They used Saint Maximin as a stronghold from which to organize their campaign against Aix and Marseille.[65]

The lords of Provence, organized by the Estates of Provence, resisted as best they could. Cities from Tarascon to Nice repaired their walls, garrisoned outlying towns, and sent reinforcements to weaker cities when possible.[66] The leaders and citizens of Marseille removed all foreign fighters from the city, solidified their ramparts, abandoned their suburbs, gathered men-at-arms and crossbowmen, and bought artillery.[67] The lords of Marseille sent crossbowmen to Aix and a galley and three hundred soldiers up the Rhône River to Avignon.[68]

In July 1357, Pope Innocent VI gave 150 florins to the marshal of the court of Avignon to repair and reconstruct the gates and walls of the city. And in August, Innocent purchased arbalests for the protection of the papal palace and city of Avignon and the materials for local officials to construct more.[69] Also in July, Innocent engaged four hundred mercenary soldiers to defend Avignon and the Comtat Venaissin. As a reflection of how ubiquitous mercenaries were, these men were referred to as *briganti* and were fighting for pay.[70]

The main focus of attack continued to be Marseille and Aix-en-Provence. The lords of these cities, often at odds with each other, as we saw in chapter 2, worked together for a time to try to drive Arnau de Cervole's troops out of this region. But when Philippe of Taranto burned Aubagne, the lords of Marseille took offense at the destruction of a city they thought of as their own.[71] In response to the burning, they removed their support from the joint action with other lords of Provence.[72] Marseille faced other threats, including attacks of opportunity by sea from Genoese, Catalan, and Pisan ships.[73]

The seneschal of Provence, Fulk d'Agoult, and Philippe of Taranto worked to face the varied threats. Philippe sold property to raise money to pay troops and sent letters to the count of Savoy, urging him to resist the attacks of opportunity. Fulk and Innocent VI accepted the count of Armagnac's offer of defense to the north, even though it meant losing important cities. They also accepted the count of Armagnac's offer of two hundred mercenaries, even though they would have to pay for these mercenary troops themselves. In late October, Fulk d'Agoult led an army made up of mercenaries and Provençal militia against the forces of Arnau de Cervole.[74]

The fighting peaked at the end of October, but the rivalry between Aix and Marseille kept Marseille's troops out of the battle, and Fulk failed to drive the mercenaries out of the Huveaune valley. As winter set in, Arnau de Cervole's troops settled into their captured towns and castles, frequently sending out sorties against the Provençal lords. One of these castles, Éguilles, was only a few miles from Aix-en-Provence and proved particularly dangerous.[75]

By February, conditions in Marseille were dire. With enemies on all sides and shipments of basic goods dwindling, the city experienced a famine.[76] But when a Marseille merchant traveled to Agde, a coastal city between Narbonne and Montpellier, to buy wheat, he was told that it was forbidden to sell food to Provence. The merchant went to Montpellier to beg the count of Poitiers, the French king's lieutenant in Languedoc, to revoke the ban, but the count replied that he supported the ban and did not revoke it.[77]

By the end of February 1358, after nearly a year of occupation, fighting, and disruption, the situation in Provence had become desperate. The Provençaux had received little outside aid, food supplies were cut off from Languedoc, and several major cities and castles had fallen. On top of this, the count of Armagnac's two hundred mercenary soldiers, reaching the end of their contract with the lords of Provence, went over to Arnau de Cervole's side.[78] Fulk d'Agoult had been unable to pay Jean of Armagnac for the soldiers, so Fulk was being held in Avignon until he paid. He was no longer able to lead the Provençal troops, and those troops would not follow Philippe of Taranto.[79]

This was a war fought with money, and Provence was feeling the strain.[80] The lords of Provence needed a different strategy. On February 24, 1358, the vice seneschal, Lord Johan de Revest, wrote a clear and moving letter to the leaders of Provençal cities still resisting the invasion. He outlined the problems they faced, explicitly stating that mercenary troops were the problem and not a solution. They were too expensive and unreliable. Instead, he called for all of Provence to send what soldiers they could to drive the mercenaries out the Huveaune valley.

Throughout the letter, he spoke to the Provençal sense of identity. He stated that the enemies of Provence rode unhindered through the county and that no outside help was coming to stop them. The Provençaux would have to defend themselves. If every community willingly sent what men they could, Johan de Revest and other military leaders could drive the mercenaries out. And, he wrote, "if this could happen, all of our land could be healthy [*salus*]."[81]

The cities and aristocracy of Provence responded well to this letter.[82] They sent what men they could spare to fight in the Huveaune valley and in the entire region between Marseille to the west, Toulon to the east, and Aix to the north. Even Marseille sent troops to Aix to help retake Éguilles.[83] The cities "mutilated themselves" even further to give the mercenaries fewer resources. Marseille dug trenches around its walls, Aix sacrificed its suburbs, and other cities further destroyed stone buildings outside their walls. Fields were not being sown at this time, so food supplies for both mercenaries and inhabitants, already running low, would not be replenished locally.[84]

Fighting continued until the end of summer 1358, but many mercenary bands left before that, drawn to more lucrative battles in other regions of Europe. Finally, in August, Arnau de Cervole left with the majority of his men to defend the Dauphin Charles against the Jacquerie in Paris.[85] The main part of "the war of the Gascons" was over.[86]

Throughout the invasion, Arnau de Cervole's mercenaries ranged far beyond the two main targets of Marseille and Aix. They made attacks of opportunity east of Marseille, including against the count of Savoy and the cities of Vintemille and Monaco. Even after the fighting stopped in most other places, at least one region still remained caught in violence. Mercenaries still held cities in the Luberon region near Apt and Ansouis where Delphine lived. Although the region lay outside the main area of fighting near Marseille and Aix, mercenaries had taken nine towns and forts in this region and refused to leave. Although local lords led sorties against these mercenaries, they were not successful. The mercenaries left only when Innocent VI agreed to pay 1,000 florins in ransom, which the seneschal and communities of Provence were supposed to reimburse by 1359.[87] In the letter to the lords, Innocent VI used the phrase "*magna societas armigerorum*," one of the earliest references to the Great Companies.[88]

The invasion left the region shaken. Buildings were destroyed or damaged, fields went unsown, captured cities and towns recovered slowly, resources had been destroyed or consumed by the mercenaries, and travel became more dangerous. Displaced populations—including religious groups and rural populations that had relocated within city walls—slowly returned to their previous locations or chose to stay in the city.[89]

Mercenaries in Delphine's Inquest: The Battle for the Luberon

The gritty details of this yearlong invasion help us understand what shaped witnesses' testimonies. Men and women, religious and lay, noble and merchant, were all affected by the mercenaries. The stories they told reflect their fear, anger, and confusion. Their lives were upended by unpredictable mercenary attacks.

The four articles of interrogation that Master Nicolau Laurens wrote capture the plight of besieged towns and inexpert defenders in this changing field of warfare. The professional soldiers, unemployed during a truce, joined local battles where they fought against inexperienced and undermanned local militias. As we see in witness testimony, local lords were often out of their depth, and they knew it. But not only the lives and souls of defenders were on the line. Mercenary companies killed defenders, stole food and materials, and captured towns and wealthy individuals and held them for personal gain. By doing so, the mercenaries risked their souls by attacking, violating, and killing Christians, including women and clergy. Defender and attacker alike were in physical and spiritual danger.

Master Nicolau Laurens and the witnesses included none of the political landscape in the articles or testimonies. Many of the witnesses were aware of the political machinations, however. Some witnesses, like Bishop Philippe Cabassole, Lord Johan de Sabran, and the noble Lord Giraud de Simiana, were involved in organizing the defense. And as we have seen, people shared stories everywhere they traveled, speaking with a diverse array of people. In the articles and testimonies to the articles, Laurens and the witnesses focused on the local stories of successful protection and transformation. These local stories had a wide audience, which emerges as witnesses described where, when, and from whom they heard the stories. Master Nicolau increased that audience in his articles to include the papal commissioners and anyone who read the documents they produced.

Although Laurens had a bird's-eye view of witness testimony, most of the witnesses told only one or two stories about this time. None of them spoke to all four articles or mentioned all of the events in their testimony to Article 1. Each witness brought his or her own perspective to the events. Unlike official letters, which used stylistized rhetoric to describe the devastation of warfare,

Master Laurens's articles and witness testimony were all stories of successful protection and spiritual transformation.[90] His articles allowed witnesses to share the solutions that people of Provence found by turning to their holy woman, Countess Delphine, even as their political leaders struggled to protect them or, worse, were part of the problem.

Before looking at the four specific articles that Master Nicolau wrote about this moment of danger, a few stories emerge from Article 1. Some of the most dramatic stories, with the greatest contrast to official letters about these events, came from women. For example, when asked about Delphine's miracles in the open-ended Article 1, Lady Catherine de Pui, a member of the local nobility and close companion of Delphine after 1343, told a remarkable story about how Delphine saved Ansouis, the ancestral home of Delphine's late husband's family, from mercenary attack. According to Catherine, "during the year the Gascons were in Provence" a terrible storm hit Ansouis.[91] Defenders on the fortifications could not see from one person to the next because of the storm and were forced to leave the fortifications.[92]

Catherine, like everyone else in Ansouis, knew this was a dangerous moment for the town. Mercenary scouts had scaled the unprotected walls of neighboring towns during storms like this, opened the gates from inside, and let in the invaders.[93] It was a tactic called escalade, commonly practiced by mercenary companies. Since mercenary forces held the nearby towns of Cabrières and Cucuron, escalade was a real threat to Ansouis during any storm.[94] According to Catherine, the people of Ansouis were fearful and sad (*timens et tristis*) that they had to leave the city walls and could not protect the town.[95]

Therefore, when Catherine brought Delphine dinner, she begged Delphine to ask God to stop the storm on behalf of the troubled people. According to Catherine, Delphine joined her hands and raised them to the sky and said, "O Lord God, have pity on these poor people!" And then Delphine spoke to the storm: "I urge you through the living God, through the holy God, and through the omnipotent God."[96] Delphine said other things that Catherine did not understand, but by the time Catherine had finished setting the table for dinner, the storm had receded, the weather was clear, and the town of Ansouis was defendable again.[97]

Catherine de Pui's miracle story gives us insight into the efforts and limitations of local lords and citizens to resist the invading mercenaries. It presents women as defenders, not just victims, during mercenary attacks. In her story, Delphine's special relationship to God protected Ansouis by quickly dispersing a storm that kept defenders from guarding the city. But her story also shows what it was like to live with mercenaries in one's region. The people of Ansouis lived in constant fear with watchers on the walls at all times. Any lapse could result in capture, looting, rape, and death for the town's inhabitants.

The relationship of combatants and noncombatants was more complex than this one miracle story shows, however. This moment of danger in 1357–1358 revealed the ambiguous place that mercenaries held in Christian society. The mercenaries were Christians themselves, but behaving in an unchristian manner, creating a kind of warfare that people like Delphine's witnesses were still trying to understand and control.[98] Unlike Catherine's story, the four articles that Master Nicolau wrote allowed witnesses to tell nuanced stories of the dangers they faced and how they turned to Delphine to protect them. At least one article also allowed Master Nicolau himself to address the skepticism surrounding the mercenaries as redeemable Christians. Neither the warfare nor healing were like what this community had encountered less than ten years earlier in the "war of the seneschals." The experience of violence and peace had changed.

Article 54: Miraculous Defense and Mercenary Informants

We see in Master Nicolau's articles that other cities had not been as lucky as Ansouis. As part of the fighting in Provence, mercenaries captured and controlled nine towns and forts in the Luberon region. According to testimonies, the mercenaries appeared to use Cucuron, about four miles from Ansouis, as a base from which to attack the rest of the region. Cucuron had substantial city walls, and once mercenaries held it, it was difficult for the lords of Provence, with their less experienced troops, to retake that town.[99]

Article 54 explains why people like Catherine de Pui were so frightened of these opportunistic attacks. According to the article, the mercenaries working for Arnau de Cervole and living in Cucuron decided to seize the town and castle of Ansouis, "seeing themselves daily injured by the people" in that place.[100] In other words, the fighters of Ansouis were resisting the invaders, and the mercenaries wanted to bring them under control.

The mercenaries sent out an invasion force under cover of darkness, then sent a small group ahead to scout the area around Ansouis's walls to find the best place to set up their equipment (*machinari*). This small group, however, saw armed, mounted soldiers carrying torches and guarding the walls. Frightened by what they saw, the small scout group met up with the larger invasion force, and they all retreated to the nearby abandoned church of St. Peter. They decided not to invade Ansouis because they believed that the town must have recently received reinforcements. When the defending lords of Ansouis later learned about the guards that the invaders saw, they believed that Delphine, who was staying in Ansouis at the time, must have produced a miracle, because they had no warhorses.[101]

In the second part of this miracle, the mercenaries decided to set an ambush for the men of Ansouis from their relatively secure position in the abandoned church. A hermit visited the church unexpectedly, however, and discovered the mercenaries. He escaped and returned to Ansouis and told the townspeople about what he had seen. In this way, no one left the walls of Ansouis, and the ambush failed.[102]

Three witnesses testified to this two-part miracle. Two witnesses had been in Ansouis at the time: Romeus Romei, a local lord, and Lord Johan de Sabran, part of the noble Sabran family, a relative of Delphine's deceased husband and the *domicellus* of Ansouis at the time of the miracle. Though neither saw the apparition of armed horsemen, they had both spoken to a captured mercenary captain, Gailhardo de Saint Germain, who claimed to have been part of the group planning to attack Ansouis at night and who saw and heard the mounted guards.[103] The third witness, Lord Guilhem Enric, heard about only the first part of the miracle long after it happened. His testimony tells us less about the event and more about the spread of the story in Provence.

Lord Johan gave more detail about the nature of the failed attack. He placed the mercenary attack in September about six years before Delphine's inquest.[104] And he stated that Gailhardo told him that there were a hundred mercenaries involved with two leaders—himself and Gailhardo of Perrinus Terreta.[105] They planned to use two ballistas, perhaps catapults or trebuchets, in a surprise night attack. Gailhardo and several others had been looking for the best place to set up the ballistas when they heard hoofbeats and saw four armed horsemen with their lances lowered. The attackers were afraid and retreated quietly back to their group. Johan emphasized the miraculous nature of the guards by explaining that the city had no armed guards that night and that "there were only three small horses, which were not large enough that armed men [could ride]."[106]

Both Romeus and Lord Johan testified about the hermit, called Brother Martin. According to Johan (who was relating the experience of Gailhardo), the mercenaries planned to use the abandoned church as a base from which to ambush anyone who tried to leave or enter the city. Here we see the danger of large stone buildings near the city walls and understand why so many cities decided to "mutilate themselves" by preemptively destroying them. The hermit, Martin, went out to the church of St. Peter to pray, though this was not something he usually did. According to Romeus, Brother Martin saw the mercenaries and fled. One of the mercenaries injured Brother Martin in the head with a sword, but the hermit reached Ansouis and told the men of the town about the mercenaries in the church.[107]

For Romeus and Lord Johan, both the appearance of guards and the hermit's unexpected visit to the church that interrupted a potential ambush were evidence of God's intercession because of the merits of Delphine. Unlike in Catherine de Pui's description of Delphine's banishing the storm, however, none of the witnesses to Article 54 described asking Delphine for help. Nor did they describe any prayers or statements Delphine might have made. Instead the witnesses assumed the miracles occurred because Delphine was in Ansouis at the time. They did not, therefore, describe Delphine's actions, but focused their testimonies on the threats to the city and castle. They described the city's poor defenses and the relative strength of the mercenaries, according to the captured mercenary captain.

These miracles made Delphine a protector of her family, her town, and Provence. As a countess and widow of Lord Elzear, Delphine was protecting her people as any noblewoman would. She had taken a vow of poverty and could not pay for protection. But her extraordinary piety resulted in divine aid in the form of a vision of mounted soldiers. The miraculous appearance of guards and the hermit's visit made sense in the picture of sanctity the organizers and witnesses developed. Both miracles made sure everyone was safe, and, more importantly, no Christian, not even the mercenaries, killed another person. In Master Nicolau's structuring of events, Delphine had physically and spiritually protected everyone involved and minimized the violence that caused her such great sadness.

In light of Article 38, which also mentioned the mercenary companies, Delphine had actually protected the mercenaries from the even more spiritually damaging practice of attacking Christians. Gailhardo of Saint Germain's participation in the miracle and his indirect reporting of it via Lord Johan de Sabran and Romeus Romei made him a part of Delphine's inquest as well as a part of a mostly peaceful solution to a physically and spiritually dangerous event. In Delphine's inquest, the mercenary acted as an informant about a miracle rather than as a brigand.

This article and testimonies to it reflect the struggle to articulate the complex social and spiritual place of mercenaries in Europe in the fourteenth century. Witnesses suffered at their hands and lived in fear of them. But without the mercenary informant, the organizers of Delphine's inquest would not have known about the failed attack. By including Gailhardo's story, the witnesses included their attackers by name in Delphine's inquest. Gailhardo, though a mercenary, was a Christian with similar cultural influences on his behavior and expectations that Delphine's witnesses experienced.[108] This story helps us understand, and perhaps take more seriously, mercenaries' attempts to negotiate with spiritual leaders for forgiveness and their desire to go on crusades to heal their souls.[109]

The third witness to Article 54 reveals less about the mercenaries and more about the *fama* of this miracle and its place in a sense of Provençal identity. Master Guilhem Enric was a sixty-year-old nobleman and had been *juge mage* in 1348 in Queen Johanna's court in Aix.[110] He recalled the miraculous vision of soldiers in his testimony to Article 1. In his version of the event, however, many men with great torches and weapons had been seen in Ansouis during the war with the Gascons. Guilhem claimed that they "struck terror in the enemy, who then did not invade the castle of Ansouis."[111]

Master Guilhem's version of the story evoked the language of Lord Johan de Revest's letter, which called the Provençaux to arms in 1358, but told a different story. In de Revest's inspiring letter, he wrote that the mercenaries rode through Provence without fear because no one dared to resist them.[112] Master Guilhem showed that Ansouis had resisted and that Delphine had inspired fear through her miraculous aid.

Master Guilhem claimed to have heard about this event in Aix in 1362 from Lord Johan Raymon, who was then the *domicellus* of Ansouis. Master Guilhem's testimony allows us to see that lords continued to recall Delphine's miracles and tell them to others in later years. They also adapted the stories to reflect later knowledge or to create a greater impact.

Article 55: The Defender's Soul and Honor

Article 55 described a failed attempt by Provençal lords to retake Cucuron, the mercenary stronghold, in May 1358, eight months after their attack on Ansouis. The article presents the experiences of Lord Ferrier of Cucuron, who as leader of his people was expected to lead this attack.[113] He ultimately failed to do so, but Delphine's miraculous intervention saved his life, honor, and soul. In this swiftly changing landscape of warfare, where local lords faced far more experienced mercenaries, Master Nicolau Laurens and Lord Ferrier found a different way to understand and present this moment of violence and failure.

The article and testimony start before the battle. Before leading his men against the mercenaries, Lord Ferrier visited Delphine in Ansouis. He had great esteem for her on account of her great devotion and sanctity. While in her presence, he commended himself to her. Perhaps this was a way of preparing his soul before an event in which he might die. While in her presence, he described the danger of the upcoming battle. She warned Ferrier that he should not go, but he did not dare to follow her warning because "he would be reproached if he stayed behind and he did not want cowardliness or shame ascribed to him."[114] Seeing that Ferrier could not retreat, Delphine "made a promise to him that he would kill no one and that she would intercede with God on his behalf."[115]

We can infer from this promise that Delphine and Lord Ferrier saw different dangers in this attack. As we saw in testimony to Article 38, for Delphine any violence, especially violence that led to the death of another person, was a great evil and danger to the immortal soul. So even though Ferrier described his situation as dangerous for either his body or his reputation, he recalled that Delphine interpreted the situation as even more dangerous for his soul.

According to the article, Ferrier left her presence greatly consoled and went to complete his task. He gathered his people at Vaugines near Lourmarin to prepare for the attack against the mercenaries, whom they could see a few miles away (see map 2). Before the battle, Ferrier "recommended himself in his heart to Delphine." Then he grasped his sword and mounted his horse, wishing to ride against the mercenaries.[116]

Almost immediately, Ferrier had trouble with his horse. His testimony and the article diverge at this point, so I will follow Ferrier's description of his horse troubles.[117] According to his testimony, he urged his horse to run, but it could not move. The horse's left leg appeared to be injured, although it had not been when he led it from the stable. Realizing he could not ride this horse, Ferrier dismounted and asked one of his associates to whom he had loaned a horse to give the horse back. The associate did so, and Ferrier readied himself again to lead the attack. He led his men about the distance of a ballista-throw from the enemy. Ferrier urged the new horse to run, but it soon lost a shoe and began to drag one foot. The horse suffered so much that eventually it could not walk.[118]

At this point, Ferrier recalled Delphine's words and began to suspect her intervention, since the horses' injuries allowed him to leave the battle without shame. He went back to Vaugines while his people continued on. A short way from the walls of Cucuron, however, his people encountered an ambush, and at least sixty men were killed.[119]

The commissioners asked Ferrier very specific questions about this event. They asked for clarification about the horses' injuries, especially about the shoeing of the second horse. Ferrier described both horses as so injured that they required several days to recover. The commissioners also asked who had heard his conversation with Delphine, and he named Lady Catherine de Pui and her sister and Lady Ugueta.[120] The commissioners asked who had seen the horses' impediments, and he named two soldiers of Cucuron and a priest named Lord Amblard. The commissioners also asked if he made any other kind of vow to Delphine than the one he testified to, and he replied that he only recommended himself as he had said.[121]

The most interesting question, however, highlighted the tension between shame and danger of death that these local lords and their men faced when fighting the mercenaries. The commissioners asked Ferrier whether, if Delphine had not said those words to him and if he had had another horse to ride, "would he have ridden against the mercenaries."[122] The commissioners' underlying question of Ferrier's intention highlights their search for a miracle, but many of Ferrier's contemporaries (as well as skeptical readers) may have been asking the same thing: Was this really a miracle, or was Ferrier trying to use his testimony in Delphine's inquest to preserve his honor after a cowardly act?

Ultimately, we cannot know. We have only Ferrier's testimony and Master Nicolau's article. But it is useful to temper our skepticism by considering factors that shaped Ferrier's actions. First, as he had stated in his testimony, he feared the repercussions if he acted in a cowardly manner and did not lead his men into battle. The historian of warfare Philippe Contamine revealed that Ferrier's fear of shame was a real one based on cultural expectations. Contamine studied "*chanson de geste*, chronicles, didactic treatises, biographies of soldiers, panegyrics and epitaphs" to flesh out the idea of courage in medieval warfare. He determined that "courage was conceived above all as an aristocratic, noble form of behavior, linked to race, blood and lineage. . . . It was necessary to avoid 'shame' which was engendered despite oneself and one's family by 'despicable actions,' 'cowardice,' and laziness."[123] Ferrier's position in society came from his lineage, his relationships to other lords, and his reputation. If he had refused to lead his men against the invaders, his reputation and social position would have suffered greatly.[124] To establish his reputation in his testimony, he presented himself as desiring to charge toward the enemy, displaying his "great ardor" for combat.[125] He was also living up to Johan de Revest's call for the men of Provence to defend their territory themselves. Had he not tried to lead the attack on Cucuron, he would have been a coward.

At the same time, however, according to Contamine, once Ferrier's horses were injured, it did not make sense for him to go into battle. In fact, it could have been construed as rash or arrogant because he would have encountered too great a risk of death or capture.[126] Ferrier's intentions to fight and attempts to go into battle secured his honor.

Ferrier told the commissioners that yes, he would have ridden against the mercenaries. His fear of shame if he did not constrained his actions. By implication he was also saying that yes, he would have been killed with his men in the ambush the mercenaries had set for them. Through his testimony, therefore, he rehabilitated his own honor. He was allowed to say that he tried to lead his men into battle and that he would have died with them, but God's grace, experienced through the holy Countess Delphine, saved his body, soul, and honor.

But there is another issue here, unstated in the questioning, but strongly implied by the story of the miracle. Because of Delphine's intercession, not only was Ferrier alive, but he did not end up in a situation where he had to kill anyone. Only those men who rushed to kill the mercenaries were themselves killed. If they had followed Ferrier, and by implication Delphine, they all would have lived. In this way, not only was Ferrier's name cleared of any shame of not being in the battle, but he is also placed in the moral right by siding with Delphine.[127] It is worth remembering that Ferrier told this story in 1363, after years of occupation by the Great Companies had shown local lords the weakness of their defenses against these mercenaries.

Ferrier's sense of identity emerges through the article and his testimony. Here is a fighting man—a *miles*—who found it appropriate to his status to describe the dangers he was about to face in battle and commend himself to a holy woman. By going to Delphine before the battle he implies both his Christian faith and his anxiety or fear of death. This is a rare presentation of a knight's awareness of danger and fear, strikingly different from what is seen in chronicles from the time.[128]

Ferrier was in a different situation than the warring lords of Provence in 1349. He did not seek Delphine as a peacemaker, but as a protector in a battle that he could not avoid. As a fighting man, he could not follow her suggestion to not participate in the attack. The shame of not participating would be as bad as dying. But he could seek out and benefit from her protection without damage to his honor.

Both Articles 54 and 55 shed light on the weakness of local militias in the face of experienced mercenary troops like those under Arnau de Cervole. In Article 54 and testimonies to it, as well as Catherine de Pui's story of the storm, we see how few resources local lords had to defend their castles. In Article 54, we see that the lords of Ansouis did not have men or horses to defend the city. In Article 55, we see the inexperience of local soldiers against the mercenaries. It took two miracles—the ghostly guards and the hermit's visit—to protect Ansouis from a force with reportedly a hundred soldiers and two large projectile weapons. Although at times local lords and townspeople succeeded against the mercenaries, as the capture of Gailhardo de Saint Germain shows, these towns were struggling in the eight months between the two miracles.

Master Nicolau Laurens and the witnesses presented various miracles that God worked through Delphine as saving both lives and souls in this time of the great company of the Gascons. They used her access to God's grace to solve new problems caused by mercenary troops. Through their testimony they presented a different picture of men at war in the fourteenth century. These were men who found a way to admit to the dangers they faced and the complex fear of not living up to expectations.

Article 56: From Mercenary to Penitent

The mercenaries—Christian men attacking other Christians and fighting outside the traditional boundaries of Christian warfare—were relatively new in Provence in the mid-fourteenth century. The Christian community, which included the mercenaries, struggled to find a place for them. The great lords of Europe needed professional soldiers for extended campaigns. But they also needed these men to stop fighting during truces. Arnau de Cervole's service to the king of France and others shows how hard this balance was to achieve.[129]

People living in the region had to make sense of mercenary actions and find ways to survive this transformation in warfare. As Master Nicolau Laurens gathered information for Delphine's inquest, one story in particular stood out: Delphine had transformed the heart of a mercenary soldier, and he became a penitent. This miracle struck a nerve in western Provence. Thirteen witnesses—an extraordinary number for a miracle in Delphine's canonization inquest (or any fourteenth-century inquest, for that matter)—described these events. This group included everyone from local soldiers to elite witnesses like Bishop Philippe de Cabassole, Bishop Anglic Grimoard, and Master Guilhem Enric.

In Article 56, Master Nicolau presented this miraculous transformation. And the testimonies to the article highlighted the possibility of transforming a mercenary from a violent attacker into a penitent. In this way, he showed how a mercenary could stop fighting and rejoin a Christian community.[130]

According Article 56 and testimony to it, the mercenary, Durand Arnau de Rupa Ayneria had been captured along with several of his fellow Gascons. The men of Ansouis decided to execute the invaders by hurling them into a dry well, throwing large stones on them, and leaving any survivors to die of exposure.[131] Therefore, Durand found himself bound with his hands behind his back, about to be thrown headfirst to his death.

Before being thrown in, however, Durand uttered a supplication to Delphine, whom he had heard about while living in Provence. Much like Lord Ferrier de Cucuron, the mercenary sought protection for his soul before what he believed was to be his death. The article described how he transformed himself in this moment. It states, "He changed the feelings [*affectibus*] of his whole heart, begging to her in his heart, and indeed pronouncing with a secret voice, that that same lady should help him in such great danger, especially because, if he escaped death, he would come to her, and whatever he would receive in advance would be fulfilled."[132]

According to Durand's testimony, God answered Durand's prayer.[133] Durand did not die from the fall or from the stones. Instead, while in the well, he saw a vision of light. This light revealed his dead companions, and a voice urged him to get up. When he regained full consciousness two days later, his bonds had disappeared and he was able to get up and shout for help. The soldiers of Ansouis, understanding this event as a miracle, hauled him out of the well. Finally free, Durand wrapped the rope used to haul him out around his neck and walked to see Delphine in Ansouis, where he lived as a penitent for at least a year.

Unlike Article 54, which included only indirect testimony from a mercenary, the witnesses for Article 56 included the mercenary, Durand Arnau. Master Nicolau Laurens traveled to Ansouis to take down witness testimony shortly after the miracle occurred. Three of the testimonies he took there, including Durand Arnau's, were reproduced in Delphine's inquest, even though those men did not appear before the commissioners in Apt in 1363. The commissioners heard and included the written testimonies in the inquest documents on the same day that an eyewitness to these events testified.[134]

The commissioners questioned witnesses about every detail of this miracle. They asked how tightly Durand had been tied, how deep the dry well was, whether or not it had any water in it, how big the rocks were that were thrown into the well after him, and even about the length of the rope used to haul him out. Eyewitness answers remained fairly consistent, though witnesses who had heard about the miracle from others exaggerated somewhat. None expressed doubt that Durand Arnau's internal transformation had allowed a miraculous protection and recovery. The man they had drawn out of the dry well was not the same person they had thrown in.

This miracle reflects the desire that mercenaries could be transformed. Papal letters sent from Avignon capture this complex attitude. Between 1356 and 1358, Innocent VI repeatedly reissued the bull *Ad reprimendas insolentias* in response to letters from abbots and bishops from Cambrai to Rodez begging for aid against the mercenaries. The language of the bull echoes twelfth-century language used to condemn violence during the Peace and Truce of God movement, similar to what we saw in chapter 2. It described the mercenaries' looting and violence against noncombatants and religious houses, excommunicated the mercenaries for this behavior, and in some cases even declared a limited crusade against them, since their violence against Christians made their acts heretical.[135]

Witnesses in Delphine's inquest appeared to be aware of this rhetoric. For example, Friar Bertran Jusbert, in his testimony to the portion of Article 38 that referred to Delphine's weeping and fever caused by the companies, referred to the men in the companies as unfaithful Christians. Not only were they making war in Provence, but they also "blasphemed the Virgin Mary by calling her a whore."[136] Friar Bertran included many witnesses close to Delphine in his depiction of the mercenaries, saying he heard about Delphine's reaction to the mercenaries from Bertranda Bertomieua, Master Nicolau Laurens, and Ugueta and Catherine de Pui. He claimed that his attitude toward the mercenaries was widespread, not just clerical rhetoric.[137]

But religious and secular leaders did not present the mercenaries as non-Christians. As we have seen, even the pope hired the mercenaries and rewarded them well for their services. Pope Innocent VI's representative in the Papal States, Gil Abornoz, had hired mercenaries as early as 1353 to retake and protect papal territory in the Italian peninsula.[138] And mercenaries had been hired to fight in crusades in Spain, Hungary, and the Levant.

Rather than present the mercenaries as non-Christian, leaders like Pope Innocent VI described them as straying sons, a problematic part of the Christian community. In a slightly later letter, Innocent VI wrote that he agreed that the mercenaries' crimes were wicked and demanded, in his words, "the serious rigor of the judges."[139] But he argued that leaders, including himself, should first guide the mercenaries through warnings and rules to leave their violent behavior and free the cities and property they had taken. Innocent VI described this plan as following in the footsteps of pious fathers "who did not seek the death of straying sons, but their health [*salutem*]."[140] Durand Arnau was a perfect example of a straying son, reformed and returned to the Christian community. His experience proved that these mercenaries could be reformed at a time when they seemed uncontrollable. This made it a powerful miracle to highlight, as Master Nicolau Laurens seemed to know.

The commissioners' questions also revealed that non-eyewitnesses heard about the event in a variety of ways and from a variety of sources. Three witnesses heard about the event shortly after it happened, but in two different cities, Apt and Avignon. Two other witnesses heard about it in 1360 in Apt. Bishop Philippe Cabassole may have heard it during the meeting of the Estates of Provence, which took place in Apt in 1360. He heard it from Lord Johan Raymon, the new *domicellus* of Ansouis and, in turn, told Friar Ysnard Risi.

Master Guilhem Enric heard it even later, in 1362, and in a third city, Aix. He also heard it from Johan Raymon. His version of the miracle is the least specific, saying only that he heard about the miraculous survival of the mercenary who had been thrown in a pit followed by rocks.

The movement of this story through its tellers shows how people from various social groups communicated with each other. Although the *domicellus* of Ansouis, Johan Raymon, did not testify in Delphine's inquest, he played an active role in spreading news of the miracle to the bishops and court officials in his social group and slightly above. In the case of Friar Ysnard Risi, we see someone in contact with multiple social groups, including religious and lay people.

Regardless of where a witness heard the story, however, this miracle resonated. For these witnesses, a prayer to Delphine had miraculously saved the life and healed the soul of a straying son. Not only had he found a way to stop fighting, but the soul of this violent attacker was returned to health through penitence, and he was reintegrated into the Christian community.

Article 57: From Mercenary to Penitent?

For Master Nicolau Laurens, however, there was an implied instability in the mercenary's transformation. Was surviving the execution attempt enough evidence that Durand Arnau had truly transformed his heart? Could he simply have been continuing to try to save his life after a lucky fall? The witnesses to Article 56 spoke as if convinced of the miracle, but the proctor, Master Nicolau Laurens, may not have been satisfied.

Article 57, which concerned Durand Arnau's encounter with Delphine in Apt, tried to deal with potential skepticism. It was not as popular as Article 56. Only two people testified to it, perhaps because there were no eyewitnesses. It did not appear in Durand's testimony, because that had been taken in Ansouis before he left for Apt. Its author, Master Laurens, seemed to know more about it than anyone else.[141]

The article stated that Durand Arnau came to the Holy Cross convent near Apt to visit Delphine and perform his penance. When the mercenary entered her presence, the article states that Delphine, "recognizing that grace had been done to him through the mercy of God, knew the heart of that man to be contrite and humble in consideration of gifts so immense."[142] According to the article, Delphine saw the internal state of the person in her presence—a common expression of sanctity in the fourteenth century. But what is less common, Master Nicolau presents Delphine as also recognizing the reconciliation between Durand and God as a priest might have in confession.[143]

After intuiting Durand Arnau's change, Delphine spoke to him. According to the article, she spoke kindly, but the words recorded in the article were not especially kind. She said, "Go and no longer wish to sin anymore. And, in the future you should choose to die before you undertake similar evil that you have reveled in until now. Now guard against the many temptations and demonic goadings that you endure."[144] Finally, Durand left Delphine's presence and became a penitent in Apt for at least a year. The article concludes by stating that this man, "having changed inside" [*mutatus interius*] entered a *hermitorium* of Blessed Mary of Claromonte and performed fasts and vigils.[145]

The article's description of Delphine's reaction to this mercenary moves beyond the tears and physical suffering in Article 38. First, she looked into Durand's heart, as she did for so many witnesses in the inquest, as we will see in chapters 5 and 6. Unlike for other witnesses, however, Delphine did not see what problems Durand struggled with. Instead she saw that God had truly transformed him. For Master Nicolau, her special relationship to God allowed her to ratify the earlier miracle that had taken place. This put to rest any fears that the mercenary had just been lucky. Second, Delphine warned Durand about how to act in the future. In the harshest words attributed to her in the inquest, she told Durand to choose to die before acting again as a mercenary—attacking Christians outside of war—and to guard against the temptation to do so.

The attitude attributed to Delphine reflected the attitude in Innocent's letter. The ideal solution against the mercenaries was redemption. But if they continued in unchristian violence, or in the case of Durand Arnau returned to it in the future, then they were excommunicated and could find themselves branded as heretics.

Through Delphine's words to the mercenary in Master Nicolau's Article 57, however, we also see the lingering fear that reform was only temporary in these men. They would appear reformed, perhaps even be reformed, but the temptation to give in to "demonic goadings" of violence would be too strong. The fact that no one knew for certain what happened to Durand Arnau after he left Apt highlights that fear of relapse.[146]

Surviving on the Fringes of the Hundred Years War

Truces in the Hundred Years War became dangerous times for the Rhône valley. The truce of Bordeaux from 1357 to 1359 released mercenary companies from their contracts with the kings of England and France and pushed their leaders to find new sources of employment, pay, and booty for their men. The mercenary leader Arnau de Cervole took the opportunity to cross the Rhône in the pay of the lords of Baux and Durazzo. Although they did not capture Marseille or Aix-en-Provence, they introduced the region to mercenary warfare.

The history of a mercenary leader like Arnau de Cervole shows how violence and warfare changed after the battle of Poitiers. The French and English kings, not to mention most other leaders in Europe, needed professional soldiers, but had little control over them. A leader like Arnau de Cervole had more control over his men, but he was not their sovereign. What war was, who fought in it, and what warriors did during times of peace changed in the mid-fourteenth century.

By exploring witnesses' testimonies to the mercenary invasion of 1357–1358, we see how people at all social levels were involved in warfare-like violence. We see their reactions and their attempts to define dangerous situations in a way that gave them some means to fix the problems they encountered. On the one side were noncombatants like Lady Catherine de Pui, who begged Delphine to banish a storm that could mask a mercenary attack. According to Pope Innocent's letter to King Jean of France, women like Delphine and Catherine had much to fear from these mercenaries.

But lords of the region had fears as well. They feared for the safety of cities that they had too few resources to protect. They feared engaging with experienced fighters who had taken so many cities. They may also have feared for their souls if they fought and killed. But they feared for their honor and *fama* if they did not fight. And, finally, while the papacy hoped to reform these mercenaries—make them Christian again—people feared that reform was only a sham or only temporary. And, after a short hiatus, as the number of mercenaries in the region grew after the Treaty of Bretigny, war remained a constant for these witnesses.

Chapter 4

Lady Andrea Raymon and the Great Companies, 1361

On November 26, 1360, Countess Delphine de Puimichel died at the age of seventy-five.[1] This was a momentous event for her close associates, the city of Apt, and the Agoult and Sabran families. Witnesses recalled many miracles that took place during Delphine's vigil, proving for them her sanctity. At least five witnesses mentioned hearing miraculous celestial music that night.[2] Many more witnesses, including her medical doctor and confessor, Master Durand Andree, recalled that Delphine's feet stayed pliable as if still living, a familiar mark of sanctity.[3] Delphine's feet were the site of several miracles at her vigil. For example, a prostitute kissed Delphine's feet and immediately changed her life, a mother wrapped Delphine's feet around the neck of her ill son and he was healed, and one witness made multiple healing objects by touching them to Delphine's feet.[4] People took advantage of this special moment of access to Delphine's body to find healing and transformation.

One month before Delphine died there had been another momentous event, one that affected many more people. On October 24 1360, King Edward III of England and King Jean II of France ratified the Treaty of Bretigny. The treaty negotiated the release of King Jean for a ransom of 3 million gold ecus and King Edward receiving the duchy of Aquitaine without the limitations of feudal obligation to the king of France.[5]

In the treaty, King Edward agreed to remove his men from occupied castles and towns in areas that remained under King Jean. But the treaty did not include any arrangements for dispersing or otherwise employing the hundreds of mercenary companies that had held these castles and towns.[6] Their removal became a complex operation that required twelve commissioners of King Edward traveling from castle to castle, helping conclude negotiations that often required cities to pay large ransoms to the departing leaders of independent mercenary companies.[7] The first region to be evacuated in this way was the duchy of Burgundy, directly north of Provence on the Saone River, which connects to the Rhône in Lyon.

These men found a new goal when they learned that the first installment of the French king's ransom would soon move up the Rhône by barge. As a result, by December 1360, a month after Delphine's vigil, a massive wave of unemployed mercenaries, far larger than the invasion three years earlier, moved into Provence. These mercenaries would disrupt trade, agriculture, and daily life for years.

After months of mercenary occupation, a second wave of plague also erupted in Provence. According to Master Guy de Chauliac, a surgeon for the popes in Avignon and author of a well-known text on surgery, plague returned to Avignon from Germany and northern regions. De Chauliac described it as waxing and waning until September, at which point it flared up and ravaged major cities like Avignon and Aix from the end of September through December.[8]

At least ten witnesses in Delphine's inquest pinpointed 1361 as a moment of danger. They told personal stories of secret prayers to Delphine, often at the moment they believed they might die. They told stories of mercenary attack, plague, and fever in this dangerous year. Although no one miracle stands out, several trends do tie these personal stories together. One trend is the experience of transformation. Witnesses sought Delphine's help in a time of crisis and experienced some type of transformation as part of that miraculous aid. These transformations took many different forms, which reveal the diverse ways these witnesses understood miraculous and medical healing, the importance of the state of the soul, and external behavior that could aid others.

Another trend, perhaps the clearest, is the active engagement of women as protectors and healers in times of war and illness. Women's miracle stories were personal stories, but at the same time, they were also stories of caring for towns, institutions, and families. These are some of the most vivid and exciting narratives in the inquest. Women described how they felt and what they did when they came under attack or fell ill. Through their testimonies about this moment of danger, we also see women of various social statuses using their holy countess to protect people and resources from mercenary depredations and heal plague and fevers that emerged in the wake of those attacks.

One witness brings together both the waves of mercenary invasion and waves of illness. In her short testimony, Lady Andrea Raymon, a fifty-one-year-old noblewoman living in Ansouis, testified to two miracles. In her answer to Article 1, she described escaping a mercenary ambush. In this moment of danger, she felt herself transformed from terrified to courageous after a prayer to Delphine. This transformation allowed her to protect her whole entourage from capture. Lady Andrea also testified to the miraculous healing of the brother of the prior of St. Peter's church in Ansouis from a deadly fever. This fever occurred not in 1361 but in 1363. This story of illness helps us see the impact on health that the mercenary invasion had, not just in the short term by possibly reintroducing the plague, but also in the long term by disrupting food production, storage, and shipment; straining energy sources and sanitation; destroying infrastructure; and bring displaced populations into contact.

Lady Andrea's testimony gives us the perspective of the upper aristocracy of Provence, a group involved in fighting the mercenaries, but also a target for mercenaries who wished to capture and ransom wealthy people. The larger context of the Hundred Years War, especially the widespread impact of treaties on disruption in food production and sanitation in areas outside the immediate zone of war, helps us better understand the many dangers everyone in Provence faced in 1361 through 1363. Witnesses were again caught in the unintended consequences of another truce, which showed the weak influence of royal and papal authority over mercenary soldiers. When facing these dangers, witnesses turned to their recently deceased holy woman who had protected them for decades. The stories that witnesses like Lady Andrea Raymon told showed how they continued making Delphine part of the survival of the region even after the holy woman's death.

Mercenaries in Provence, 1360–1362

As King Edward's commissioners removed mercenary troops from the Burgundy region, those unemployed mercenaries looked for new opportunities. Like the mercenaries working for Arnau de Cervole in 1357–1358, these were semiautonomous bands of professional soldiers under experienced captains.

A few returned home, but most instead started seeking a new employer or source of income.[9]

It was at this moment in 1360, from September to December, that the course of the Hundred Years War entered what historian Kenneth Fowler identifies as a turning point. Warfare in Europe—large-scale and local—was conducted by mercenary companies. There were tens of thousands of mercenaries in Europe. These men did not fight for the Christian God, a king, a country, or a chivalric identity. They were professionals, and they fought for pay. As they left their captured castles and cities in Burgundy, more and more of these unemployed, displaced mercenaries reformed into companies under their previous captains.[10] These bands of twenty to two hundred men then merged into larger companies, which included up to ten thousand, under successful mercenary leaders.[11] Historians refer to these much larger companies as the Great Companies.

Unluckily for the people of Provence, just as the mercenaries were leaving Burgundy, they found a new goal to the south. The first installment of King Jean's ransom was being collected in Toulouse, Carcassone, and Nîmes. It would move north up the Rhône from Avignon in December. Learning this, a large group of mercenaries moved south, hoping to capture the ransom money. This was not a war in any sense of the word for fourteenth-century Christians. The mercenaries had not been hired to defeat an enemy. Instead they were sustaining and enriching themselves until they were hired again. To put it bluntly, this was looting. Few rules of warfare applied.[12]

On the night of December 28, a large group of mercenaries attacked Pont-Saint-Esprit, twenty-five miles north of Avignon. The mercenaries had timed their attack to intercept the seneschal of Beaucaire, Jean Souvain, who had the task of overseeing the ransom transport.[13] Unlike in the attack led by Arnau de Cervole, this attack, which occurred in 1357–1358, had not been long planned. Pope Innocent VI had only a few weeks' notice of the mercenaries' plans and probably did not have a clear idea of the magnitude of the attacking force.[14] There was also no clear leader to whom Innocent could write for mercy.

The agents of the French crown, hearing rumors of the mercenaries, stopped in Avignon. Jean Souvain went to Pont-Saint-Esprit on schedule, but did not have the money with him. Hearing that Souvain had arrived, however, the mercenaries attacked. Souvain tried to lead the defense of Pont-Saint-Esprit, but the town was not well defended and not completely enclosed by walls.[15] Souvain was killed, and the surviving defenders retreated to a fortified church and held it for six days. Finally, they paid the mercenaries 6,000 florins for safe conduct out of the church and the town, but several chronicles indicate that even after payment, men were killed and women were raped.[16] Once mercenaries held Pont-Saint-Esprit, the agents of the French crown sent the ransom money back to Nîmes for safekeeping and did not reattempt transport for almost a year.[17]

Although this Great Company did not capture the French king's ransom, they found themselves in control of one of only four bridges across the Rhône. This placed them near the papal court, which was the wealthiest bureaucracy in Europe, receiving tithes and important visitors from around Europe. It also placed them above Marseille, a major Mediterranean port. Avignon and Marseille had been rebuilding city defenses since Arnau de Cervole's occupation two years earlier, but the region was still not well defended.[18]

In the first days of the attack and occupation, bands of mercenaries captured Roquemaure and the village of Chuslan, both of which were pillaged and burned, and the inhabitants ransomed. They also seized the village of Codolet. After they were in control of Pont-Saint-Esprit and the immediate region, groups of mercenaries moved outward on either side of the Rhône, setting up bases in Carpentras in the east and near Montpellier in the west.[19] From Pont-Saint-Esprit, they stopped food shipments by land and water and ransomed wealthy travelers. On the eastern side of the Rhône, they raided the poorly defended towns of the Comtat Venaissin. Inhabitants of the region, who were still trying to rebuild, lost everything again. People living in the countryside or even city suburbs withdrew again inside fortified towns and stayed there if they could.[20]

Local and papal defenders did not have the forces to stop the mercenaries. They had struggled against Arnau de Cervole's four thousand mercenaries. In the face of the Great Companies, local defenders were completely overwhelmed. Even fortified towns and cities struggled. La Motte and Montaigu were burned. The Franciscans lost houses outside Bagnol and Uzès and had to look for refuge in walled cities. As in 1357–1358, other religious houses were abandoned and destroyed by order of nearby cities. The Cistercians of Valsauve and Goudargues, for example, were pillaged.[21] In Avignon, the defenses begun in 1357–1358 were not complete and had to be supplemented with wooden barricades.[22]

Drawn by the strategic location, unemployed mercenaries continued to move south as King Edward's commissioners gradually evacuated the duchy of Burgundy. By January 1361, companies also started arriving from war-depleted Gascony and the kingdom of Aragon, swelling this Great Company to what Fowler calls "mega-proportions."[23] Ultimately, five Great Companies made up of tens of thousands of experienced soldiers found their way to the lower Rhône valley in 1361.[24]

Unlike the companies of Arnau de Cervole in 1357–1358, this collection of Great Companies was constantly expanding, and had no single leader, no single goal, and no legitimate reason to be in the region.[25] In January and February 1361, several mercenary leaders, including such well-known mercenaries as John Hawkwood and Bernard de Sorgues, established themselves in Carpentras, roughly fifteen miles from Avignon.[26] This was a messy, unpredictable occupation. Even the changes in military organization that occurred in Provence in 1359 in response to Cervole's invasion could not cope.[27]

In an attempt to stop more companies from joining those already in Provence, Pope Innocent VI contacted the duke of Burgundy, the king of France, Emperor Charles IV of Bohemia, the duke of Austria, the doge of Genoa, and many other lords, archbishops, bishops, and communes, begging them to oppose the movement of mercenaries through their regions.[28] This was a difficult request, since most of these areas had few resources to stop the mercenaries. They also did not want the mercenaries in their own territory, so they had a strong incentive to not hinder the mercenaries.

Unlike in the battle against Arnau de Cervole, Innocent VI did receive aid, partly because outside leaders did not perceive this event as linked to Queen Johanna or King Louis of Naples. The hospitaller Juan Fernandez de Heredia led troops from the king of Aragon. Lords from Languedoc under the king of France sent some aid to try to drive the mercenaries out.[29] King Louis of Naples also offered to send aid, but since he was at war with the king of Aragon, and Aragon had already sent troops, Pope Innocent did not accept King Louis's offer.[30]

Also, to raise troops against the companies already in Provence, Innocent VI preached a crusade against these invaders, promising indulgences for those who fought and for those who paid someone to fight.[31] The crusaders on the eastern and western sides of the Rhône attacked smaller mercenary strongholds with some success. Finally, they laid siege to Pont-Saint-Esprit, but their leaders avoided direct attack against the main mercenary force. Contemporary sources suggest that since Innocent VI expected the crusaders to fight without pay, there was no surety that they would not quit or join the mercenary forces.[32]

By mid-February, with the crusaders' siege weakening, Innocent and the crusade leaders decided to pay the mercenaries to leave and fight somewhere else. After a brief negotiation with representatives from several of the largest companies, most agreed to leave Pont-Saint-Esprit and the region of the lower Rhône.[33]

Here again the splintered nature of the Great Companies caused new problems. By April, one group of mercenaries agreed to leave Pont-Saint-Esprit in return for absolution for their crimes and 14,500 florins. They agreed to follow the marquis de Montferrat through the Alps and join the war with the dukes of Milan. Innocent negotiated a safe-conduct from the seneschal of Provence in order to allow Jean de Montferrat and the mercenaries to leave.[34] The safe-conduct was jeopardized, however, when Marseille, still recovering from a famine the mercenaries caused, refused to sell the departing mercenaries food. The mercenaries set fire to the suburbs in retaliation.[35]

Another group of mercenaries negotiated a separate agreement with the French king's representatives on April 22. They agreed to leave the lower Rhône and fight for the king of Aragon against Castile.[36] The mercenaries were paid and left Pont-Saint-Esprit, but when the kings of Aragon and Castile negotiated a peace treaty, this group of mercenaries, led by Seguin de Badefol, continued to attack Languedoc around Montpellier and Perpignan.[37]

Spiritual Reaction to the Great Companies

The defenders, including the papacy and the people of Provence and the Comtat Venaissin, struggled to organize against this new and overwhelming violent threat. Pope Innocent VI's call for crusade shows the changing reactions to these mercenaries as they moved beyond the confines of any kind of legitimate warfare. The language of healing still appeared in papal letters addressing these events. Innocent VI's crusade preaching at the beginning of the invasion sounded much like the language of Article 38 in Delphine's inquest. Like Article 38, this letter emphasized the health of men's souls—attackers and defenders alike.[38] In the letter, the pope criticized the invaders. He identified them as "many iniquitous sons, who come from diverse nations into a group" and as "a deep evil, impious set assembled to disturb the interests and serenity of the community and the peace of Christ."[39] He described their acts as sins and crimes, saying that, in the manner of thieves and enemies they seize goods through hostile action and keep what they take. The pope desired to advance against these men both spiritually and temporally in order to heal them.[40] As we saw in chapter 3, the first goal was applying the "serious rigor of the judges."[41] These men should be warned and led back to proper Christian behavior. As Innocent put it, they should first be called to penitence in the manner of the fathers, who did not seek the death of straying sons, but their health (*salutem*).[42]

But after experiencing the attack of Arnau de Cervole in 1357–1358, Pope Innocent knew that "warnings and rules," while ideal, were not likely to be effective. Therefore he identified another group within the invading mercenaries. These men were "too proud." In many sources, including the perennially influential Gregory the Great, pride was depicted as the chief deadly sin.[43] Those who were prideful placed themselves above God. Unlike Durand Arnau de Rupa Ayneria—the mercenary who saw a vision of holy light inspired by Delphine and became a penitent—these men refused the warnings and rules and persisted in their wickedness. They were not changed by lessons for their soul's health (*salutem*) and wished to join themselves to evil. These are the men Friar Bertran Jusbert described in his testimony to Article 38 as blaspheming the Virgin Mary, separating themselves from the Christian community.[44] While Innocent's separate category of mercenaries likely held little visible distinction within the Great Companies, it made these men non-Christian and therefore an appropriate subject for a crusade.[45]

Against these men, Innocent called local and distant defenders to arms. To them he offered an indulgence, which he referred to as both "health-giving and glorious," for fighting or equipping others to fight and carry out God's business.[46] While we tend to think of indulgences from the perspective of the Protestant Revolution, in which they were depicted negatively, in the fourteenth century they were diverse and popular. For example, Pope Innocent VI had also offered an indulgence for all those who made a pilgrimage to Rome in 1360. Both of the holy women, Dorothy of Montau and Birgitta of Sweden, made the journey. Birgitta even had visions of both Jesus and Mary extolling the virtues of indulgences.[47]

For the pope and those fighting the mercenaries, 1361 was a moment of crusade and indulgence. The rhetoric emphasized the health of men's souls, both those attacking and those defending. But the defenders also understood that this was a different kind of invasion than they had faced only a few years earlier. Pope Innocent's letter pointed out the practical difficulties introduced by thousands of mercenaries holding Pont-Saint-Esprit. The pope and cardinals living in Avignon experienced the type of famine that Marseille had faced in 1358. Papal officials especially found it difficult to bring in the "many goods and necessary and useful for the court."[48] In the months after the ratification of the Treaty of Bretigny, daily life in Provence became unpredictable. Mercenary bands roamed the countryside for months after the main mercenary groups left, complicating travel, food production, and sanitation for years.

Noncombatants in a Leaderless Invasion

This invasion was even less like traditional warfare than the attacks of 1357–1358.[49] In 1361, there was no dramatic call to arms by the seneschal of Provence.

This was not a moment when the lords of Provence stood alone against an invading army that attacked as part of the protracted battle for the Crown of Naples. And witnesses felt the impact of the large number of mercenaries in the region in different ways. Most testimony described vows to Delphine made in secret during sudden, unexpected attacks or during acute bouts of illness.

Witness testimonies give us a different vantage point to understand how people survived this leaderless invasion. They did not speak of a kiss of peace that would end unhealthy violence. Nor did they speak of organized attacks with specific goals as they had when Arnau de Cervole's soldiers had invaded. No witnesses spoke of military men leading sorties to retake captured towns. Instead people spoke of surviving sudden, unexpected danger.

Women's testimony in particular allows us to see women actively engaged in their own and others' protection. Like Catherine de Pui, who had begged Delphine to pray for the end of the storm that could have let the mercenaries attack Ansouis, the women attesting to miracles in 1361 turned to their holy woman for the good of a larger group. And like Catherine de Pui, they took an active approach to their safety and well-being. Their miracle stories give us insight into women's protective and leadership roles in their communities and how those roles could expand during times of heightened violence.

Lady Andrea Raymon was one of those active women. Lady Andrea was wife of Lord Johan Raymon, the *domicellus* of Ansouis, whom we met in chapter 3 as an active teller of the story of the reformed mercenary. He was a member of the household of noble Lord Guilhem de Sabran. Through her husband's position as *domicellus*, she had links to Lady Delphine's extended family, though her testimony does not indicate she knew Delphine personally. Lady Andrea testified on June 15 before the papal commissioners in the cathedral in Apt. Her testimony sheds light on two of Delphine's postmortem miracles. One she experienced and one she heard about. She spoke about both in response to Article 1.

The miracle Lady Andrea Raymon experienced was her transformation from terrified to courageous.[50] This transformation helped her protect herself and members of her family and household when they were ambushed by mercenaries. Lady Andrea was traveling in late November 1361 near the castle of Meyrargues, located about ten miles north of Aix-en-Provence on the main road connecting Pertuis to Aix. She rode on horseback, as did her son Peter and several knights traveling with them, including Raymon of Rustrel. At least one servant traveling on foot accompanied them.

When her group neared the church of the Blessed John outside Meyrargues, they saw thirty men on horseback and many others on foot. There were two groups—one appeared behind Lady Andrea's group, and one appeared to the left. All were armed and moving swiftly to capture Lady Andrea's group. Lady Andrea and everyone with her were greatly terrified (*valde terruerant*) and full of confusion and fear (*in magna perplexitate et timore*). They could not retreat because of the horsemen behind them, and they did not see any other place to turn. They feared they would fall into the hands of the armed men.[51]

Stunned (*stupefacta*) and without any remedy (*remedio*), Andrea hastened to Lady Delphine in her heart. She asked Delphine to pray to God that the armed men not capture her and her group. If Andrea obtained God's grace, she promised that she would go on pilgrimage to Delphine's sepulcher.[52] Immediately after making the vow, Lady Andrea's heart changed. She became confident (*assumpsit audaciam*) and experienced consolation in her heart (*consolacionem in corde suo*). She noticed the same effect in her son. With this new confidence, she and the others were able to save themselves. They rode across the bridge of Meyrargues and to the castle, which rests on a hill above the town.

Lady Andrea told the commissioners that their escape was particularly miraculous for two reasons. First, as she rode, part of her horse's tackle broke. This increased her fear and disturbance and made her ride more slowly. Second, in her estimation the armed men should have reached the bridge twice as quickly as her group. They should have crossed it and cut off access to the castle. In fact, she feared that armed men were already on the other side of the bridge and had perhaps spent the night in the town of Meyrargues at the foot of the castle.

But by the time she and her group reached the bridge, the armed men had only moved "through the space of one long lance or glaive."[53] Seeing that they could barely move, the armed men shouted at them, "Go in evil hour!," and Lady Andrea shouted back, "And you remain in evil hour!"[54] No other armed men attacked after they crossed the bridge, and they entered the castle in safety.

Lady Andrea felt transformed from terrified to courageous and attributed this change to Delphine's intercession. She received the confidence and consolation to ride away just as the attackers were miraculously hindered. She received so much confidence, in fact, that she was able to ride with broken harness and return the attackers' taunts. In addition to transformation, here again we see a woman protecting herself and the people around her by asking for Delphine's aid. Like Catherine de Pui, who begged Delphine to protect Ansouis, Andrea turned in her heart to Delphine and prayed for a "remedy" through God's grace. In this way she protected not only herself, but her son and retinue.

Andrea's presentation of herself differs dramatically from the presentation of women in official letters concerning the mercenaries. Of course, it would have been very lucrative for the mercenaries to capture a noblewoman and her son. And with capture, Andrea faced the likelihood of rape and injury. She greatly feared falling into their hands. But Andrea did not depict herself as a victim. Instead, she presented herself actively resisting the real danger these men posed. Andrea's whole group reached the safety of the castle of Meyrargues because Andrea—from her own perspective—thought on her feet, quickly prayed to her holy woman, and was worthy of the miracle she begged for.

The inquest includes a second miracle concerning the mercenaries in 1361. This miracle involves a transformation of sorts, but it better highlights the indirect dangers that the companies posed and the active steps that women in authority took to protect those in their care. This miracle takes more contextualization to fully understand. But its implications help us see how women protected their communities during the mercenary invasion, second wave of plague, and multiple waves of illness that spread through Provence.

Article 78 described the experience of the forty-year-old Lady Ayselena d'Apt—a member of the local aristocracy of Apt and abbess of the Holy Cross convent. She prayed to Delphine for the protection of the convent's and the lord of Apt's property during an unexpected mercenary raid.[55] The events took place in September 1361, again months after the mercenaries were supposed to have left and just as plague erupted in Avignon.

According to the article, at the time when the companies of Spain were in Provence, Abbess Ayselena heard the market bell ring and was told that mercenaries had raided the castle of Gargas, less than two miles away.[56] Like many other local nobles, Ayselena kept the convent's livestock there—six cows used for plowing—under the care of a herdsman. Fearing that the cows would be taken, she immediately converted her heart to the merits of the holy countess and begged Delphine to ease the needs of the convent as the holy countess had so frequently done during her lifetime. If the cows were saved, Ayselena would bring a wax cow to Delphine's tomb.

The events depicted in Article 78 are somewhat unclear, since no one person (especially Ayselena) could have seen them, and no mercenary, like Gailhardo of Saint-Germain in 1358, described them. Ayselena said she heard about the cows' intriguing behavior from Bonopari, the *bailie* of Gargas, who was a relative of one of the nuns. No one heard Ayselena make the vow, but many saw the returned cows. The article and Ayselena's testimony, therefore, reflect how Ayselena understood the event and chose to describe it.

The article roughly explains that the cows belonging to the convent and to Lord Giraud de Simiana, the lord of Apt, were seized from their caretaker by mercenaries. But the convent's six cows, acting "as if they were rational participants," led themselves and all the other cows away from the fortifications of Gargas at a run, thereby escaping the mercenaries.[57] Afterward, one of the convent's cows and all the other cows were seemingly recaptured by the mercenaries, but the convent's remaining cows appeared at the convent's hayloft the next day. To make a complicated story short, Abbess Ayselena turned to Delphine for help, and the recently deceased holy woman answered her prayer.

The miracle shows Delphine and the women she interacted with during life acting as protectors. Ayselena described Delphine as someone who had eased the cares of the Holy Cross convent during her life. She had certainly produced miracles there, including protecting the convent from fire. It made sense to Ayselena to call on Delphine to protect the cows and therefore sustain the productivity of the convent's lands. To stretch the point just a bit farther, Ayselena also claimed that her cows had attempted to aid Lord Giraud de Simiana's cows, thus making them protectors and leaders of others in this dangerous situation.

The quaintness of this miracle, with its rational cows leading their bovine compatriots away from the mercenaries, can mask the real danger to Ayselena's community. The miracle sheds light on the experience of devastation that invading mercenaries caused for towns and religious institutions.[58] Towns like Gargas in the hills around Apt produced grain not just for their own consumption but also for larger towns, like Apt and Ansouis, and cities like Avignon and Aix.[59] With the region recovering from the 1357–1358 depredations, the loss of six animals engaged in plowing and, perhaps, transportation would have been a significant blow to local grain production.

The experiences of both Lady Andrea Raymon and Abbess Ayselena reveal the long-term impact of the Treaty of Bretigny. The mercenaries drawn by the wealth of the lower Rhône did not all leave in orderly groups after the negotiations in April. This was not a unified army with a specific goal, but many semiautonomous bands supporting themselves through violence. They became a fact of life in this region after 1361. This was no longer described as a war, with the Gascons or anyone else, but simply as a time when the companies were in Provence. In many small instances, most lost to history, women like Lady Andrea and Abbess Ayselena had to find whatever means they could to overcome their own fears, save themselves, and protect those in their care.

Problems of Sanitation, Food Production, and Energy Sources during the Mercenary Occupation

The witnesses testifying to war, plague, and fever give us none of the context of their lives. They did not feel they had to tell the papal commissioners, who had lived through the same events, so a modern audience has to build the context that the witnesses and inquest organizers experienced. The arrival of multiple Great Companies, tens of thousands of mercenaries, in this one region certainly influenced living conditions and food production. It complicated communication and travel, displaced groups of people, and intensified contact with disease vectors in the region.

The Great Companies meant the movement of many bands of soldiers from all over Europe into one region. At least one physician, Master Guy de Chauliac, who served the popes of Avignon and was the author of a well-known text on surgery, observed that plague returned to Avignon from Germany and northern regions.[60] Although he did not specify that mercenaries were responsible, the mercenaries were the main group coming into the region from the north. While we do not have definitive evidence to claim they brought the plague with them from another region or caused it to resurface, they certainly provided contact between diverse regions and exacerbated conditions that supported epidemic illnesses (not just plague).[61] Although we have few statistics for deaths caused by this invasion and wave of plague, there are accounts of the deaths of at least nine cardinals and ninety-seven dignitaries, and roughly seventeen thousand people in Avignon.[62] This was not all from plague, but plague was a factor.

While the miraculous protection of the Holy Cross convent's cows gives us insight into the increasing food pressures, the presence of large numbers of soldiers introduced sanitation issues as well. On a simplistic level, the mercenaries not only had to eat, they also had to excrete. To get a very rough idea of the waste produced by the Great Companies, we can consider the approach that John W. I. Lee—a historian of ancient Greece—used when exploring the quotidian experiences of soldiers in Xenophon's *Anabasis*. He found that an ancient Greek army of roughly ten thousand men (eating the foods they would have eaten and in the proportions they would have had at the time) produced an estimated average of about 4,400 pounds of feces daily.[63]

If we put these relatively low numbers, useful for considering an army with limited resources, into the context of the mercenary invasion of Provence, the amount of feces is significant.[64] There were far more than ten thousand mercenaries in Provence. According to Fowler, one Great Company had roughly twelve thousand men. There were five Great Companies in Provence at this time, so the number was closer to fifty thousand (to be conservative). That's over twenty-two thousand pounds of feces a day, just for the people. While some of the mercenaries spread out into the countryside in small bands, lessening the impact of sanitation issues, many others lived in captured towns and cities.

Human waste in the countryside, even on a large scale, likely had no significant impact on health. However, occupation and sieges were a different matter. In terms of occupation, it was common practice for mercenary groups to live in large monasteries or captured towns, especially during winter months, as we saw in chapter 3. In early 1361, mercenary leaders captured many towns like Pont-Saint-Esprit and set up bases in cities as large as Carpentras and Montpellier. Occupation added several hundred more people to a town's population. It also significantly added to the distress and danger of the people who lived in the town and had nowhere else to go. Added people and limited control over the behavior of that displaced community could dramatically impact the regular sanitation habits of a town or city.[65]

To help us understand the pressure of displaced populations, it is helpful to consider sanitation efforts in cities in the Italian peninsula, which had a long history of intense urbanization. Guy Geltner's study of Pistoian city statutes on hygiene shows long-standing concern and attempts to regulate market and labor activities, town walls and boundaries, burial and funeral practices, waste disposal, air and water pollution, and food production.[66] All of these came under special scrutiny, especially when illness threatened the city. But all of these efforts were strained during an occupation, whether the invaders were outside or inside the city walls.

While all aspects of sanitation were important, looking at human waste disposal highlights the difficulties towns and cities faced. According to historian Richard Hoffmann, "If an average adult produces about 150 grams of feces and 1 to 1.5 liters of urine each day, a modest medieval urban center of five thousand had annually to dispose of some 250 tons of solids and 2500 tons of liquid human wastes or sewage."[67] By the fourteenth century, cities and towns had protocols and laws to manage human waste.[68] Most had a combination of burying household waste and flushing it, along with manufacturing waste, out of town along waterways.[69] Even in times without undue pressure, cities challenged the surrounding ecosystems. With larger populations, including occupying forces and other displaced populations who may not have had access to household waste disposal options, sanitation suffered, and the likelihood of disease, especially acute and epidemic disease, increased.

Sieges were far worse. A siege brought many thousands of soldiers, defenders, and noncombatants into one area for an extended period of time.[70] Although plague is not transferred by contact with feces, other diseases, which can weaken a population and heighten the impact of plague, are. Dysentery, for example, was a particular danger during sieges like the one at Pont-Saint-Esprit, even though it occurred in winter.[71] Since the defenders and others fighting for papal indulgences were not a cohesive army, there may have been little coordination for setting up camp in a healthier area, establishing latrines, and caring for the sick and injured.[72]

As we saw in Lady Andrea's testimony, however, occupation and active sieges were only part of the problem. The constant threat of the Great Companies meant the retreat of the population into smaller spaces within city walls.[73] Two communities in Delphine's canonization inquest—the Holy Cross convent, whose abbess prayed to save the cows, and the convent of St. Catherine—give us some insight into displaced groups. The Holy Cross convent was originally outside the city walls but was threatened by mercenaries in 1358 and destroyed in 1361.[74] The nuns moved temporarily inside the city walls of Apt.[75] Although there were plans to rebuild their convent, by 1372 they had moved into Apt permanently.[76] A notarial document from 1357 lists twenty-one nuns by name, most of them officials in the convent, and mentions that there were others.[77] This was a sizable addition to the population of Apt.

St. Catherine's convent is a slightly different story. This convent, located in Apt, was supposed to maintain fifty-two nuns or less at any time. It was not supposed to get any larger than this, on pain of excommunication.[78] A notarial document from 1360 lists thirty-seven names of nuns associated with St. Catherine's.[79] However, this number could fluctuate. After the first wave of plague in 1348, convents at this time often housed women who were not officially nuns. Delphine and her ladies, such as Catherine de Pui and Bertranda Bertomieua, are examples. Testimonies in Delphine's inquest, which we will explore in chapter 5, give us some idea of the many widows from the region who may have swelled the convent's community. This evidence gives insight into how specific kinds of communities could absorb a moving population.

Increased population due to refugees, who often stayed for long periods of time, overwhelmed walled cities' sanitation measures. But refugees also strained food supplies, disrupted production, and limited energy resources. The constant danger of mercenary attack also spurred the construction of stronger city walls and the destruction of suburbs and outbuildings. Along with the burning of towns by mercenaries, this disruption of town and city infrastructure increased pressures on inhabitants and likely displaced rodent populations, a major disease vector of plague.

In addition to the loss of animals that Abbess Ayselena described, the fact that these raids were happening in September, when people would be finishing the harvest, processing summer crops, and planting winter crops, reveals another impact of the mercenaries on food production.[80] Bands of armed men foraging for food in the countryside made going out into the fields to harvest grain and other produce dangerous. Preparing and transporting grain from the fields after it was harvested also left people working in the fields exposed. There is also evidence that the mercenaries, or those in their employ, might take the harvestable grain for themselves. Mercenary companies were known to employ looters, who would steal foodstuffs as well as goods.[81] Finally, on top of this, the harvest was threatened by the loss of humans to illness, especially the second wave of plague, because epidemic illness limited the number of people available to work in the fields.

Mercenary activity also limited the storage of harvested grain. Cities and towns had limited granaries that had to store food for both humans and animals during times of siege or, in this case, long-term uncertainty. A market town like Apt, in a grain-growing region, would have had one or more warehouses for grain. But even in Apt (let alone a perched village like Ansouis where other witnesses lived), warehouses within town walls were very expensive compared to those outside and using them could raise the price of grain. Many larger storage facilities existed outside of town walls. These were risky to use, however, since mercenaries could capture them. With large numbers of mercenaries in the region, few of the larger, more exposed granaries were used, and some were preemptively destroyed. This meant that less of what people managed to harvest could be stored. This would be disastrous in the spring months, when communities traditionally relied on their stored grain for food and as seed grain for a new crop.[82]

Grain shipments for larger cities like Avignon and Aix were blocked or stolen by the mercenaries. Three letters from Pope Innocent VI in February 1361 describe missing or stolen shipments of grain from northern Italy and Burgundy.[83] For example, in a letter to the town of Embrun in which Innocent VI had preached a crusade against the mercenaries, he pointed out (among other things) the practical difficulties introduced by mercenaries holding Pont-Saint-Esprit.[84]

Most people in Provence depended on grain, primarily in the form of bread, as a large part of their daily diet.[85] People like the lord of Apt and Abbess Ayselena, who owned land and supported civic or religious institutions, would most likely have had to buy grain in the short term to support those who depended on them. In the long term, they would have had to buy more plow animals to replace those stolen. Both grain and oxen would be far more expensive due to their scarcity.[86] They would also need to be bought by people who were also paying higher taxes to cover the 14,500 florins and more that the pope and local lords paid the main body of mercenaries to leave. In a region beset by multiple disasters between 1348 and 1361, the economic impact, especially for the convent, might have been too great to overcome. Some of the religious institutions in this region ceased to exist by the end of the fourteenth century due to war, plague, and other illnesses.[87]

Towns and cities' inability to store large supplies of grain and other dried foods inside the city walls restricted the normal food intake of all those inside the city. In average years, the daily diet of ordinary townspeople in Provence usually consisted of soup and bread.[88] The soup might be a cabbage soup with legumes, especially those that could be dried and stored, such as peas, lentils, chickpeas, or beans. The soup could also be a meat broth with small pieces of salted pork. Townspeople preferred wheat bread, and wheat was the most commonly grown grain in Provence, but they could also eat bread made from other grains, including rye, barley, oats, and millet. The primary sources of animal protein were eggs and fish, but these were not everyday foods. Consumption patterns of foods like milk, cheese, and fruit were regional. Those in the mountains ate more cheese, while those near the coast ate more fruit. Peasants living in the countryside usually had more access to fresh foods, but even in towns, people owned sheep and poultry, and had kitchen gardens.[89]

Disrupted food shipments combined with a higher population meant that people were eating less, eating strange foods, and competing for food with domesticated animals and rodents. Over many months, poor nutrition would make everyone in town more susceptible to disease. Delphine's inquest gives us a glimpse of these food pressures. According to witness Raybaud St. Mitri, part of the celebration of Delphine's burial in 1360 included feeding lunch to poor people who had taken part in the ceremony.[90] They were to be fed at the hospice (*hospicio*) in which Delphine had died. Raybaud St. Mitri had been asked by the city council to organize and pay for Delphine's burial, including this lunch for the poor. When he saw the number of poor people gathered at the hospice, however, he realized that the amount of chickpeas he had was far short of what would be needed. He would need more than three times as much as he had planned on. They handed out the chickpeas, however, and at the end of the lunch a large jar of chickpeas remained. Many people in the town saw this and considered it a miracle.[91]

Delphine's reputation for sanctity was widespread, her family's wealth was reknowned, and feeding the poor was a common event at fourteenth-century funerals. Raybaud had expected a large crowd. But the event occurred in a region still recovering from the mercenary attacks in 1358. The extraordinary size of the crowd looking for food within the safety of Apt's walls may reflect the long-term impact of those attacks. The miracle certainly reflected the care that the people of Provence would expect from their "holy countess."

Food would not have been the only scarce necessity. Energy sources, especially firewood for cooking, heating, and crafts, would have been limited too.[92] To give some idea of firewood needs in the fourteenth century, a large city like London needed on average eighty-eight thousand tons of firewood, which it could not produce for itself. Cities and towns often transported firewood from long distances.[93] Even a much smaller market town like Apt would need significant amounts of firewood. With mercenaries in the countryside, this would have been dangerous. Townspeople would also have been in competition with the mercenaries for firewood, especially in winter and spring months. Lack of firewood would have made baking bread and heating houses difficult. Both would have had an impact on human health.

With armed bands in the countryside or camped nearby, people could not leave towns and cities for a place with healthier air, fewer people, and fewer rodents. They often could not even live in a city's suburbs just outside the walls. As we saw above, mercenaries burned and pillaged towns. But as the Great Companies lingered and then disintegrated back into smaller, decentralized military bands that continued to live in the area, city leaders also had to disrupt the city, especially by the construction of walls and destruction of outbuildings.

It is hard to know the impact of fire, destruction, and rebuilding city walls and infrastructure, though it likely dislocated both human and rodent populations, forcing them into closer contact. This could facilitate the spread of a disease like plague in a community that was undernourished, overpopulated, and under stress. The mercenary presence forced people to stay in close proximity to one another and to the rodent and flea populations most often seen as the main vectors for *Yersinia pestis* and other wartime infectious diseases.[94] At the same time, food pressures also caused rodents to compete more heavily with the human populations in towns, increasing contact with fleas and flea-borne illnesses. And while we think of the black rat and the *Xenopsylla cheopis* flea as the vectors of plague, they were not the only ones. Nearly all mammals are susceptible to *Yersina pestis*, and over eighty species of flea can spread the bacteria.[95]

Disruption of food production and crop cycles; limited food storage options; increased population in cities and towns; the physical and psychological pressures of siege warfare; theft of livestock; capture, rape, and ransom—witnesses in Delphine's inquest faced all of these and more in 1361. While these pressures appeared only in glimpses in witness testimony, they lay behind every story that every witness told. In the late spring and summer of 1363 as witnesses testified, they were still navigating the long-term effects of occupation by the Great Companies. Nowhere was this clearer than in stories of plague and fever.

Plague and Fever in 1361 and Beyond

At least sixteen witnesses testified to plague and fever that they experienced or saw between Delphine's vigil in December 1360 and her inquest in the summer of 1363. These illnesses affected a diverse group of men, women, and especially children of various social statuses. In their stories we see the two trends of transformation and women's protection.

Delphine's witnesses, when discussing healing during the second wave of plague, considered this a sickness with causes and treatments.[96] When witnesses contracted the illness, they turned to doctors and medical procedures first. When they could not get effective medical treatment, then they turned to their holy woman for miraculous care.[97] Asking for a miracle was not the same as asking for medicine, however. One had to be worthy of a miracle. Transformation was an important part of miraculous healing and could take diverse forms. As we saw with the mercenary Durand Arnau de Rupa Ayneria, who converted his whole heart to the love of Delphine before being thrown into the well, a person who wanted a miracle had to transform his or her interior self in order to be worthy of it. Or, in the case of sudden illness or danger, a supplicant had to hope that they already were worthy.

Transformation of one's interior self appears clearly in the testimony of Master Laurens of Florence. Master Laurens was a legal professional in the royal court in Aix. In response to Article 1, he described his experience of plague.[98] In the month of May or June, when the great mortality thrived in Aix (earlier than Guy de Chauliac claimed), Laurens experienced a severe fever, called in the common tongue *lo cat*.[99] He knew that anyone suffering this fever died because no remedy healed the illness. When he first sensed the illness in himself, however, Laurens searched for remedies (*remedia sanitatis*) anyway. A woman in his neighborhood suggested that he make a vow to Countess Delphine because Delphine had made many miracles. Laurens may also have heard stories of miracles occurring through Delphine, since both he and his colleague Master Guilhem Enric were at her vigil.[100] At this event, they may have heard about the miraculous cure of Lord Giraud de Simiana during the first wave of plague.

According to his testimony, Laurens acted on his neighbor's advice. Spurred by great devotion (*magna devocione compunctus*), Laurens made a vow to Countess Delphine to bring wax to her tomb if he were freed from the fever. After making the vow, Laurens was seized by sleep and slept deeply in peace throughout the night. The next morning when he woke, the fever and illness were completely gone.

Laurens ultimately received a miracle through the experience of compunction of great devotion to Delphine. This phrase, especially the concept of compunction, would have had a strong resonance with the papal commissioners and pious Christians at the time. The experience of compunction was usually one found in people preparing for confession, as we will see in chapter 5. Compunction—an internal drive often described as a spur—was part of an ideal confession, since it showed that a person confessed not out of fear or duty, but out of desire to repair one's relationship to God. For Laurens, part of achieving a miracle was experiencing great devotion toward Delphine, and through her, for God. His description of his internal change fit the way people spoke of transforming their internal selves to heal their souls. The compunction of great devotion made a healing miracle through Delphine's intercession possible.

This miracle helps us understand how witnesses conceived of illness, health, medicine, and healing. For Christians in the fourteenth century, medicine and miracle were not strictly separate healing methods. We see this in the details of Master Laurens's experience, particularly the deep sleep. Sleep was a familiar part of any healing regimen for people in the fourteenth century and had clear medical overtones. Sleep was one of the six nonnaturals known and manipulated by any doctor and familiar to many educated individuals through regimens of health.[101] As we saw in chapter 2, the nonnaturals were not "natural" to the body in the way that blood, organs, or limbs were natural. But they were necessary for the body to survive and be healthy. The nonnaturals included air and breathing, food and drink, sleep and waking, motion and rest, excretion and repletion, and the passions or accidents of the soul. Regimens of health had become increasingly popular texts for lay people over the course of the fourteenth century. While these regimens considered a healthy person one who experienced a balance of humors, the regimens were not profound theoretical texts. They focused on basic explanations of ways to manipulate one's health through the six nonnaturals. Regimens like that for the king of Aragon, which was copied in various regions of Mediterranean Europe, recommended diet, exercise, and daily habits for improved health.[102] The deep sleep that Laurens experienced was an increasingly familiar way that healing practitioners manipulated the body to restore its balance. Master Laurens's experience of transforming himself through great devotion and experiencing a miraculous healing through deep sleep fit well with ideas about healing at the time.

Master Laurens's healing from plague was not the only one that included internal transformation. Article 77 described the experience of Raymon of

Ansouis, a twenty-eight-year-old priest living in Marseille in the parish church of St. Martin. Raymon was gravely ill of fever and tumor in early June 1361.[103] Raymon said that, when the people serving him despaired of his life and he sensed a weakening (*defectum nature*) that seemed to him the approach of death, he imagined (*habuit imaginacionem*) that he saw before him two ladies, one of whom seemed to be Delphine. After this imagining, he converted his heart to the sanctity and merits of Delphine with the greatest devotion that he could. "He invoked her with his whole affect and his whole heart and mind."[104] He could not speak, but instead begged in his mind that Delphine intercede for him with God, and he vowed to visit her tomb with an image of wax if he survived.

Having made the vow in his mind and emitted it through his heart, he immediately sensed himself somewhat better. After five days he was free of the fever, and after fifteen days he was fully free of the tumor and the illness and could walk. Although no one heard his vow, several people, including Bishop Elzear of Ansouis and Lord Raymon Laugier, who was vicar of the church of St. Martin in Marseille, saw his miraculous recovery.[105]

Raymon's description of his transformation reflects his education as a priest, but also perhaps some medical knowledge. Raymon described the experience of his vision of Delphine as "having an imagination" (*habuit ymaginacionem*). This was an interesting choice of words, particularly in light of his emphasis on emotion, heart, and mind throughout his testimony.[106] He did not say he saw Delphine in a dream, but that he had an *imaginatio* when he was awake and sensed himself drawing near death. For the educated in the fourteenth century, the imagination could refer to the "image-making power" of the brain that could produce phantasms—the embodiment of the thing imagined.[107] He did not physically see Delphine and another woman, but he had their image in his mind.

In his testimony, Raymon then reacted to his *imaginatio* by devoting all of his affect, heart, and mind to Delphine. In this way he suggests the idea that *imaginatio*, like memory, was an affection or motion of the soul. His testimony conflates two ideas about *imaginatio*, as a thing like a *phantasia* and a power of the mind that involves the soul.[108] His healing *phantasia* of Delphine, therefore, involved his body in a transformative process of mind and soul.

The *imaginatio* was an important element in medical regimens written specifically for plague, which Raymon may have known.[109] As we saw in chapter 2, in the first wave of plague in 1348, the physician Jacme d'Agramont wrote a plague regimen for the city of Lerida and helped disseminate it before the plague arrived. D'Agramont spent as much time on the moral workings of epidemic as the physical. For him, the dangers of *imaginatio* were part of the epidemic illness.[110] His regimen urged sufferers to avoid excessive fear and sorrow during an epidemic because of their impact on the *imaginatio*. He urged people to avoid despair and suggested that cities and churches avoid ringing death bells to help people maintain hope.[111]

Jacme d'Agramont emphasized that the sufferer's *imaginatio* directly influenced his or her health.[112] Witnesses' experiences supported his statement, particularly the emphasis on spiritual transformation and seeking consolation. Through testimonies like theirs, we see from the sufferers' point of view how they sought out and implemented changes in their thoughts and emotional states in order to return to health. Raymon's testimony shows that by the second wave in 1361, not only could *imaginatio* cause the illness from which everyone died, but *imaginatio* in the form of a saint, could also heal it by helping someone like Raymon the priest use the moment to completely devote himself to Delphine.

His was not a simple vow, an exchange of wax for healing. This was a bodily process of devotion—a vow made mentally and heartfully (*mentaliter et cordialiter emisso*).[113] Mind and heart proved instrumental tools with power over flesh and illness.[114] He transformed his internal self to save his physical body. This healing method was an extension of Delphine's well-known ability to transform the hearts of those around her. Raymon's encounter with the *imaginatio* of Delphine gave him the inspiration and ability to devote his heart and mind to Delphine and thereby find healing of this illness.

Another testimony reveals that transforming one's self in order to be worthy of a miracle could also heal others. Lady Monna de Mauriaco and her husband, Lord Rigo, both testified to the miraculous healing of their son, Anthonet, in August 1361. At the time of the inquest, Lord Rigo had the title *miles* and was a papal representative.[115] They rank among the highest status witnesses in the inquest. They were both invited to testify directly by the papal commissioners rather than by the proctor, Master Nicolau Laurens.

According to Article 74, Anthonet developed a continual fever, buboes, and another type of swelling above the buboes.[116] According to his mother, he was sick for seven days, during which time he did not eat and drank only a little milk. After seven days, his bones had begun to show through his skin, and he was showing several signs of death, including loss of speech and vision.[117] Lady Monna, believing her son was dead, felt great sadness.

With the affect of her whole heart, she transformed her heart to the merits of Lady Delphine and made a rather elaborate vow. Like many others who made vows, Lady Monna promised to walk barefoot to Delphine's tomb and bring a wax image of her son. But then she offered more. She promised that for the rest of her life she would show her reverence to God and Lady Delphine by saying the Pater Noster and the Ave Maria seven times daily. She would also visit Delphine's tomb on a different day with bread and wine. She would feed everyone at the tomb, but she herself would fast. She would also fast for the journey to and from Delphine's tomb. After making her vow, her son was healed.[118]

In this miracle story we see the trends that weave through the many testimonies to illness and mercenary attack in 1361. Lady Monna experienced two different types of transformation. She transformed her heart, as we saw both Master Laurens and Raymon the priest do, but she also transformed her behavior, becoming a more pious person. Unlike other witnesses, however, she also vowed to imitate Delphine if she received this miracle. She vowed to pray each day, to give food to others, and to fast. At the same time, Lady Monna was also protecting her family. She was not praying for her own health, but for her son's. Her husband, Lord Rigo, recognized this by attesting to her vow and agreeing that this was a miraculous healing.[119] His wife had saved his son and heir by praying for Delphine's intercessory aid.

Other witness testimonies to plague in 1361 show how women could work together to organize and provide health care. The testimony of Alazays Mesellano helps us see the many ways that women could manage health care for themselves and their family members. Alazays was not a member of the aristocracy of Provence. She was a fifty-year-old widow of a cloth merchant. But from her lengthy testimony we see that she was a wealthy, well-traveled woman who considered herself to have a close relationship to Countess Delphine. While we do not know how Delphine understood their relationship, Alazays Mesellano felt that she could visit with and speak to Delphine. For example, Alazays described how she had chatted with Delphine as they walked to mass. Countess Delphine was not a distant saint for Alazays, but someone she could turn to for help when crisis struck in the form of plague in 1361. Through Alazays Mesellano's testimony, we see several sources of healing that she turned to during the second wave of plague. We also see her actively pursuing health care for her family and herself.

In her response to Article 1, Alazays indicated that in July 1361 her two-year-old granddaughter Dalphineta (namesake and goddaughter of Delphine) suffered from a continual fever and had a tumor. Alazays specified that at that time all who had such a tumor were considered dead. A Jewish doctor in Apt, Master Unias, who had been called in to treat Dalphineta, had in fact declared her dead.[120]

In the middle of the night, Alazays's daughter Catherina, who was a nun at the Holy Cross convent, brought some of Delphine's hair to Alazays's home, where Dalphineta's mother and Alazays were caring for the girl. Around the time of vespers, Catherina wrapped the hair in fine cloth and tied it to Dalphineta's arm. After five days, Dalphineta was totally cured of the fever and tumor, neither of which returned.[121]

In this miracle, Dalphineta's grandmother, mother, aunt, and godmother come together to save her from the epidemic illness. Alazays presented herself as leading these efforts by caring for the girl in her home and calling in a doctor. Catherina, Dalphineta's aunt, also shares the healing authority by bringing a relic of Delphine, preparing it, and administering it to the dying girl. The women circumvent human authority and limitations by turning to Delphine, whom they had interacted with through the Holy Cross convent. Delphine, the girl's godmother, ultimately saved her through miraculous intercession.[122]

After describing the survival of her granddaughter, Alazays described her own near-death experience during the 1361 epidemic. She also suffered the fever and tumor from which all died. The doctors did not believe she would survive, and she received extreme unction. But she did not have a good memory at that time, and, because of the fever, she spoke as if mad. Nuns took her in, and though she did not specify, it was likely the nuns of the Holy Cross convent.[123]

At this point, Alazays "hastened to Delphine, who had cared for her, so that she could petition God on Alazays's behalf."[124] Alazays made a vow, including an offering of wax, after which she began to speak intelligibly and recover from the fever. After eight days, the fever was gone, and she did not experience the crisis or usual end of this illness. In this miracle, as in the miraculous healing of her granddaughter, Alazays turned to Delphine only after trying to find an earthly remedy for her illness. After exhausting other alternatives, she turned to Delphine for divine intercession.

Alazays's near-death experience was made even more dangerous by her inability to speak rationally. This would have hindered dictating a will and would have kept her from making a general confession, which was part of extreme unction by the fourteenth century. At this moment, Alazays's body and soul were in danger. The first impact of the vow was regaining her ability to speak, which would have allowed her to confess. Even if she had not survived the illness, her soul would have been healthy at death.

The Holy Cross convent served as a place of healing women during the second wave of plague that moved through Provence in 1361. Several nuns had been close associates of Delphine and held relics such as her veil and strands of her hair. The convent remained a place that those who had been close to the deceased holy countess could turn for help. Alazays Mesellano, a woman who fully believed in visiting doctors when sick, also found healing at the Holy Cross convent.

If we look at testimonies about illness after 1361, acute illnesses stand out. Seventeen witness described their own and others' illnesses occurring from 1362 through the spring of 1363 and the opening of Delphine's inquest. All but four of the illnesses they described were acute illnesses including fever, stomach flux, aborting a fetus, and swelling.

Lady Andrea Raymon's testimony helps us see one of those miracles, but also how people wove stories about Delphine's aid into the larger stories of plague and war. Lady Andrea described a case of continual fever in the spring of 1363. In this miracle, Lord Peire Alexi, the prior of the church of St. Peter in Ansouis, had a vision of Lady Delphine. During a profound sleep, Lord Peire saw Delphine with a large retinue in a chapel of St. Peter's church, where, as he explained, many masses had been celebrated. Delphine and her retinue wore beautiful clothing, and a great light illuminated them. Shortly after this vision, Lord Peire's brother, Guilhem, fell ill with a continual fever. There was no hope that he would survive. So Lord Peire, with the greatest devotion, transformed his whole heart to the merits of Delphine and begged her to intercede with God on his brother's behalf. His brother, who was near death, became healthy again.[125]

In her testimony, Lady Andrea supported Lord Peire's testimony. She too had seen Guilhem so ill that no one believed that he could escape death. She had also seen Guilhem after his brother had made the vow and he had been miraculously healed.[126]

Her testimony wove these more recent eruptions of fever into the earlier moments of danger in Delphine's inquest. It is helpful here to think about who Lady Andrea was and the links she had to the Provençal community. Although Lady Andrea's husband was not *domicellus* during the events of 1358, including the miraculous protection of Ansouis from mercenary capture and the transformation of the mercenary thrown in the well, he had publicized those events. As we saw in chapter 3, when witnesses told papal commissioners where they heard about those miracles, they mentioned Lord Johan Raymon. Lady Andrea's husband shared stories about Delphine's protection of his town, showing how this Provençal woman had never abandoned her community, but instead protected it against many dangers.

Lady Andrea's testimony to her miraculous protection through prayers to Delphine continued the story of Delphine's protection of the people of Ansouis beyond that city's walls. It also wove Lady Andrea and her husband into the narrative of earlier, more famous events. Finally, her testimony to the miraculous healing of the brother of the prior of St. Peter's church wove this physical space into a story of healing after mercenary invasion. As we saw in chapter 3, St. Peter's church had been captured by mercenaries in 1358 and used as a base of ambush. At least one holy man was gravely injured there. The vision of Countess Delphine in St. Peter's church, illuminated with celestial light, healed not just one man from fever, but the institution from its grim association with violent invasion.

The Repercussions of Mercenary Occupation beyond 1361

For modern audiences, the testimonies describing miraculous healing of plague can seem separate from the stories of mercenary attack. But for witnesses they were deeply linked. The year 1361 was a devastating one for the people of Provence. The ratification of the Treaty of Bretigny in 1360 unexpectedly transformed life at the mouth of the Rhône River for years. Mercenaries and disease followed the Rhône south to a region little prepared for either. This moment was less about their political relationship with Queen Johanna and King Louis and more about the ramifications of large-scale warfare in the fourteenth century. Life was changing for everyone in Europe as mercenaries became the primary soldiers that all leaders relied on.

The impact of the Great Companies did not end in 1361, however. The disruption of crop cycles, planting, food production and transportation, along with the stresses of living with the threat of constant attack, appeared in other ways in the inquest. We get some indication of the overall impact of the Great Companies and the subsequent plague from an economic inquiry conducted by Bishop Philippe Cabassole in 1363. This witness in Delphine's inquest also served Pope Urban V as the rector of the Comtat Venaissin.[127] In an attempt to recoup the money spent to pay the mercenaries to leave, the pope levied a special tax on the Comtat Venaissin. When representatives of the region begged to postpone the tax, however, Cabassole's inquiry discovered that the damage had been so significant to crops, farmland, orchards, vineyards, and livestock that the people could not pay the new tax and could only pay a reduced amount of their previous taxes.[128]

Even though witnesses in Delphine's inquest had not had much time to share their stories of protection and healing in 1361 before they testified in 1363, their stories reflected a swiftly changing world. The new epidemic illness had gone from a watershed event that other sources described as a punishment from God to an illness interpretable by physicians, if not yet treatable. Warfare had changed from quasi-civil war among local lords to an overwhelming wave of mercenaries. Witnesses' stories of attack, protection, and peace had transformed in response.

CHAPTER 5

Master Durand Andree and the Sacrament of Penance as a Moment of Danger

I have allowed moments of danger to emerge organically from witness testimony. Rather than impose my sense of what the dangerous moments were, I have searched for moments when five or more witnesses described a specific time or event when they were in danger. It is easy to see how mercenary attacks and waves of plague are dangerous moments. But using these criteria, one of the most dangerous moments Delphine's witnesses faced was the sacrament of penance. Over half of the sixty-eight witnesses mentioned some element of the sacrament in their testimonies. At least eight witnesses described difficulties with a specific confession they made. While they would all have encountered this "moment of danger" at different times chronologically, as pious Christians they all encountered it. And if their testimonies are any indication, the sacrament was a moment when they believed that things could go terribly wrong.[1]

When modern audiences consider the changes in the sacrament of penance in the fourteenth and fifteenth centuries, we can be swayed by the extremes presented in the writings of reformers of the Catholic Church. Corrupt clergy—ignorant of theology, lax in their duties, and charging to perform the sacraments—held sway over a vulnerable laity. Or we have penitential literature and sermon collections produced for the clergy, which can present an equally one-sided picture of a corrupt, resistant laity.[2]

Delphine's witnesses give us a different view. How they spoke about their experiences reveals the stresses of the sacrament of penance on pious people who had access to trained confessors, or might even be confessors themselves. Their testimonies show that it was difficult for them to understand the proliferation of sins and the role of penitential acts in forgiveness. And it could be difficult to achieve the physical requirements of the sacrament when sick, perhaps dying.

But how witnesses spoke—the stories they told about this sacrament—also reveal what they expected from this sacrament and often did not get. They did not feel reassured about their souls by the sacrament, though they seem to have expected to feel that way. Long before the Protestant Reformation, these pious Christians understood that the sacrament of penance could unsettle more than console.[3]

The demands of the sacrament of penance, combined with the heightened physical and spiritual dangers between 1343 and 1363, made the moment of confession a difficult one for witnesses in Delphine's inquest. Witness testimonies give an intriguing perspective on distress that pious people felt in a time of crisis. Queen Johanna's tumultuous early reign, the mercenary invasions, and the waves of plague were not only physical threats. They were also spiritual threats. As we have seen, Delphine's witnesses understood violence as a spiritual sickness for everyone involved, aggressors and defenders alike. It was also a potential source of God's wrath, which according to people like Louis Heyligen, friend of Bishop Philippe Cabassole, may have caused God to punish people in the form of plague. The spiritual as well as the physical dangers had to be addressed.[4]

The heightened physical danger during this time increased the number of confessions. One of Delphine's confessors, Friar Bertran Jusbert, recalled that Delphine made a full confession to him in 1348. This was the moment he learned many things about her life, because she tried to remember all the sins she had ever committed.[5] Delphine would not have been the only person repairing her soul during a time of epidemic. Although we have little way of knowing the exact number of confessions made, we do have surviving testaments, of which confession was often a part. Louis Stouff estimates the number of surviving testaments in Provence from the mid-fourteenth to the mid-fifteenth century at thirty-five thousand to forty thousand. He indicates that many of these were made just before and just after waves of plague or at times of increased warfare.[6] While the sacrament of penance protected the living soul, testaments protected the soul after death. The person making the will allocated resources for prayers, alms, and works of mercy to aid their soul's journey to purgatory, or perhaps heaven.[7]

One witness, Master Durand Andree, is a helpful guide through issues of penance. Master Durand was a cathedral canon in Apt, one of Delphine's confessors, and a medical doctor who treated Delphine, her ladies, and other members of the Apt community.[8] All three roles would give him different perspectives on the sacrament of penance in fourteenth-century Provence. As a cathedral canon who helped in the administration and running of the bishop of Apt's cathedral, Master Durand knew the needs of the religious and lay communities in the town. As Delphine's confessor—and perhaps a confessor for others, though he does not say—he helped people understand the sacrament and heard the confessions they made. As a medical doctor, especially one trained as a confessor, he had a special awareness of the impact that confession and penance could have on health. Finally, another identity emerges through Master Durand's testimony. Like all other Christians, he too had to confess his sins. Just like everyone else, he was a confessee, a penitent. He experienced and spoke about both sides of the confession experience in his testimony.

Master Durand also provides the perspective of a politically connected person in Provence. He was part of Delphine's entourage in Apt between 1350 and 1360. This brought him into contact with many politically connected women and their families. For example, a surviving notarial register shows him interacting with Abbess Ayselena and the nuns of the Holy Cross convent in Apt.[9] In his testimony he mentioned hearing stories from and telling stories to members of the Catholic hierarchy from Avignon and other cities. And he also interacted with the papal court in Avignon. He and Master Nicolau Laurens traveled to Avignon and met with Bishop Anglic Grimaud, Pope Urban V's brother, in support of Delphine's inquest.[10] He was not as politically and socially well connected as Bishop Philippe Cabassole, but his sphere of knowledge and influence was broader than Apt.

Master Durand's testimony reflects the spiritual needs and expectations of the aristocracy of Provence and the Catholic ideals of the sacrament of penance. His testimony provides multiple vantage points to help modern audiences understand the difficulties inherent in the sacrament of penance, especially making a confession, but also doing penance. The difficulties that this group of relatively wealthy, educated, and politically connected witnesses faced made it a moment of danger, especially when they thought the confession might be their last.

Difficulties in Making the Ideal Confession

The Fourth Lateran Council decree in 1215 required Catholic Christians to confess their sins at least once a year. By the fourteenth century, there are many indications that Christians did so, often during Lent, but many confessed more frequently.[11] Confession was part of the pious person's life and offered significant benefits for the health of the immortal soul.[12] There was an increasing understanding among pious Christians, however, that a person had to confess correctly. Christians received guidance about sin, confession, and penance in a variety of ways, especially sermons.[13]

Ideally, at each confession the penitent made a complete or perfect confession, which required three main elements. First, inspired by compunction, penitents should desire to confess. Compunction was an internal desire rather than a sense of duty or fear. Second, confession required penitents to feel real and appropriate sorrow for their sins and to speak all of their sins aloud to a priest. And finally, confession required penitents to intend not to sin this way again.[14] The lack of any of these elements could make confession impossible or unsuccessful.

These three requirements reveal the physical labor and internal investigation involved in making a perfect confession. This was not a simple process. Physically, every penitent needed to have the ability to speak clearly and coherently. Internally, penitents needed to know what was sinful behavior, remember their life events, desire to confess, feel real sorrow about their sins, and intend to change their behavior. This sacrament was a complex physical and spiritual task.

We see elements of the perfect confession in the testimony of Master Durand Andree.[15] In his testimony to Article 35, Master Durand said that while Delphine was speaking healing words (*verba salutis*), he and several other men, including the priest Gaspert of Capite Pini and Lord Guilhem of Gordes, who was the commander of Carpentras, were moved in their hearts: "They were changed to penitence, contrition, compunction, and effusive tears. And they began suffering for their offenses to God. All the sins of their lives were restored to their memories, as if they had all been written, and they felt a great desire to confess."[16]

Master Durand and these men experienced the appropriate internal state for a successful confession, nicely articulated by someone usually hearing the confessions of others. They changed on the inside by feeling penitence, contrition, and compunction.[17] Their appropriate sorrow showed on the outside through their spiritually cleansing tears.[18] They remembered all of their sins as if they were written, which would have allowed them to state their sins aloud to a confessor. They suffered for their offenses and desired to confess. Their compunction and sorrow suggest their desire to not commit the same sins again.

The wondrous power of Delphine's voice helped them in this difficult sacrament. Just because the sacrament was difficult, however, does not mean that it was inherently dangerous. To understand this as a moment of danger, we have to think about what was at stake in this sacrament, not just for Delphine's witnesses but for all pious Christians. The short answer was eternal life or eternal damnation. The sacrament of penance was the process through which medieval Christians repaired their relationship with God. They had damaged their relationship through sinful behavior—such as the violence we saw in chapters 1 through 4—and this was the moment they regained God's love and the chance at eternal life. If they did not engage in the sacrament correctly, they risked eternal damnation. As we have seen, they took this risk seriously.

If we take each of the elements separately, we can see how each element could be difficult for people to achieve. We can also see how war and plague could introduce obstacles and make the sacrament more difficult or perhaps even impossible. Witnesses' stories show that they valued the benefits of the sacrament of penance, but did not always have the ideal experience that Master Durand Andree described.

Compunction to Confess

What is clear in Master Durand's testimony, and in much of the penitential literature, is that the sacrament of penance started before priest and penitent met. The internal state of the penitent before confession mattered, and ideally, a penitent should feel compunction. Compunction was not a gentle emotion. Theologians described it as "a puncture provoked by the thorns of sins; it was like the spur in the flank of the ox or horse in order to drive it free of the mud."[19] Witness testimony captured this intensity and the overwhelming experience of this emotion or internal state.

Bertranda Bertomieua, in her testimony to Article 39, provided an example of how people experienced compunction through the power of Delphine's voice. The events took place in the court of Naples in either 1342 or early 1343.[20] Bertranda attested to the article, but was not present at the event. She related the experiences of two ladies of Queen Sanxia's court who had described to her what they saw and felt.[21] In her testimony, Bertranda agreed with the text of the article as it was read to her. It describes a gathering led by Delphine and Queen Sanxia, which included the "noble lords and magnificent associates" of Sanxia's court.[22] At this gathering, they asked Delphine to speak of God, and she did so with such great devotion and ardor that they saw "sparks of fire emerge from her mouth."[23] The noble ladies who had gathered to pray, "having been pierced on the inside, wished to confess immediately, without any delay; and they made confession of their sins."[24]

According to Bertranda's secondhand account, hearing Delphine's words and seeing the sparkling fire inspired an irresistible desire to confess. Bertranda did not use the word *compunctio*, but the papal commissioners who questioned her and the officials reading the inquest documents likely understood the interior piercing Bertranda described as compunction. The sparkling fire, evidence of Delphine's ardor for God, spurred her audience in Naples by producing an ideal internal state for confession. Bertranda's testimony suggests that in the midst of a sinful court, compunction may have been difficult to achieve, and people needed wondrous inspiration for it.

Understanding Sin

After compunction brought penitents to confession, they had to speak their sins aloud to a priest. The encounter with the confessor required several elements, including memory, understanding sin, and speaking clearly. All three could be surprisingly difficult. For these pious witnesses, however, understanding sin could be the trickiest element. This may come as a surprise to modern audiences, since the witnesses were testifying in a canonization inquest and shared a faith in Delphine's sanctity. If anyone should understand sin, it was these pious people. But for many, their lifestyles and social roles obscured their sin from them. Some witnesses described only becoming aware of their sinful behavior when they spoke to Delphine. Her words and example gave them a new perspective, which allowed them to investigate their inner selves and their outward behavior in a different light.

This is not to say that witnesses were ignorant about sin. They did not have to be theologians, priests, or bishops to have a sense of the benefits of being a good Christian and the dangers of being a bad one.[25] The relatively wealthy, socially elite, pious people testifying about Delphine's life and miracles were the product of years of Christian education about sin and its remediation.[26] The men and women in Delphine's inquest would have been the target audience of sermons, books of hours, books of vices and virtues, poetry, and courtesy books that described dangers to the soul and how to avoid them through pious behavior and prayer.[27] People also read saints' lives for models to follow and for inspiration in difficult times.[28]

A small, beautifully illuminated fourteenth-century book of hours—identified as Delphine's and until recently held in a bank vault in the Church of St. Anne in Apt—gives us an idea about what the wealthy, pious, educated women in Delphine's inquest were reading.[29] It contains the expected prayers to Mary and a long list of saints to emulate. But the first ten folios contain prayers about avoiding worldliness (especially *gula* and *luxuria*) and seeking out the spiritual health that comes through confession. Several of the noblewomen who testified in Delphine's inquest, like Maria d'Evenos and Tiburga and Rossolina d'Agoult, would have had the status and means to own the beautiful books of hours popular in the fourteenth century.

The proliferation of books of hours shows the interest in personal care of the soul. But another text written for the laity, *The Breviary of Love*, helps us put in perspective the messages emerging from the thirteenth-century explosion of education and preaching led by the mendicant orders and spreading to every part of Europe.[30] *The Breviary of Love*, a roughly thirty-five-thousand-line poem written in Occitan, provides a representative, though also quite creative, example of the literature that both shaped and reflected lay understandings of sin, especially in fourteenth-century southern Europe. The book is particularly useful for the many miniatures it included, most of which were produced for the text. It reveals the spread of Franciscan ideas about love, the physical and spiritual works of mercy, and the importance of correct confession.[31]

The poem was written by Matfre Ermengaud, a master of civil law in Bezier. Matfre was likely influenced by Franciscan ideas during his training in law and theology at the university in Bezier.[32] His poem was meant to be informative but also entertaining for educated lay people. He consciously chose to write in the vernacular and focus on the concept of love in order to imitate troubadour poetry, which was gaining renewed popularity among the wealthy and the nobility. The poem had two parts. The first covered a range of topics, including biblical exegesis, Aristotelian understanding of plants and animals, penance, confession, and the relationship between God and man through faith. The second was a group of short poems gathered together in what Ermengaud called the "Perilhos Tractaz d'Amor"—"A Treatise on the Dangers of Love."[33]

Ermengaud's *Breviary of Love* includes common ideas of sinful behaviors and the dangers they posed. These could easily have been shared by many of Delphine's witnesses. It reflects what was written before the Black Death and the Hundred Years War and already spreading throughout the wealthy, aristocratic Mediterranean community. It is a leap, but not a large one, to imagine that the advice and images took on new resonances in the later fourteenth century, becoming behaviors people could avoid or follow in order to protect their bodies and souls during a time when threatened by larger dangers that they could not control, such as plague and mercenary violence. Delphine's witnesses may have been familiar with this text or at the very least familiar with the ideas informing it.[34]

Though meant for the laity, this text consciously drew from Gregory the Great's *Cura pastoralis*, a popular text for preachers.[35] The first part of *The Breviary of Love* highlighted the dangers of pride and the importance of humility. It also explored preaching and described how a preacher should use different emotional emphases to reach different audiences. Matfre criticized overly harsh preachers, likening their voices to those of demons.[36] This text suggests that the laity had expectations for sermons and the impact on spiritual health of the voice of a person speaking holy words.[37] These texts provide scholars with indirect evidence of what audiences, particularly in southern France and Provence, took away from confession, public sermons, or romance stories.[38]

Both the text and physical presentation of *The Breviary of Love* could inform people about their sin and reinforce moral ideas they likely already knew. The images drove home ideas concerning sin, but were also entertaining. A copy of the poem, likely produced in Toulouse in the early fourteenth century and now held by the British Library, contains images of demons engaging men and women through fighting, dancing, kissing, and admiring beautiful clothing. According to the text, these were activities that allowed demons to distance the individual soul from God. For the historian Federico Botana, the dangers of sinful love in this text emerge from lust and its pursuit. The miniature cycle depicting the dangers of love begins with two figures in bed, seen in figure 5.1, and continues through images of adorning the body, hunting, feasting, fighting, and dancing (figure 5.2). All of these were behaviors the wealthy and noble would engage in and find appropriate, even if they likely knew they were sinful. Here the language of "demonic goadings" attributed to Delphine as she warned the mercenary Durand Arnau de Rupa Ayneria appears in images. Their placement together on consecutive pages related all of the behaviors to each other for the reader.

If we consider a text like this one, in which the sinfulness of socially common and enjoyable behavior is highlighted in an entertaining way, we can see how sin might be tricky to grasp even for the pious. For example, the draper's widow Alazays Mesellano, who survived the second wave of plague through prayers to Delphine, experienced a moment of awareness of worldly sins straight from the pages of the *Breviary*. Though she remembered hearing

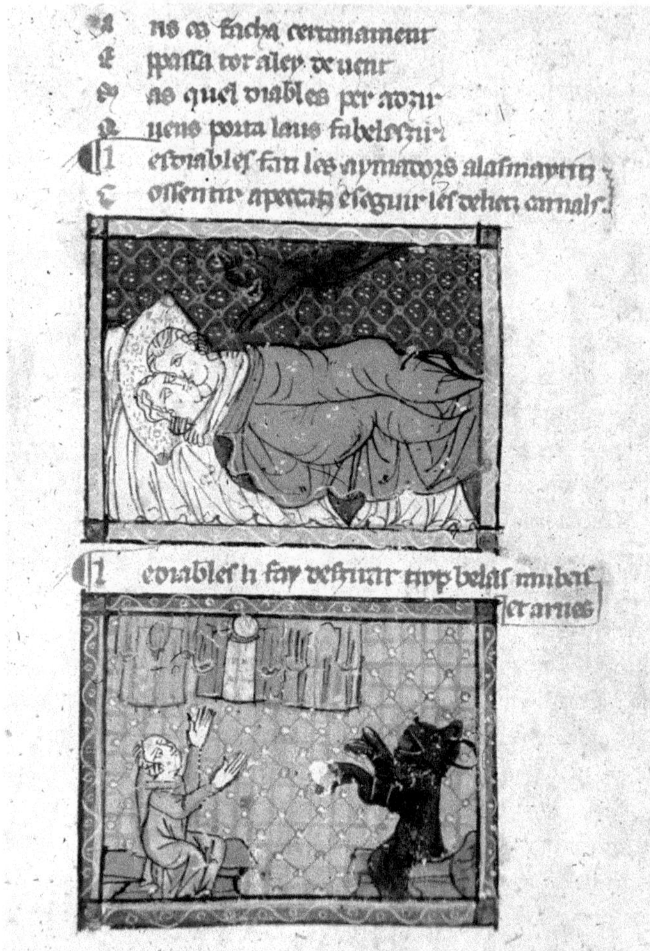

Figure 5.1. Image from *The Breviary of Love* by Matfre Ermengaud. © The British Library Board, MS Royal 19 C1 203v–204v.

Delphine speak in many places and as early as 1343, she recalled becoming aware of sinful behavior in reference to a specific day—the vigil of Saint Francis. While she walked with Delphine to the church of the Friars Minor in Apt, Delphine said many good words about God, contempt of the world, that all things would come to an end, and many other good words and good examples. On account of this, Alazays was much consoled in her soul (*fuit in animo suo consolata multum*), and it seemed to her that Delphine touched all internal things of her conscience. And suddenly she renounced the pretty gilded ornaments and other things she wore, such as tiaras with pearls and precious stones and expensive luxurious clothes. "From then on she wore

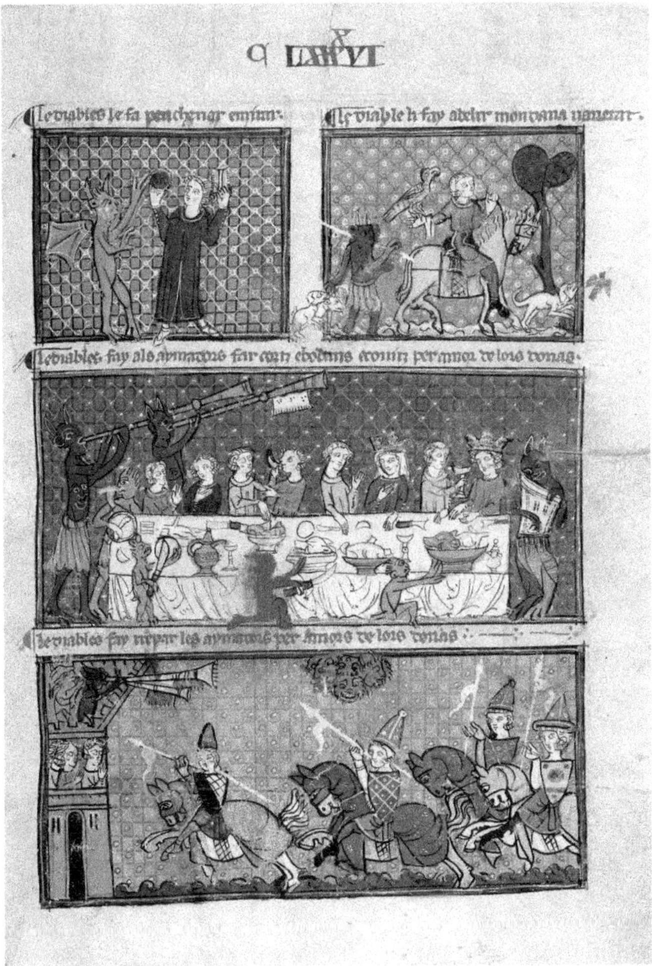

Figure 5.2. Image from *The Breviary of Love* by Matfre Ermengaud. © The British Library Board, MS Royal 19 C1 203v–204v.

humble clothes and changed her life for the better. And through the inducement of Delphine, Alazays made a general confession of all her sins many times."[39] While Alazays might have felt that tiaras and expensive clothes were appropriate to wear to the vigil of an important saint, Delphine's words helped her understand their sinfulness.

The final image of the miniature cycle of the dangers of love makes clear the results of engaging in sinful behavior. In figure 5.3, a demon carries off the soul of the sinner at death. The familial concern for the soul at death that we see in this image appeared in Delphine's inquest as well. As we saw in chapter 2,

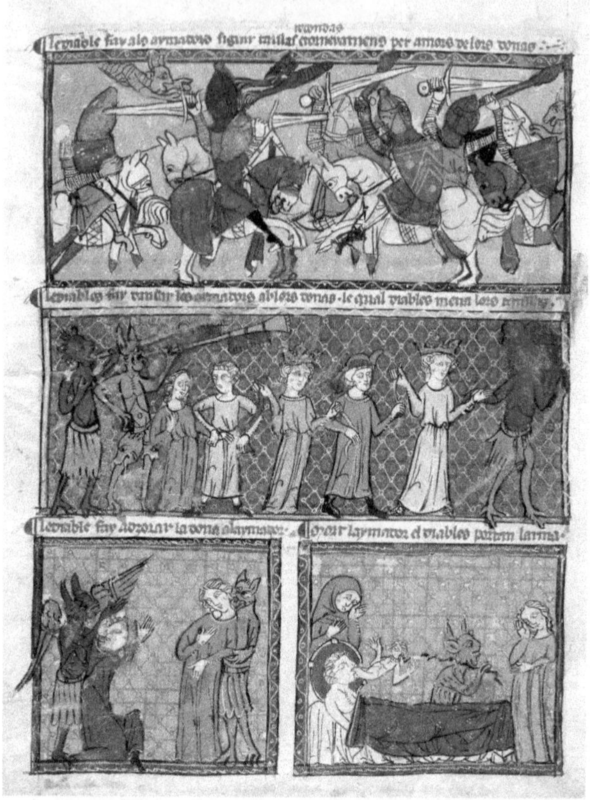

Figure 5.3. Image from *The Breviary of Love* by Matfre Ermengaud.
© The British Library Board, MS Royal 19 C1 203v–204v.

Lord Raymon d'Agoult's daughters, Tiburga and Rossolina, asked Delphine about the state of their father's soul at his death. Delphine consoled them by saying that this dire fate—a demon carrying off the departing soul—had not happened to him.

The beautifully illuminated book itself can reveal the difficulty of being aware of sin. Owning a book like this, or like Delphine's book of hours for that matter, might indicate the readers' interest in spiritual health and paths to it.[40] But this book was also a luxury item that displayed an individual's wealth even as it described sinful behavior. The dangers of pleasurable activities and beautiful objects were being reinforced through the lavishly illuminated pages of an expensive book. A list of goods provided by Abbess Ayselena d'Apt shows how nuns listening to Delphine's words became aware of their luxury and sold their beautiful spiritual objects in order to give the money away as alms. According to Ayselena, she and the nuns of the Holy Cross convent "renounced excessively elaborate and expensive clothing, rings, silver cups and spoons, an Agnus Dei of silver, and many other pleasures which they had. They sold [these things] and gave the money to the poor."[41] For late medieval preachers, one of the main dangers of vanity, especially in the form of extravagant ornament, was that it kept money from the poor. Whether consciously or not, these women addressed sermon writers' criticism of vanity by selling their goods and giving the money as alms.[42]

Objects and clothing, even ones for a spiritual purpose like an Agnus Dei, are easy to understand as potentially sinful. But a brief story told by Catherine Giraud, the sixty-year-old abbess of St. Catherine's convent, gives insight into how witnesses' daily lives and social roles might make it difficult to identify sinful behavior and change it. Abbess Catherine remembered hearing Delphine speak first in 1336 in Apt and many times afterward in St. Catherine's convent. Delphine's words caused her to reconsider her own piety.

Abbess Catherine stated that she once heard the lady Delphine say that "when God made grace and consolation for someone in confession, that person ought to attribute all to God and humble herself. From these words, Catherine carefully assessed that lady Delphine touched the interior of her heart, because whenever she had been occupied with prayer and prayed with devotion, she had given herself over to vainglory and attributed to herself all and attributed nothing to God with humility, from whom all proceeded. And on account of Delphine's words from then on, however much grace God gave her, she corrected herself from the previous vainglory and attributed that grace to God."[43]

This behavior was not an obvious sin, like wearing a pearl tiara, but it was still a version of the sin of pride. Avoiding pride in one's own piety was a common message for clergy in the thirteenth and fourteenth centuries and one that Delphine, her inquest organizers, and witnesses like Catherine addressed.[44] After considering Delphine's words about God's grace, Abbess Catherine understood true humility. In other words, she understood that she was sinning every time she confessed. Delphine's words allowed her to correct the way she thought about prayer and humility and therefore confess effectively. Abbess Catherine's experience of pride in her own humility reveals that sin was not always the direct experience that the pictures in *The Breviary of Love* show. Many of Delphine's witnesses were aware of the obvious sins and avoided them. But the non-obvious sins, especially involving one's internal state rather than outward behavior, could be just as dangerous.

A final example shows how even trying to do a pious act could damage the soul. Master Durand remembered a moment in 1355 when Lord Raymon d'Agoult and his entourage wished to see Delphine and speak to her in Apt.

When they announced their intention, Delphine replied, "O what false and perverse sights that do not lead the soul, except to harmful worldly honors, fame, and favor!"[45] She said that she would become ill if they visited her.[46]

On the surface, Lord Raymon's desire to visit does not seem problematic. Delphine was a holy person through whom he had found spiritual aid in his dispute with Lord Uguo de Baux. Delphine's refusal shows the worldly nature of such visits, however. Lord Raymon's very public intention to see and speak to her *because* she was a holy woman undermined their humility. For Delphine, if she had accepted the visit (and therefore in essence accepted a reward for her holiness in the shape of public honor), it would have damaged the health of her soul. Lord Raymon, by seeking the public honor of meeting with a holy person, risked damaging his soul.

The way Delphine, Master Durand, and Lord Guido de Cavaillon, a member of Lord Raymon's entourage, navigated this event shows that they understood the danger of worldly fame and favor. Master Durand and Lord Guido met with Delphine to see if she would change her mind. In response, Delphine set conditions for a visit. She only agreed to see Lord Raymon, or members of his entourage, if they truly wished to speak to her about things that "touched the health of their souls" and if they came in secret and in small numbers.[47] Otherwise, they would find no cure (*aliter non curaret*) for the illnesses (*discrasiata*) that weighed them down.[48] According to Master Durand, Delphine's statement to Lord Raymon made him and many others aware of behavior that they did not before perceive as sinful and thereby brought them joy and health. It was not sinful to visit a holy woman, but it was vainglorious to do so publicly with an entourage. This small story shows how complex sinfulness, and therefore confession and caring for the health of one's soul, could be. It was difficult to understand sin.

Remembering One's Sins

The soul risked damnation even for sins a person did not remember, since this constituted an incomplete or imperfect confession. As historian Thomas Tentler states, "To exaggerate the importance of completeness seems hardly possible. It was and has remained indispensable to forgiveness in the Roman Catholic Sacrament of Penance."[49] Confessors' manuals discussed the problem of faulty memory and confession.[50] One popular manual that would have been available in Provence in the mid-fourteenth century is the *Manipulus curatorum* by Guido of Monte Rochen. This text reflects a collection of common advice for those engaged in pastoral care and can serve the modern reader as a representative example of confessors' manuals.[51] In this text, forgetting sins appears in several sections.

The author of the *Manipulus curatorum* considered honest forgetfulness of mortal and venial sins as less damaging than conscious secrecy or refusal to confess. Honest forgetfulness did not necessarily damn the individual, but to avoid damnation, the author urged a certain internal state. "A person ought to believe that he has probably offended God in many ways that he does not remember, and so under this estimation, let him sorrow and repent as if he were certain."[52] In other words, a person should live in a state of constant contrition and penitence. People, especially priests, should also make a general confession of sins in the assumption that forgotten sins exist.[53]

The language of Master Durand Andree's ideal experience of confession resonates in light of this advice. It highlights what penitents and their confessors feared and what they hoped would happen. They feared depending on a possibly faulty memory and thereby making an imperfect confession and risking damnation. They also seemed uncomfortable with feeling perpetually contrite and penitent. Instead Master Durand and the men with him heard Delphine's voice and remembered all of their sins as if they were written. They did not risk damnation or experience the perpetual uncertainty described in the *Manipulus curatorum*. They knew their sins and, therefore, knew they had confessed them.

Speaking Sins Aloud

Once penitents understood and remembered their sin, they had to speak their sins aloud to a priest. In the *Manipulus curatorum*, this was where forgiveness happened, since priests had the ability to absolve sin.[54] Handbooks of behavior written for an aristocratic audience, like those derived from *Le somme le roi*, included detailed information about how one behaved in confession.[55] This included considerations even of small details such as where to sit with the confessor in the church (the confessional booth did not exist in the fourteenth century), where to keep one's gaze as one confessed, and the words to use to indicate one's sorrow at offending God.

Speaking sins aloud in the fourteenth century was a dialogue between penitent and confessor. The confessor asked questions about categories of sin based on the seven deadly sins. Those questions could be about sinful behavior or thought.[56] The penitent answered those questions and asked for God's mercy.

This physical element of confession could also introduce dangers. We saw this in the experience of Alazays Mesellano, the wealthy draper's widow, who contracted plague in 1361. The fever she experienced made her "speak as if mad," which meant she could not make the necessary confession that was part of extreme unction. A person who could not speak coherently could not confess and risked dying with unconfessed sins. Alazays, therefore, faced not just death, but also damnation. As a pious Christian, she would have been very aware of both dangers. In her testimony, she described this miracle that she received through God's grace channeled through the merits of Delphine as saving both her body and soul.

Even when not on one's potential deathbed, speaking one's sins aloud could be difficult. When questioning the fifty-year-old Lady Rossolina d'Agoult, the noble widow of Uguo of Garda, about her testimony to Article 35, the commissioners asked her "in what way she sensed in her heart that lady Delphine knew her interior conscience."[57] Rossolina tried to capture the experience by describing a particular day before the feast of Palm Sunday in 1360. "She had been waiting for a confessor and was anxious in her mind about a certain sin that she wished to confess. Delphine was there with her, but on account of Rossolina's anxiety, she did not pay attention to Delphine's words."[58] Delphine, however, knew how much Rossolina was disturbed even though Rossolina had not understood what Delphine said and had said nothing to Delphine.

The interaction between Rossolina and Delphine was not particularly wondrous or miraculous, but it does reveal the anxiety that this demanding sacrament could cause. Speaking one's sins aloud to a confessor required preparation and the courage to undertake a difficult task.[59]

Master Durand Andree's testimony shows how the confessor's dialogue with a person confessing could be difficult for the confessor as well. As one of Delphine's confessors, he struggled with the holy woman's sense of her own sinfulness. As he stated, her confession of sins often became a statement of virtues. Listening to her state what she considered her offenses to God seemed to him "as if he were collecting a handful of diverse flowers."[60] But according to his testimony, she did not see her actions as virtuous. She thought of herself as a sinful person, and therefore did not feel that her confessors were being rigorous enough. Master Durand remembered a specific confession event when Delphine rebuked him, saying, "What kind of confessor are you, who does not hold me accountable for my sins, which I confess to you!"[61] After saying this, she began to confess a series of sins. As he listened to them, he was thunderstruck, because they were *his* sins, not hers. Not just at that moment, but in general Master Durand said that he found hearing her confession to be edifying for him, rather than for her.[62]

Hearing a proto-saint's confession was not a common occurrence for a confessor. Master Durand's experience, however, suggests how confessors could struggle with the confession process, too. Navigating penitents' expectations of confession, as well as the act of educating penitents about sin, could be difficult for the confessor. Confessors were expected to teach and console as the penitent spoke their sins aloud. This could be challenging in unexpected ways and risk the souls of both parties.

Didactic texts appearing in the thirteenth and fourteenth centuries indicate that not every community had confessors like Master Durand. Many confessors may have lacked a sophisticated knowledge of sin, questioned confessees clumsily, or were not caring nurturers of the faithful.[63] Confessors' manuals also had to give advice for a range of confessees—from the ignorant and resistant to the pious and sensitive. As a later medieval manual advised, "Let him [the confessor] speak with caution so that he may thus frighten and soften the hardhearted, but so that he may not cause the weak to despair of forgiveness."[64] It might have been difficult for less skilled confessors to do both. Finally, scholars point out that those providing pastoral care were fallible humans and might not inspire confidence.[65]

Contrition and Intending Not to Sin Again

For a perfect confession, a person needed to feel proper contrition and intend not to sin in these ways again. For some of the witnesses in Delphine's inquest, this could be almost impossible. Lord Ferrier of Cucuron, for example, certainly did not feel that he could avoid spiritually damaging violence, even though Delphine urged him to do so. This potentially sinful behavior was too much a part of his social role. Leading his men against the mercenaries was not frivolous violence, like participating in a tournament, as we saw in the image from *The Breviary of Love*. This was his duty, and he would have experienced shame and potentially a loss of social status if he had refused. So, even though he was a pious man—he had thought it appropriate to visit a holy woman before a major battle—he could never intend to not sin this way again.

And Lord Ferrier was not alone. As we saw in chapter 2, from Queen Johanna of Naples to individual mercenary attackers, everyone engaged in violence risked the damnation of their immortal soul to a certain extent, and they knew it. Political leaders engaged in violent behavior and warfare were especially spiritually dangerous, since they also risked the bodies and souls of those who had sworn oaths to them. The risk of damnation weighed heavily even on some mercenaries. Although warfare was their profession, as we saw in chapter 4, mercenary leaders like John Hawkwood negotiated forgiveness of sins along with ransom money when leaving Provence. They had engaged in inappropriate violence against Christians for which many were excommunicated.

Violence was not the only problematic behavior, however. Some of the pious people in Delphine's community could not control their reactions to carnal temptation. They described feeling continuous sinful desire. This continuing desire can be seen as difficulty with contrition—one of the main requirements of confession. For Guido of Monte Rochen, contrition was profoundly important to the sacrament of penance. He wrote seven chapters informing confessors what contrition was, what they and others should be contrite about, and the proper way to express contrition. As we saw above, Guido of Monte Rochen believed people should be in an almost constant state of contrition.[66]

Several of Delphine's witnesses found carnal and worldly desire particularly difficult to control. They knew their behavior was sinful, but they did not want to stop or could not. People who could not control carnal desire would not have been experiencing the proper sorrow for their sins. Instead of a sorrow of contrition that helped the penitent repair their relationship with God, they would have experienced a sorrow that continued to separate them from God, since they continued to desire the sinful behavior.

One story shows a person struggling with the social expectations that we see in the miniature cycle at the top of figure 5.2. Catherine de Pui a close associate of Delphine's for decades, told the papal commissioners about her sister Ugueta's experience with vanity. When Ugueta was about fifteen years old, she had beautiful hair, which induced pride and worldly vanity. Ugueta's mother was not able to convince her that this was a problem, however. Then Ugueta and her mother visited Delphine, who asked Ugueta, "Do you wish to serve God and are you my daughter?," and Ugueta replied, "Freely!" To this statement, Delphine replied, "Remove your hair which impedes your soul."[67] According to Catherine, Ugueta told her that she immediately "changed the spirit which she had had at first concerning her hair," and she had her mother remove her hair.[68] After this, she changed her soul to good, humility, and devotion and made a vow of virginity on the altar of the blessed Mary in the church of St. Salvator in Bonnieux. From this point until her death, Ugueta wore humble clothes and sought alms.[69]

Ugueta likely knew that her vanity about her hair could be sinful. She had likely heard *contra-vanitatem* sermons directed at wealthy young women.[70] And according to Catherine de Pui she had been told by their mother. But she did not want to stop her worldly behavior. It took a conversation with Delphine to change her soul to humility.

One of the most startling stories of this trouble with the desire to stop sinning came from Lady Rossolina d'Agoult and her sister Lady Tiburga. Like

Rossolina, Tiburga was from the upper level of Provençal aristocracy.[71] Tiburgia was forty-seven and married to the lord of La Motte d'Aigues just outside Cabrières in the diocese of Aix. From their testimonies, however, it is clear that they spent time at St. Catherine's convent and knew many women in the Apt diocese, including Ugueta and Catherine de Pui. They also visited Apt frequently enough to notice changes in the behavior and dress of the bishop, Bertran Meissenier, when he led mass there.[72]

In their testimonies, Tiburga and Rossolina both recalled the experience of Jordana de Viens, a nun at St. Catherine's convent.[73] According to the noble sisters, Jordana suffered for a long time from carnal temptation.[74] She tried to free herself from this temptation through humble confessions, fasts, disciplines, and other punishments of the body, but they did not work. The continuing temptation caused her to feel sorrow.[75] Since Jordana could not control her temptation, she could not feel truly contrite. This would have caused her to experience a dangerous kind of sadness—a despair that drew her away from God rather than a healing sadness that helped her repair her relationship with God.[76]

After other methods, including confession, did not work, Jordana recalled Delphine's zeal and love for chastity and purity, but she could not be in Delphine's presence because Delphine was not at St. Catherine's convent at that time. So instead, Jordana went to the isolated room where Delphine stayed when she visited the convent.[77] Only Delphine had slept in the bed in that room, and it had taken on a relic-like quality for the nuns. Not only had it healed several people (including Lord Giraud de Simiana, as we saw in chapter 2), but when that wing of the convent burned, Delphine's bed did not.[78]

Jordana knelt before Delphine's bed and crawled on her bare knees around it, thinking constantly about Delphine's purity and chastity and begging Delphine to help her. According to Article 61, on which Rossolina and Tiburga agreed, her prayers were answered. "She was suddenly freed from temptation internally and completely. Jordana could not think about those things, which caused her such grave temptation."[79] She could finally make a perfect confession.

The Danger of Deathbed Confession

Confession on the deathbed was an obviously dangerous moment. All of the difficulties of confession we have seen were especially severe in this moment. The testimony of noble Lady Maria d'Evenos captures the difficulty of deathbed confession and the danger those difficulties imposed on the immortal soul.

She experienced problems with several elements of confession with the added pressure that she faced eternal damnation if she did not succeed.

Article 41, which described Lady Maria's experience, stated that beginning around 1346, Maria became increasingly disgusted by food, and she had trouble eating.[80] Maria suffered with this difficulty for seven years, and by 1353 she became seriously ill. Hoping to recuperate from her illness and regain her ability to eat, she visited Delphine in Cabrières, outside Ansouis, where Delphine lived in a hermitage. When Maria did not recover the ability to eat, however, she felt that she was about to die and desired to confess her sins to one of Delphine's confessors. Maria, however, "could not find in herself a way to make a perfect confession in either form or manner, and she could not remember her sins as she wished. She was saddened, because she considered herself to be damned."[81]

Lady Maria's language shows that she had a sophisticated understanding of confession. She understood what a perfect confession required and that she was incapable of making one. Unable to make a perfect confession, Maria sought out Delphine, who intuited her anxieties and spoke to her about the sacrament of confession. Maria laid her head in Delphine's lap (a gesture strongly suggestive of both consolation and confession) and listened to her words.[82] According to the article, Delphine told Maria that "purity, humility, and true confession removed God's indignation and reconciled the soul with its Creator."[83] In response, Maria experienced compunction, and after leaving Delphine's presence she entered another room, and with divine grace she began to cry. At the same time, all the sins she had committed since the age of seven to that day came clearly to her mind, "as if they were described in one book."[84] In other words, she experienced two of the necessary elements of confession—compunction and contrition—and remembered all of her sins starting from the age of reason.

After weeping, Maria felt wonder and joy and was filled with the sorrow of devotion (*merore devocionis repleta*).[85] Because of Delphine's merits and having heard her voice, not only was Maria able to confess her sins to a confessor, but she also regained her ability to eat, and her health improved. For Maria, confession was a cathartic moment. Experiencing a range of spiritual states—from compunction all the way through joy—healed her soul and healed her body, returning her from "the gates of death."[86]

The two main witnesses to this article, noble lady Maria d'Evenos and Friar Bertran Jusbert, both agreed to the basic story in Article 41, but added more information. Maria declared the article to be true.[87] In her short testimony she did not restate the whole sequence of events. She did specify, however, that after hearing Delphine speak about confession, she did not immediately confess. Instead, she waited until the following morning to confess to Friar Bertran in the parish church of Cabrières.[88]

Friar Bertran, who was not present when Delphine spoke to Maria, focused instead on his own attempts to help. After Maria failed to make a perfect confession, he had made a vow to God through Delphine. For Friar Bertran, his prayer caused Maria's memory to return. Although his testimony challenged the power of Delphine's voice, he still highlighted the importance of memory.[89]

All three sources of the events surrounding Maria's wondrous confession and return to health highlighted the difficulties in the elements of confession. Loss of memory, just like the inability to speak that Alazays Mesellano experienced, limited witnesses' ability to repair their relationship with God, and in Maria's case nearly led to her dying without making a complete confession.

The Danger of Unfinished Penance

For many confessors and many devout Christians, the performance of penance after making a perfect confession was a crucial part of the sacrament. Although by the fourteenth century the soul was forgiven through the act of confession, penance was considered a spiritually healthy way to show one's appropriate sorrow and desire to not sin the same way again. But it could also be perceived as a source of danger to the soul, especially if people were unable to complete the penance assigned them.

We see this danger in the testimony of Lady Catherine de Pui the close associate of Delphine who had begged the holy woman to protect Ansouis during the mercenary invasion of 1357–1358. According to her testimony to Article 35, Catherine "experienced great sadness on account of her sins, because she feared that she would not have sufficient time to do penance and therefore could be damned."[90] According to Catherine, Delphine knew her sadness even before she could say anything. Delphine spoke good words and gave consoling examples.

The commissioners asked Catherine what Delphine said that caused her sadness to withdraw. Catherine replied that Delphine told her that she had knowledge of her sins, but she did not have confidence in God. To clarify, Delphine "gave an example of two millstones: one above and one below. The upper millstone stood for the confidence in God, and the lower millstone stood for the knowledge of sins."[91] Delphine explained to Catherine, "When you consider only the lower millstone, which is the knowledge of sins, and do not consider the upper millstone, which is confidence in God, and just as the inferior millstone without the superior one cannot grind wheat, so it is with you. Simply consider the upper millstone and you have confidence in God, and thus you are consoled from sadness in this way!"[92] This explanation immediately consoled Catherine.

In Catherine de Pui's testimony, we see that she believed that the physical part of her penance, what some theologians called satisfaction through deeds or what Raymon Penyaforte, who wrote one of the most famous manuals of confession, called "exterior penance," was the crucial part of the forgiveness of sins.[93] Therefore, if she did not have enough time to complete her penance before her death, her confession was incomplete and she would be damned. She did not specify what her sins were or what satisfaction she had been told to perform, but even in the new literature of confession some penances could last for years and include prayer, alms, fasting, vigils, and disciplining the body.[94] In Catherine's understanding before talking to Delphine, she had to complete the whole satisfaction in order to be forgiven by God.

Delphine's metaphor helps us see how Catherine understood the working of the sacrament of penance.[95] The idea that the priest absolved a person from sin when the penitent confessed had not taken root in Catherine's understanding of sacramental confession.[96] What had taken root instead was the idea that she would be absolved only when she completed satisfaction.

Catherine's confusion is understandable. The relationship between confession and penance was evolving in the fourteenth century. Theologians at this time had a two-part view of the punishment of sin, especially mortal sins. First, the confessing sinner avoided eternal punishment by experiencing heartfelt sorrow. This was interior satisfaction. Second, since medieval Christians were part of a visible, temporal Christian community, they also performed exterior satisfaction in response to temporal punishment for sin. If this were incomplete, the sinner might face time in purgatory. Overall, most theologians considered satisfaction part of a sinner's healthy expression of humility, but not part of God's forgiveness per se nor part of absolution.[97]

Delphine's metaphor, therefore, informed Catherine that she had been trying to do the whole process of forgiveness by herself—that is, trying to grind grain with one millstone. While Catherine's soul was not in danger of damnation the way she feared, her ideas about confession caused the internal distress that Catherine described as *tristitia*, or sadness.[98] By explaining that trust in God is the other half of forgiveness, Delphine calmed Catherine's anxiety about not having time to finish her physical acts of penitence.[99]

This exploration of the main elements of the sacrament of penance as they appeared in witness testimony helps a modern audience understand how this was not just a difficult moment, but a dangerous one for these pious people.

The testimonies of Master Durand and others show how difficult it could be for a penitent to do and feel all the elements of a perfect confession. Penitents needed to have the appropriate internal state to confess, remember all of their sins, be able to say them aloud, and intend not to sin again. Even in times of peace, these were all potential stumbling blocks, especially for the wealthy or socially elite, and the stakes were high. The fourteenth century, however, was not a time of peace. The profound transition in warfare and the emergence of an epidemic illness that many felt was a divine punishment for sinful behavior likely made the stakes feel even higher, while the requirements of confession and penance could be unattainable. The testimonies in Delphine's inquest show that witnesses were aware of this problem. They knew what they had to do to confess effectively, but also that their lifestyles or immediate circumstances might prohibit them from doing so. In their stories we see how their interactions with Delphine helped them overcome difficulties in this dangerous moment.

Chapter 6

Sister Resens de Insula and the Desire for Certainty

Chapter 5 showed that witnesses in Delphine's inquest saw the sacrament of penance as a potentially dangerous moment for their souls. Their experiences raise interesting questions. What did witnesses expect from the sacrament of penance and why? How did witnesses describe healing encounters with Delphine in relation to the sacrament, and what can that tell us about how they understood the sacrament? The article of interrogation they responded to and the stories they shared help us understand their expectations and fears about the sacrament of penance and other spiritually dangerous moments.

In general, these testimonies reveal that witnesses wanted and, more importantly, expected to feel an internal transformation when they took part in the sacrament of penance. As we saw for witnesses like Maria d'Evenos and Master Durand Andree, they were experiencing the compunction, contrition, and sorrow of the sacrament and, through what they perceived as divine grace through Delphine's voice, experienced consolation, certainty about their sins and the state of their souls, and clarity about spiritual issues. When people engaged in all of the elements of the sacrament of penance, however, and remained sorrowful, uncertain, or confused, they experienced an unhealthy internal state. Their experience with Delphine, with her voice in particular, helped them experience what they expected from the sacrament of penance, but apparently sometimes did not get.

The experience of Sister Resens de Insula, a thirty-seven-year-old nun at the Holy Cross convent, captures the limitations of the sacrament of penance succinctly. The inquest documents tell us little about Sister Resens. Like other women in the convents of Apt, she had lived through the first and second mortalities, the mercenary invasions, and manifestations of the political unrest linked to the transfer of power from King Robert I of Naples to Queen Johanna I.[1] As we saw in chapter 4, these events had an impact on the daily lives of the nuns and visitors of the Holy Cross convent. Some of these women lost husbands to illness and war. And as mercenaries attacked, the convent had to move from outside the walls into a hospice within the city.[2] The complex politics of the Agoult, Simiane, Sabran, and Baux families influenced these women directly. In these turbulent decades of the fourteenth century, from 1343 to 1363, women like Resens found that Delphine's words resonated with the people who gathered to listen at the Holy Cross convent.

Resens remembered being present when Delphine spoke divine words at the Holy Cross convent in 1351.[3] At that time, as Sister Resens explained to the commissioners, "she experienced sadness and suffering in her heart because of doubts of conscience that she could not remove even though she had confessed many times."[4] Delphine recognized Resens's sadness and called her over. Resens told Delphine the cause of her sadness, but she also believed that Delphine already knew it. "Delphine said good and consoling words to Resens on account of which she was consoled and no longer felt the sadness she had before."[5]

Resens's description of her experience shows that she expected confession to console her doubts of conscience. In other words, she expected not to feel doubts of conscience after completing the sacrament. Resens even repeated the sacrament to get this result. When this did not happen, she experienced sadness and suffering because of these doubts. It is difficult to know exactly why this individual woman might have expected confession to remove her doubts of conscience. Sister Resens and the other witnesses do not answer this question directly. But the language that surrounds confession in many pastoral care manuals, especially the *Manipulus curatorum*, may have led witnesses to believe that they would feel different after confession. The care of soul, mind, and conscience was an important part of pastoral care, so much so that the care of souls through confession was often presented as medicine. Confessors healed the ills of the soul as a physician healed the ills of the body.[6] As Thomas Tentler pointed out, "The penitent is supposed to derive profound psychological benefits from sacramental confession, and authorities try to ensure that this forum offers consolation as well as discipline."[7] Guido of Monte Rochen, the author of the *Manipulus curatorum*, wrote, "Although one ought to sorrow over the sins one has committed, yet one ought also to rejoice on account of the life which one recovers."[8] The language in pastoral care manuals suggests that people like Delphine's witnesses were receiving a message that confession would console them.

But sermons and texts about sin and the soul frequently assumed an audience reluctant or unknowledgeable about sin.[9] This could limit the benefits for people who were already trying to live spiritually healthy lives. Sister Resens's expectations and experience show that pious people knew what they should do and the contrition and sorrow they should feel in order to make a successful confession. Just before describing her experiences with Delphine, for example, Sister Resens described how she had changed her behavior. She had changed her delicate, expensive clothing for humble, inexpensive clothing. She had also engaged in the correct emotions to undertake the sacrament. When she did not experience consolation through the sacrament, however, it opened the door to her extended sadness and suffering of heart. And as we have already seen in the *Manipulus curatorum*, the author also expected people to experience an almost perpetual state of contrition and sorrow for sin. So Resens's experience may not have been as unexpected for her confessor as it was for her. But for this nun who was also living through the crises of plague and mercenary violence, constant doubts of conscience may have been very difficult to live with.

Sister Resens's testimony, as with most of the testimony about witnesses' experiences of the sacrament of penance, appeared in response to Article 35. It is worth exploring the language of Article 35 in order to understand how internal transformation was presented to Delphine's witnesses. The language of the article also helps us see how their responses both agreed with it and slightly reinterpreted it in order to tell other kinds of stories.

The language of the article was flexible enough to capture different experience, though, as we will see, witnesses still described internal transformations that differed from what the article lays out. The article states:

> Moreover, by common statement, common opinion, common assertion and reputation, and public voice and reputation in parts of Provence and other areas it was and is well known that the said lady Delphine, from her great devotion and fervor of spirit towards God, brought forth many and almost continuous words of God from her mouth. And through her words, the people hearing were often and wondrously moved to change their lives and do penitence. And they said they had never heard words concerning changing life and repenting and correcting their sins so greatly persuasive and enticing as the words of the said lady. And because

> God endowed the said lady Delphine wondrously and uniquely in this thing and gave her grace that whoever, seeing her and hearing her words, said and sensed that the said lady knew and touched the individual and interior conscience, no matter the position and life of those hearing and seeing. And no matter which person, hearing her and desiring to take in her lesson, each one was recalled to his mind and consoled in his spirit and reassured from his doubts of conscience, although those doubts had not been revealed through any person to that lady. On the contrary, the thing that was most wondrous was that in a certain assembly or discussion speaking about God, with her words she spiritually refreshed and educated many people in attendance listening to her, even though the listeners had diverse worries and wishes and various scruples and doubts. And each person listening reported that for him the work was from the words of that lady. And for that reason many and many persons, husbands and wives, seculars as much as regulars and the religious, even children were wondrously changed from a pompous, lustful, and deceitful secular life to a good, holy, and honest life and turned themselves over to a humble and penitent status.[10]

After Article 1, witnesses spoke to Article 35 the most frequently. Twenty people testified to it—ten men and ten women—from various ages and backgrounds. The youngest witness was twenty-three (one of the youngest in the entire inquest), and the oldest witness was seventy. Twelve of the witnesses were religious, including Franciscan friars, priests, abbesses, nuns, and two bishops. The lay witnesses included everyone from servants, merchants, and legal professionals to the highest nobility in Provence. This combination of witnesses cuts through common dichotomies such as lay/cleric or men/women. It reveals a shared sense of concern about the state of one's soul and the search for a way to heal sicknesses of the soul and provide certainty that one's soul is healthy.

Article 35 described how Delphine healed sufferers' doubts and worries of conscience and moved people to penitence when she spoke words of God. According to the article, witnesses sensed an internal touch, and through this internal touch, witnesses felt Delphine's influence. This experience, in other words, was not one-sided. Both Delphine and the individual witness actively participated in the transformation. Delphine spoke, but listeners had to want to hear what she had to say in order to feel restored in mind, consoled in spirit, and reassured about their doubts of conscience.

What appeared particularly wondrous to witnesses, according to the article, was that even when Delphine spoke to groups of people with diverse worries and doubts, each one felt spiritually refreshed and educated. Even when Delphine spoke in a general way to a group, each person felt that the words were specifically targeting his or her individual doubt. As a result, diverse people changed from spiritually damaging internal states reflected by worldly pride and lust to spiritually healthy internal states emphasizing humility and penitence. Through Delphine's words of God, witnesses escaped dangers to the health of their souls.

In many ways, this article had surprising similarities to Article 38, discussed in chapters 2 through 4, which described Delphine's response to the "war of the seneschals" and the waves of mercenary invaders. For example, in Article 38, Delphine's great affection and desire for the health of men's souls let her suffering transform them. In Article 35, Delphine's great devotion and spiritual fervor emerged through her holy words. These words then had the power to wondrously move people to contrition and penitence, change their lives, and heal their souls. Finally, like the dangers of violence to men's souls in Article 38, the "diverse worries, and wishes, various scruples and doubts" described in Article 35 threatened the health of witnesses' souls.

Through witness testimonies, Delphine's voice emerged as a kind of aural body relic, something that poured out of her that was less tangible than blood or milk, but still touched and healed the sufferers.[11] Witnesses used the tactile verb *tangere* and said her voice touched them inside, transformed them, and consoled their doubts of conscience.[12] Her voice changed them internally. In some cases this transformation was then revealed when their outward behavior changed from pompous, lustful, and violent to humble, chaste, and peaceful.

Some witnesses, like Sister Resens, however, had already made the external and internal changes required of the sacrament. Their experiences differed from the description in Article 35, but they testified to it anyway. In these cases, Delphine's voice helped them feel differently after they had already felt contrition and changed their behavior. For Resens, God's grace through Delphine's voice helped her experience the consolation she had hoped to receive from the sacrament of penance.

Sister Cecilia Baussana and the Nuns of the Holy Cross Convent

Not every witness had the same experience as Sister Resens, however. Sister Cecilia Baussana of the Holy Cross convent experienced Delphine's voice in a way that more closely reflected the order of events that appeared in Article 35.

Sister Cecilia was one of seven widows—a significant number for one year in a relatively small convent—who took holy orders in 1349. Testimonies about and by these witnesses give us the chance to consider the spiritual and emotional impact of the first mortality on women widowed during that year.[13]

Testimony gives insight into two widows in particular—Lauduna d'Apt and Cecilia Baussana. Lauduna died before the inquest, so we learn most about her from her aunt, Abbess Ayselena of the Holy Cross convent.[14] Cecilia Baussana testified about her own experience after the first mortality. According to the witnesses' testimonies, these two women had different experiences of becoming nuns after the first wave of plague. Their stories help us see how crisis might make the experience of internal distress and the sacrament of penance more difficult and potentially dangerous.

According to Abbess Ayselena, Lauduna's husband died when she was seventeen. He died in 1348, perhaps during the first mortality, but Ayselena did not specify. After his death, Lauduna came to live at her aunt's convent, where she heard Delphine speak. Ayselena remarked that Lauduna had had a rich dowry. And before she heard Delphine speak, Lauduna may have greatly desired to enter into a relationship with a man and remain in the secular world.[15] After hearing Delphine, however, Lauduna scorned and abandoned the people and goods of the world. She desired to be received by the nuns, and in the convent she learned her duty, religiously and devotedly.

Abbess Ayselena accepted her niece only as an ancillary who served the nuns of the convent, however. She was not certain that Lauduna's desire to enter the convent would last. When Lauduna finally took her vow of chastity with "many other widowed women in the city of Apt," Abbess Ayselena was present.[16] Lauduna remained with the nuns and devoted herself to God until her death.[17]

Lauduna's story, told by her aunt, shows a relatively positive experience of Lauduna's reaction to widowhood in the year after the first mortality. Delphine's words consoled and inspired Lauduna in the immediate aftermath of the epidemic, but Ayselena made her niece wait to become a nun. Ayselena knew her niece had the means and opportunity to remarry, as many did in the years after, and did not want her niece to make a hasty decision. Ultimately, Lauduna's choice was successful.

Not all of the widows made the transition as successfully as Lauduna. Other testimonies reveal that conflicting emotions surfaced in the year after the first mortality, causing debilitating emotional suffering for some. One sufferer in particular, Cecilia Baussana, a thirty-five-year-old nun at the Holy Cross convent, was surprisingly candid about her struggles. She too decided to become a nun in 1349 after hearing Delphine speak. According to Cecilia's testimony, the bishop at the time warned the women about the difficulties of the life they had chosen and urged them to reconsider.

Cecilia went ahead and took holy orders. But after about a year, she began to have many diverse carnal temptations. She could not seem to have any consolation, and "she was led into desperation."[18] To end her desperation, she considered breaking her vow to God and instead following her family's wishes for her to remarry.

She described her emotional state while she struggled with the temptation to leave as "confused." She "could not have any happiness but she remained in great sadness and suffering."[19] A relative, who was also a nun at the convent, saw her sadness and asked her what caused it. Cecilia was too ashamed to say, so her relative took her to Delphine. According to Cecilia's testimony, Delphine saw into her heart and began to speak about how others, like the Apostle Paul for example, had resisted temptation. After leaving Delphine's presence, Cecilia was transformed inside. As she put it, "All sadness withdrew from her heart, and indeed all improper thought; and she did not feel the various and diverse temptations which she had had before, but she remained cheerful and steady in her vow, just as she remains."[20]

Cecilia's testimony follows Article 35 relatively directly. Sister Cecilia felt a strong desire to sin, but resisted this and wanted to hear what Delphine had to say. After hearing Delphine's voice, she was transformed from sinful to penitent and from sad to joyful. Although she did not mention the sacrament of penance, she had finally stopped desiring to sin and therefore could have made an effective confession.

Even beyond the sacrament, however, her experience can show modern audiences the slowly emerging emotional impact of the first mortality that stayed with these witnesses through subsequent crises. After the first impact of the epidemic, Cecilia experienced a complex series of transformations. She became a widow, joined a group of women suffering in a similar way, and then soon after became a nun. In the year after making her vow, however, her internal state changed. She began to be tempted by carnal desire and considered returning to her family and remarrying. This temptation and wishing to remarry were serious sins for a nun to commit. She was essentially sinning against Christ, who was her husband. The inability to stop desiring to sin trapped Cecilia in conflicting emotions. Her desperation and sadness changed her behavior in the eyes of those who knew her. Delphine healed that distress by seeing into Cecilia's heart and speaking words of consolation, which allowed Cecilia to feel untempted and cheerful. Cecilia's testimony shows how survivors made choices in the aftermath of the first mortality that they might not otherwise have made. Her reactions help us understand how the first mortality was a transformative moment that increased the danger individuals perceived for their souls.

Lauduna's and Cecilia's long-term reactions provide counterpoints to the immediate desperation presented in Louis Heyligen's letter, discussed in chapter 2. Heyligen described intense, alienating reactions to the epidemic. People processed "with burning lamentation and tears, with hair trailing, they beat themselves with piercing whips until the blood ran."[21] Lauduna and Cecilia, too, reacted strongly to the first mortality by choosing to become nuns. Lauduna experienced consolation at this point, but Cecilia suffered longer. After many transformations, she gradually found cheerfulness again. But neither described beating themselves in the street.

The link between healing and emotion in Cecilia's testimony brings us to the liminal ground between body and soul in a similar way that violence did in chapters 2 through 4. Cecilia described the causal links clearly. Temptation to sin caused desperation and sorrow and removed her ability to feel the healthy emotions of peacefulness and cheerfulness. In other words, her spiritual state had an impact on her health. And though she never used the term "melancholy" and did not seek a doctor, her cycle of negative emotion strongly evoked the way that fourteenth-century doctors explained melancholy.[22]

This cycle of negative emotion was even clearer in the experiences of Sister Jordana de Viens that we saw in chapter 5. Sister Jordana's story, as told by Tiburga and Rossolina d'Agoult, revealed desperation brought on by being unable to resist temptation. As a nun, Jordana was supposed to be thinking of Christ's suffering on the cross, not her own carnal desires.[23] Like Sister Cecilia Baussana's, Sister Jordana's thoughts were deeply sinful and separated her from God and the community of nuns.

The list of things Sister Jordana did to feel differently provides an interesting look at how a pious woman would attempt to control her internal self in order to stop the temptation that caused her to suffer. In her case we do see an extreme effort that evokes the flagellants. Through fasts and punishments she tried to control her physical self in order to have an impact on her internal self. She also tried confession, like Sister Resens, which did not provide an internal change for her either.

Unlike Sister Cecilia, Sister Jordana could not hear Delphine speak or feel the holy woman's touch. Instead she found another way to enter Delphine's presence by creating a type of personal ceremony, a last attempt to control behavior that threatened her place in her community and her self-identity as a nun. According to the Agoult sisters, Sister Jordana's prayers to Delphine succeeded where confession, fasting, and self-discipline had failed.

Providing Consolation and Assurance

Other testimonies to Article 35 do not have the physical extremes of those of Sister Resens and Sister Cecilia. Master Durand Andree's testimony about the experiences of others reveals a widespread desire for consolation and assurance about one's sins. As we saw in chapter 5, Master Durand was a cathedral canon of Apt, one of Delphine's confessors, and a medical doctor. In these capacities, he provided physical and pastoral care to people in Apt. In his testimony to Article 35, he described encountering people suffering from sadness and confusion about the state of their souls. After experiencing the transformative power of Delphine's voice for himself, he found a way to harness that healing for others. His testimony shows how important this concept of internal transformation was to the sacrament of penance and the health of the soul.

According to Master Durand's testimony, many men and women came to see Delphine. The visitors included religious and secular people who came to see her in Apt, Avignon, and other places. They came in small groups or large groups of up to twenty.[24] These men and women asked Durand to allow them to speak to Delphine for the health of their souls (*pro salute animarum suarum*). They told him that they desired to be instructed about their consciences and to be assured about their doubts of conscience.[25] When describing the assurance they sought, Master Durand used the same word as the article—*certificari*—which suggests a sense of guarantee.

According to his testimony, Durand introduced these visitors to Delphine and situated them in her presence in a group. They did not speak to her at this time about their individual doubts of conscience. Then Delphine said general words of God and made a general discussion (*collacionem*), speaking sometimes about the lives of the saints, sometimes about vices and virtues, sometimes about the Ten Commandments, articles of faith, and detesting sin. Master Durand summed up these encounters by saying that Delphine said many generally instructive and edifying things to her audience.[26]

After the general discussion, Master Durand described the sufferers leaving Delphine's presence having been consoled of their doubts of conscience and assured. Though they never told her about their individual doubts, each one told Durand that it seemed that Delphine's words were spoken for him or her alone. And when Durand asked them again later why they did not speak to Delphine (presumably individually) when they had wished to speak to her before, they told him that their doubts were sufficiently clear (*clare satisfactum*) now after the group encounter.[27]

Durand gives us a rare glimpse of a healing practitioner trained in both medical and pastoral care. Having experienced the positive effects of Delphine's voice, and knowing—as a doctor and confessor—the physical and spiritual damage that doubt and anxiety could cause, he took it upon himself to organize these group meetings. He then followed up with these sufferers and found that Delphine's voice and words had been effective. While he does not give hard numbers for the groups that saw Delphine, he indicates that people outside of those questioned by the commissioners experienced long-term doubts of conscience and sought Delphine out for her ability to speak healing words.

By organizing these meetings, Durand was modifying, consciously or not, a familiar type of miracle often called "clear sight." In this type of miracle, a holy person looked into others' hearts, saw what troubled them, and consoled their desperation.[28] But in other canonization inquests, miracle collections, and saints' lives this transformation was presented as a personal, mostly individual encounter. Durand's description of a variety of people with doubts of conscience listening to Delphine in groups shows Durand and the other sufferers repurposing a familiar type of miracle to solve their problem and navigate the dangers of the sacrament of penance.

The Desire to Be Transformed

Sister Resens de Insula's experience and these group encounters that Master Durand described reveal that some people in the fourteenth century wanted to be assured that their souls were healthy. They did not want to be constantly contrite and sorrowful, as Guido of Monte Rochen suggested. Instead, they wanted to feel that they had a healthy relationship with God. This appeared to be an important internal state for Delphine's witnesses, but a tough one to achieve. Didactic literature such as sermons, books of vices and virtues, and saints' lives addressed other kinds of issues—what was a sin, how and when to confess sins—but they did not directly address assurance about one's immortal soul. In fact, as we have seen, they often presented an ideal penitent as one who constantly worried about the state of his or her soul.

We can use Delphine herself as an example. Everyone around her, including Master Durand, who heard her confession and observed the way she lived, considered her saintly. In contrast, she considered herself a sinner to the moment of her death. On her deathbed, this holy woman did not consider herself worthy of heaven, but she trusted that God would show her mercy. Uncertainty, therefore, was the ideal state, as the author of the *Manipulus curatorum* and testimony and articles in Delphine's inquest suggested.

As Sister Resens's and Master Durand's testimony shows, however, not everyone could live with that uncertainty. Not everyone was saint material.

These people wanted certainty about the state of their soul. They wanted not just an end to sadness and suffering. They wanted certainty or assurance—what Article 35 referred to as "*certificati*."

Theologians and *summa* writers knew about the problem of uncertainty.[29] Consolation should have come from the sacrament of penance through the sense of a person returning to the Christian community through a process of internal transformation. The author of the *Manipulus curatorum* suggested that the sacrament of penance could cause people to rejoice for this reason. Sinful persons, whether violent mercenaries or vain girls, were separate from the Christian community, since they were enemies of God while they sinned. This separation could cause anxiety for the sinner.[30] Testimonies from Delphine's inquest show that witnesses expected to change internally, to feel consolation and assurance, which indicated that they had once again become friends of God and rejoined the Christian community. Sister Resens's testimony and Master Durand's description of people visiting Delphine for the health of their souls reveal that people were not experiencing the assurance and consolation they expected and that it caused concern.

While issues of assurance about one's sins appeared as early as St. Augustine's writings, *certificare* may have had special resonance for the communities around Delphine.[31] Witnesses remembered Delphine reading about and speaking of the lives of the saints as part of her words of God. Although none of the witnesses specifically mentioned Delphine speaking about St. Francis, her devotion to that saint and her lifestyle suggest she may have done so.[32]

In St. Bonaventure's *Legenda Maior*, which was a widely accepted version of St. Francis's life, the idea of *certificare* was linked with the consideration of sin. Chapter 3, section 6 described a time when Francis was in a solitary place reflecting bitterly and weeping about his sins committed over the years. The Holy Spirit came to him with joy (*laetitia*) and "assured him of the full remission of all his sins."[33] Immediately after this experience, St. Francis experienced an ecstasy and a vision in which he and his brothers gazed at a wondrous light. After this, he comforted his brothers and urged them not to fear God, but instead to take joy in him. This statement provided an example of *certificare* and how it felt and worked. For St. Francis, the distress of sinfulness was transformed into assurance and joy.

It took the Holy Spirit to assure St. Francis and cause an internal transformation in him. While not everyone had access to the Holy Spirit, Master Durand's testimony shows how people burdened by doubts of conscience received this transformation by God's grace expressed through Delphine's voice. Though likely not as devout as St. Francis, the groups Master Durand described were an educated audience who had internalized the messages about sin and how one should feel about it.

Master Durand's testimony also brings to mind debates about introspection in the later Middle Ages, which emphasized God's role in the forgiveness of sin. The debate centered on Ecclesiastes 9:1: "No one knows whether he is worthy of God's love or hatred." By the mid-fourteenth century, many theologians argued that a sinner must "do his best" to be truly contrite and therefore deserve God's grace. This did not solve the problem of introspection, however, which for some scholars lies at the root of the Reformation.[34]

While few of Delphine's witnesses were theologians, they struggled to understand and deal with this problem of whether they were doing their best. Sister Resens's and Master Durand's testimonies help us understand this from the perspective of pious Christians rather than theologians or saints.[35] Instead of focusing on the *fact* of absolution, these witnesses or the people they described wanted a *feeling*. They wanted to experience assurance—*certificare*. Until people had that feeling, they experienced doubts of conscience. This kind of source does not let us argue that confession was supposed to induce anxiety and thereby allowed the Church to practice a form of social control.[36] But it does show that these pious, informed confessees wanted and expected to feel some kind of certainty about the state of their souls and that they were not receiving that internal transformation from the sacrament of penance. Otherwise they would not have had to turn to Delphine. Master Durand—as a confessor, medical doctor, and associate of Delphine—found a way to mediate Delphine's wondrous voice to transform the doubt of potentially hundreds of sufferers.

Another place we see a desire for transformation is in the many ways that witnesses described the transformations of others. We have already seen several. Catherine de Pui described her sister cutting off her hair. Ladies Rossolina and Tiburga described how Sister Jordana finally conquered her carnal temptation.

Describing others' transformations was a common way that witnesses responded to Article 35. Witnesses described thirty-six women and twenty-two men, most of whom did not testify to the article, as having been transformed.[37] Although we know much less about this group, since their ages were not given, there were a few famous names. Witnesses spoke of Bertran Messenier, the popular bishop of Apt who later became the bishop of Naples. They mentioned Master Nicolau Laurens, the inquest proctor, witness organizer, and writer of the articles. Several spoke about a Lord Guido de Cavaillon, who founded a hospice in which Delphine stayed as she negotiated peace between

Raymon d'Agoult and Uguo de Baux. They also added family members, prominent citizens of Apt, and various *milites* and religious of Provence.

Witnesses saw these people change their lives after hearing Delphine, which was how they knew these people had been transformed by her voice. For example, several witnesses commented on wealthy merchant couples, including Bartholomeo and Beatriz de Pertuis and Raymon and Ugueta Chieusa, who wore humble clothing, ate simple foods, and donated money to the poor after hearing Delphine speak.[38] According to Catherine de Pui, Bartholomeo and Beatritz made a particularly dramatic change, since they were wealthy drapers who dealt in fine cloth. They gave up their business and dressed only in humble cloth.[39] Bertranda Bertomieua was more critical, saying that Bartholomeo de Pertuis "had acquired many goods wrongly."[40] Regardless of how critical the individual witness was, each testimony unearthed another story about a desire for change.

Where Delphine Spoke and What She Said

In looking at these transformations, the main way that people experienced the consolation or assurance they desired was through listening to Delphine speak. They described how her words touched their hearts and caused their internal states to change. If we look at their descriptions of this encounter, we see how the stories they told framed her speaking for the papal commissioners and those who would consider her canonization. Inquest organizers and witnesses indicated that Delphine spoke about predictable topics, such as saints' lives and the Ten Commandments. And, more importantly, the articles and testimonies show that her speaking was sanctioned by Church authorities, including Pope Clement VI.

One of the most thorough descriptions of where and when Delphine spoke came from Ayselena d'Apt, the abbess of the Holy Cross convent. In her testimony to Article 35, Ayselena heard Delphine commonly speaking words of God as she conversed with them (*collacionem ipsis faciendo*) at least twice a day: early in the morning, after mass; and after a daily rest period, and sometimes after meals.[41]

Through Ayselena, we get a sense that at certain times of the day people in the convent gathered and spoke with Delphine. We know from other testimonies that this group often included more than nuns. For example, Ayselena's niece, Lauduna d'Apt, Lady Cecilia Baussana, Lady Resens de Insula, the draper's widow Alazays Mesellano, and others all testified to hearing Delphine speak at the Holy Cross convent.[42] This was a place where women spoke with and listened to Delphine.[43]

Ayselena's testimony also included details concerning what Delphine spoke about. Ayselena explained that when Delphine instructed her listeners about how they ought to serve God in humility and virginity, she emphasized that they should serve Christ as their spouse. And they should have no affection or love (*affectionem sive amorem*) for things of the world, not even friends or themselves. They should love only God. Not only should they avoid fine garments, food, and playthings, but they should avoid taking pride in their good works. They should pray, fast, and do good works to the end of their days. To reinforce this, Delphine recited many examples of male and female saints.[44]

Nothing in this list was startling or new. One would expect all of these from a woman who had taken vows of chastity and poverty and who tried to live up to the ideals of earlier saints. It is a list strongly influenced by Franciscan ideals.[45] But the detachment not only from worldly objects but also friends recalls the difficult events that Delphine and these nuns had lived through. The list reflects the ideas of sin that have emerged in these chapters.

In response to a question from the commissioners, Abbess Ayselena stated that she never heard, while she lived, any person, through words or example, better induce people to change their lives or complete penitence.[46] For Abbess Ayselena, as with many witnesses, the message was not exceptional. They had likely heard what Delphine said many times from many speakers. Instead, what stood out was how she said it. We are reminded of the sparkling fire that Queen Sanxia's court saw emerge from Delphine's mouth—a physical manifestation of God's grace acting through Delphine's voice.

Abbess Ayselena's testimony helps us see that sometimes Delphine's speaking bore a passing resemblance to preaching, which might have made papal audiences uncomfortable. The construction of Article 35, however, did not use the verb *praedico*, which might indicate the *ars praedicandi* or preaching. Instead the article highlighted the fact that listeners who desired to take in Delphine's lesson received individual consolation and assurance regardless of the way in which they spoke to her.[47] The article also specifies that Delphine spoke words of God (*verba de Deo*), another phrase indicative of preaching.[48] Witness testimony, however, framed Delphine's speaking as conversation and appropriate female teaching, attributing the astonishing transformative power of her voice to God's grace bestowed on Delphine through her devotion.[49]

For several witnesses, Delphine's speaking also reflected the actions of Mary Magdalene. The *Golden Legend* described Mary Magdalene as one of the rudderless boat saints that washed up in Provence. Historian Nicole Bériou points out that in Provence, Mary Magdalene was well known as the "apostle of the apostles" for converting the pagans of Marseille with her preaching.[50]

After Charles II of Naples discovered Mary Magdalene's relics in Provence in 1297, Mary Magdalene became even more prominent there because she was linked to the saintly family line of the Angevins of Naples.[51] She became a source of healing and protection miracles in the region, and people visited St. Maximin, where her relics were believed to be housed. The Sainte Baume, a grotto in the face of a massif where Mary Magdalene was believed to have lived as a penitent, was already a pilgrimage site but became more popular.

None of the witnesses directly compared Delphine to Mary Magdalene, but Mary Magdalene would have been a model in their minds for understanding how a holy woman could heal souls through her speaking. Bishop Philippe Cabassole, one of the most politically connected witnesses in Delphine's inquest, was also a strong advocate for the local cult of Mary Magdalene. As we saw in chapter 2, Cabassole wrote a history of the cult of Mary Magdalene.[52] This book, one of many histories of the discovery of the Magdalene's relics, was the only one to tell the complete story of the relics' survival and discovery, and one of two based on personal experience. In it, Bishop Philippe represented Mary's proficiency as a speaker and preacher with a palm frond growing from the mouth of the skull discovered by King Charles II of Naples in St. Maximin.[53] The miracle tradition surrounding Mary Magdalene presented her as one who made people aware of their sins, chastised sinners, and helped those who could not stop sinning.[54] These were the things the witnesses wanted, and it likely made sense to seek them from a holy woman.

As we have seen in several witness testimonies, people did not hear Delphine only in convents. She spoke with them as they walked to mass, during group prayers, in confession, or in gatherings like those organized by Master Durand Andree. Witness testimony and Article 35 presented Delphine as speaking words of God almost continuously. Witnesses' experience of healing through Delphine's speaking was further described and sanctioned in Articles 36 and 37. These articles did not describe moments of danger, but I include them and witness testimony to them to show why witnesses would find it appropriate to speak to Delphine when they were in danger.

These two articles, coming directly after Article 35, described related topics. Article 36 described how, in 1352, Delphine met twice with the court of Pope Clement VI to support the canonization of her husband, Elzear de Sabran. Article 37 described her meeting with the theologian and sermon writer Francis Meyronne and how she impressed him with her clear language about scripture.[55]

Six men and women testified to Article 36, either hearing about the event from others or seeing it for themselves. They focused on the reaction of Pope Clement VI. Witnesses described how the papal audience was struck by the clarity of Delphine's language as she spoke about her late husband Elzear, especially about his visions concerning the incarnation of the Word. As witnesses spoke of these meetings, they linked Delphine's speaking to the papal curia and to Elzear, who had a local cult. Their stories showed Delphine being a devoted widow and respectful to the papacy through her ability to speak.

The most developed testimony to Article 36 came not from a religious man, but from a military man. Lord Giraud de Simiana, the thirty-four-year-old noble lord of Apt and Casaneuve, given the title *miles* in Delphine's inquest, accompanied Delphine to Avignon and Villeneuve (directly across the Rhone from Avignon), where the meetings took place.[56] The meetings occurred in 1351, after the first mortality but before the invasion of Arnau de Cervole. Lord Giraud would have been twenty-two years old at the time.

Lord Giraud was a figure with multiple identities who therefore adds multiple perspectives to help us understand this article. As a noble lord, he participated in the Estates of Provence and would become seneschal of Provence in the late 1360s.[57] He was Delphine's escort to Avignon and entered the papal court with her. At the same time, as the lord of Apt, he was part of the community, sharing their danger. As we saw in chapter 4, his cows were stolen by mercenaries.

According to Giraud's testimony, he did not hear what Pope Clement VI said to Delphine at the first meeting in the papal palace in Avignon.[58] But at the second meeting in the papal consistory in Villeneuve, he did hear. In a room full of cardinals, important bishops, and lords, Pope Clement declared that what Delphine said to him was so profound concerning divinity that he had never heard any person speaking so loftily of divinity, not even Brother Francis Meyronne, who was Clement's associate. This could not be unless it came "from an infusion of the Holy Spirit."[59]

Clement VI's reaction—that her words were so "profunde" and "alte" that they seemed to come from an infusion of the Holy Spirit—sanctioned Delphine's speaking.[60] This is the only place that the Holy Spirit is invoked to explain Delphine's speaking, but it is also the only instance included in the inquest in which Delphine spoke to a large group of learned men in a quasi-church setting. This story, coming after testimony to Article 35, would have made Delphine's speaking appropriate for a potentially skeptical or hostile audience.

A different presentation of Delphine's speaking appeared in testimonies to Article 37. Article 37 stated that Delphine spoke individually with Master

Francis Meyronne, a famous theologian associated with the court of King Robert of Naples. From her, he heard lofty and wondrous words (*verba alta et mirabilia*), on account of which many of his doubts and many secrets in the knowledge of theology "were rendered clear, lucid, and settled."[61] Five men and women testified to Article 37, though all but one used Meyronne's name as a place-holder and spoke instead about themselves or other literate clerics who experienced insight from Delphine that removed their doubt.[62]

Witnesses provided significant detail about what Delphine said in response to this article. For example, Friar Bertran Jusbert said nothing about Meyronne. Instead he spoke of the experience of Friar Peire Michel of Sundria, from the diocese of Nîmes, who spoke with Delphine "before the first mortality."[63] He described Friar Peire as "a greatly reputed cleric in *sacra pagina*" in the Franciscan order and reported speaking to the man before and after his conversation with Delphine.[64] According to Friar Bertran, Friar Peire admired Delphine's ability to speak clearly and without ambiguity. He had questioned her about "three great doubts in holy scripture" that he had, and when he withdrew from her presence, those doubts were gone.[65] Friar Bertran did not describe Friar Peire as having doubts of conscience, which were so difficult for the witnesses to Article 35. Regardless of this, Friar Bertran's testimony shows the efficacy of Delphine's words and voice to transform through clarifying speech.

Master Durand Andree presented his own experience of Delphine removing his theological doubts. According to his testimony, he and Delphine spoke frequently over the years between 1350 and 1360. He described one memorable occasion when Delphine helped him better understand Psalm 90, which was recited in the office of Compline and began with the words "Who dwells in the aid of the Highest."[66] They spoke together about this and other scriptural issues for much of a night, and he left her presence with a greater understanding. He also described himself after this discussion as "*certificata*," or reassured, just like those witnesses who suffered doubts of conscience.

Bishop Philippe Cabassole mentioned Francis Meyronne by name, but like Master Durand, he focused on how Delphine clarified his own doubts. According to his testimony, he heard that Meyronne and many great literate clerics spoke of the great knowledge of Lady Delphine. Philippe had had a discussion (*habuit collacionem*) with Lady Delphine about the incarnation of the Word of God, and about virginity and poverty and continence.[67] He found Delphine's words more clear than any of his own study in his books, especially "how, in the incarnation of the Word of God, the innate, infused, and uncreated virtues come together, and at the same time it was one man."[68] Philippe made no mention of the Holy Spirit or special visions to support her explanation.

Instead, God's grace worked through her words to make complex issues understandable and remove the doubt of those whose task it was to understand those issues.

According to the witnesses to Articles 36 and 37, Delphine healed doubt with her words of God. These witnesses described doubts not of their own consciences, but about their understanding of sacred texts. According to witnesses, her words were clear, lucid, and Catholic. They impressed Pope Clement VI and clarified difficult theological issues, which helped her listeners experience an internal state unimpeded by confusion.

What the articles and testimony in Delphine's inquest show is that people experienced internal transformations when they heard Delphine speak about God. Some even actively used Delphine's voice for internal transformation. This search for transformation helps modern audiences see that most people wanted to feel consolation, joy, or simply a release from doubts of conscience and confusion. Very holy people like Delphine may have been comfortable with continuous uncertainty, contrition, and sorrow, but most people who engaged in the sacrament of penance were not proto-saints.

A woman speaking to groups of people like this could have been perceived as problematic in the mid-fourteenth century. But there were good models for women's preaching, like Mary Magdalene, that the papal commissioners and others in the Catholic hierarchy would know. And the inquest organizers and witnesses worked to present Delphine's speaking in a positive light.[69] Article 35 carefully did not describe Delphine as preaching, and inquest organizers and witnesses made sure to show in various ways that her words were valued and sanctioned by the highest Christian authorities.

We cannot know what Delphine had thought of this. She did not testify, of course, and she did not write about her own experiences. We do not have letters or any other texts written by her. Instead we have the articles and witnesses' words. And those sources inform us that her words transformed her listeners. Whether she spoke to them individually or as part of a group, witnesses felt that Delphine's voice touched them inside and transformed their temptation, lust, and worldliness into penitence and humility. This internal transformation often appeared in their behavior as they changed the clothes they wore and the food they ate.

Some of the internal transformations were linked to the events of these difficult twenty years. Survivors of the waves of epidemic, like survivors of any catastrophe, had to cope with the emotional pain and practical difficulties caused by the loss of loved ones. Witness testimony in Delphine's inquest allows us to see both immediate and longer-term reactions to crisis. For a witness like Cecilia Baussana, grappling with the death of her husband and her choice to become a nun in the wake of the first mortality, transformation meant moving from paralyzing confusion and temptation to the ability to feel cheerful again. Resens de Insula also remembered a time after the first mortality when she could not be consoled even with repeated confession. The consolation of Delphine's words helped witnesses face the spiritual disasters of the first and second mortality and waves of mercenary invasion.

Conclusion

Lord Giraud de Simiana and the Health of Body and Soul

This book has explored moments of danger identified by witnesses in the canonization inquest for Countess Delphine de Puimichel. Those moments of danger, occurring between 1343 and 1363, were diverse. Witnesses turned to their holy woman at specific chronological moments. In 1349, they asked her to travel and speak to feuding local lords who threatened peace in Provence. In 1357, they prayed for miraculous intercession when a first wave of mercenaries invaded the county. In 1361, during a plague outbreak and a far larger mercenary invasion, witnesses turned to Delphine for aid. Witnesses also sought help from their holy woman at individual moments of danger that they encountered when they struggled with the physical and mental demands of the sacrament of penance. The witnesses saw danger in the possibility of eternal damnation.

In witnesses' stories of miraculous intercession, they did not strictly mark some dangers as physical and others as spiritual. The cultural influences they shared blurred the boundaries between body and soul. For them, violence against Christians was both a physical and a spiritual danger. And the sacrament of penance had equally challenging physical and spiritual demands. When taken together, the stories of witnesses reveal a concept of health that included body and soul equally. Health was just as much about peace and safety as it was about physical robustness. This view was reflected in the diverse healing methods witnesses used to achieve health. For witnesses, saints and doctors provided health care.

We have seen in these chapters that witness testimony was shaped by time, place, and the special demands of a canonization inquest. The witnesses testified in Provence before papal commissioners in 1363. Their political world was changing rapidly. Perhaps one of the strongest influences was the death of King Louis of Naples in 1362. Many witnesses were aware that relations between lords of Provence and Queen Johanna were in a moment of possible renegotiation. Witnesses chose their words carefully during this time.

In the day-to-day procedure of the inquest, witnesses responded to the articles of interrogation written by Master Nicolau Laurens. These articles had been constructed from Master Nicolau's experiences and his conversations with the community around Delphine. He had also allowed for significant flexibility in the articles so that witnesses could add their own stories to the inquest. Article 1 in particular—which asked witnesses to describe anything they had seen, heard, or experienced in regards to Delphine's life, living miracles, or posthumous miracles—invited new stories. As witnesses recalled earlier events, they shaped narratives that wove various dangers together. These narratives ultimately reflected their moral world view. Witnesses' search for solutions from their local holy woman revealed their understanding of the dangers they faced and ways they had to heal the sicknesses they perceived.

One witness helps us bring together the chronological and individual moments of danger that this pious group identified. Lord Giraud de Simiana was a member of the highest nobility of Provence. He and his wife, Lady Maria d'Evenos, were the lord and lady of Apt and Casaneuve, just as Elzear and Delphine had been.[1] In 1363, Lord Giraud was thirty-four years old and had shared the experiences of many in Provence. He was miraculously saved by Delphine's bed from the first mortality. Mercenaries stole his cattle when the Great Companies invaded in 1361. He witnessed Pope Clement VI's reaction to Delphine's voice and words. He has appeared in almost every chapter of this book.

Lord Giraud's identity as a political and military leader, like many of those facing danger in Delphine's inquest, is important here. In 1363 Lord Giraud became the vice seneschal of Provence, entering the service of Queen Johanna.[2] Similar to other witnesses, Lord Giraud never mentioned Queen Johanna by name. In his silence, we encounter the ambiguity of Lord Giraud's experiences with the Crown of Naples.

As with many other witnesses, Lord Giraud's stories about Delphine described how her words touched his soul and transformed him. He made his clearest statement of transformation in response to the articles about Delphine's death. Lord Giraud was one of many family members and associates present at Delphine's deathbed, staying near her during the days that she was gravely ill. While he stood beside her bed, she grabbed his hand and spoke to him, saying, "You ought to see, son, how the world compensates us. You see in what state I am. You will be in great danger and infirmity, that I see, and there is no hope that you will be healed from these things; and you ought not be ungrateful to God for the graces which he made to you; because, when you will wish to do many good things, you will be at the end of your days."[3] Lord Giraud heard this warning about how death comes for everyone, and how, on his deathbed, it would be too late to prepare his soul. It made him anxious in his mind (*anxie mente*) because, like so many others in this inquest, he became aware of his sinfulness.[4] In order to alleviate this anxiety, he left Delphine and confessed his sins. When he returned to her bedside he "was much more pleased to stand joined to the lady Delphine than at first."[5] The sacrament of penance appeared to console him.

Lord Giraud was also present when Friar Peire Clodi, a priest of Apt, saw Delphine in agony and told her that she should not fear death. Delphine responded that she did not have fear. According to his testimony, this small moment had an impact on him. It caused him to change his life for the better "on account of the words of the said lady Delphine and her sanctity."[6] Giraud gave alms to the poor of Christ more than he was accustomed to. And he had a higher regard for the poor and lived more in love and fear of God.[7]

His reaction gives insight into the complex mesh of body and soul that made up his concept of health. Seeing and listening to this holy woman on her deathbed caused the noble lord Giraud to consider his own future physical deathbed. This would not have been abstract for him. According to his wife, Lord Giraud was so close to death in 1348 that his family had already bought the candles and winding sheet for his funeral. What had been abstract for him was sin. Before hearing and seeing Delphine on her deathbed, he may have faced death, but he had not perceived his own sinfulness. As we saw in regards to Article 38, Delphine's words and suffering could heal those around her. In Lord Giraud's case, healing took the form of feeling anxious about the state of his soul and the sinfulness of his day-to-day behavior. This caused him to confess and change his opinion about the poor and his behavior toward them. This ultimately changed his affective relationship to God. For him, respect for the poor could improve the health of his soul and his prospects for eternal life. His behavior encapsulates how Delphine's witnesses understood the dangers to body and soul and one way they had found to face those dangers.

Lord Giraud's experience of Delphine's deathbed calls to mind another text by Francis Petrarch, the friend of Bishop Philippe Cabassole. In *Remedies for*

Fortune Fair and Foul, Petrarch had much to say about reactions to death.[8] In a section about the fear of dying in a state of sin, the poet eloquently described the power of confession to remove the "poisonous, deadly baggage" of sin.[9] The section presented confession as a healing method for the soul. As with most other literature on the topic, however, Petrarch focused on the reluctant penitent. He criticized those who neglected confession or thought their sins too great to forgive.[10] A witness like Lord Giraud expands our view of the late medieval penitent. Like others in this inquest, Lord Giraud was not reluctant to confess but he was not always aware of what was sinful. For political leaders like Lord Giraud, even visiting Delphine in the wrong way could have been a sign of vainglory. According to Lord Giraud's testimony, Delphine's words transformed his perception of himself and allowed him to make an effective confession.

As we have seen in chapters 5 and 6, witnesses seemed to perceive the sacrament of penance as an important healing moment. But unlike Lord Giraud, who felt less anxious after his confession, other witnesses did not find the sacrament consoling. They struggled to achieve each element of a complete confession, which caused several witnesses to experience more anxiety. And most importantly, they expected to feel different after they confessed. When this did not happen, they felt anxiety or even despair. Witnesses did not embrace uncertainty about their souls like Petrarch, Delphine, or the author of the *Manipulus curatorum* suggested they should. The witnesses were not saints or philosophers. In a time of warfare and plague, they wanted consolation and certainty about their souls. And through Delphine's voice they found both.

Testimonies have shown that internal transformation was not limited to the sacrament of penance. It infused witnesses' lives. Warring Provençal lords transformed from hatred to friendship. The mercenary Durand Arnau de Rupa Ayneria transformed from a violent attacker into a devoted penitent. The terrified noblewoman Lady Andrea Raymon became a courageous resister of attack. The priest Raymon d'Ansouis transformed his heart with the greatest devotion to Delphine and invoked her with his whole affect and his whole heart and mind in an effort to survive the epidemic illness of 1361. And Lord Giraud de Simiana transformed his understanding of sin. In every transformation we see the witnesses' understanding of the world they lived in. Internal transformation healed spiritually damaging violence, gave the sufferer of epidemic illness an opportunity for miraculous healing, and prepared a person for the sacrament of penance.

Witnesses did not just talk about feeling different after hearing Delphine. Like Lord Giraud, they described changes in behavior. In many of these moments, external behavior revealed internal change and became a key element in witness stories of healing.[11] Lords Raymon and Uguo exchanged the kiss of peace. Durand Arnau de Rupa Ayneria walked from Ansouis to Apt with the rope used to draw him from the well where his failed execution took place wrapped around his neck. Lady Andrea rode for miles with broken harness and exchanged taunts with her attackers when she reached safety. Father Raymon did not die of plague. For the witnesses, all of these actions revealed an internal change. Witnesses' changed behavior was the physical evidence of God's grace. Changed behavior—spiritually healthy behavior—revealed God's grace as much as a physically healthy body did.

The testimonies to Article 35 list an array of transformations that people experienced and saw. Friar Giraud Raybaud saw aristocratic women give up their ornaments and fine clothes and become paupers.[12] Noble lady Maria d'Evenos spoke of the luxuries she renounced after hearing Delphine and being transformed by her voice. Lord Johan de Sabran saw changes in the noblemen in his household.[13] Master Guilhem Enric, the legal professional, also saw changes in the men with whom he interacted.[14] The nuns of the Holy Cross convent sold silver cups and coral devotional objects and gave the money to the poor.[15] Sister Cecilia Baussana sold her goods and gave them to the Holy Cross convent.[16] Master Durand Andree changed his life for the better and gave up a benefice.[17] All twenty witnesses who testified to Article 35 listed the names of others they had seen change. According to these testimonies, over a hundred people changed what they wore, what they ate, the work they did, and the things they owned because they had experienced internal transformation through Delphine's voice. Testimonies to Article 35 register a powerful reaction to the events of 1343–1363. During a time of plague, war, and political upheaval, these witnesses told stories about transformation. They described how they changed themselves and watched people at the highest social levels of Provence change fundamental aspects of their lives as an outgrowth of internal transformations for the health of their souls.

By contextualizing their testimonies, we can understand their internal transformations as reactions to the spiritually damaging violence surrounding them. In these twenty years, one locus of spiritual ambiguity was the Countess of Provence—Queen Johanna I of Naples. She had been accused of assassinating her first husband. She and her second husband had been involved in the "war of the seneschals." In their testimonies, witnesses like Bertranda Bertomieua highlighted their holy woman's links to King Robert, but created no links to Queen Johanna I. Through their testimonies they critiqued the violence they encountered and praised the peace that Delphine created. Their stories of internal and external transformations, shared at political or spiritual gatherings large and small, had a political context.

These transformations were not simply reactions to politics, however. They were also attempted remedies. The witnesses attempted to heal the spiritual sickness of violence, and through this to restore their relationship to God. The witnesses had a strong sense of the importance of their relationship to God. As we saw in chapter 2, at least some in this social circle framed the first wave of plague as God's punishment for the assassination of Andrew of Hungary. The difficulties they encountered with the sacrament of penance, including not feeling consoled or assured, made this an especially dangerous moment for them. Making an incomplete confession risked their immortal souls. Delphine's voice was a remedy that many experienced.

One way to understand this is through the concept of moral sanitation. This phrase is used by modern scholars who study later reactions to the plague. It often describes the efforts of city governments to improve a city's health by regulating the use and cleaning of streets and sewers, but also by regulating and even removing problematic groups of people, like prostitutes or violent men.[18] The experiences of witnesses in Delphine's inquest suggest that efforts of moral sanitation can be considered in a far more personal way. The "epidemic" of plague and war caused many pious people to engage in a personal moral sanitation, reevaluating themselves as Lord Giraud did, transforming problematic behavior, and searching for certainty in their relationship with God. This way of understanding moral sanitation helps us see how witnesses connected all of the events they lived through. It also helps us consider the changing need for the sacrament of penance to be transformative.

If we are not careful, the ways that sufferers in the fourteenth century linked body and soul in the midst of crises can seem superfluous to modern readers. But scholars of medieval history, especially medieval medicine and healing, have emphasized the importance of not ignoring what seems different. In 1995, David Lindberg offered a compelling plea to investigate medieval biomedical subjects without avoiding those fields—such as astrology—marginalized by modern scientific disciplines and without avoiding the involvement of the Catholic Church.[19] In 2009, Monica Green made a subtly different plea that thoughtful arguments about medicine and health are left out of major political, social, and religious narratives (often out of ignorance about how to approach the history of medicine), to the detriment of both the subfield of history of medicine and major fields.[20]

Several historians of medicine have addressed these problems, using canonization inquest testimony and miracle stories. Katharine Park used the fourteenth-century inquest for Clare of Montefalco to explore knowledge about and use of surgery.[21] Joseph Ziegler analyzed the testimony of doctors who testified in medieval canonization inquests in part to show that there was no antipathy between medical and miracle practitioners.[22] Sara Ritchey has used hagiography to reveal the links between health and salvation.[23] And Jacalyn Duffin studied five centuries of miracles and witness testimonies to explore how cutting-edge medical evidence has been used to prove miracles.[24] Social historians like Sari Katajala-Peltomaa and Sharon Farmer have been using information from canonization inquests and miracle stories to study things like medieval women's daily lives and health care options for the poor.[25]

Through deep contextualizing of canonization inquest testimonies, *Souls under Siege* has joined this thread of medieval history. One useful method has been by exploring the words and expression of emotion. In these testimonies, emotion words have overlapping legal, political, and medical meaning. Hatred expressed through warfare was a scandal and a sickness of the soul that could be healed with love and affection.[26] Witnesses also used emotion words to describe their reaction to extreme experiences.[27] Mercenaries, plague, and the complexities of confession inspired fear, confusion, and sadness.[28] Through protection, physical healing, and clear explanation, the witnesses perceived that Delphine transformed their internal, negative emotional states.

As witnesses testified to Delphine's holy life and miracles in 1363, the stories about how she protected Ansouis, transformed a mercenary into a penitent, and inspired consolation in those who listened to her fell on appreciative ears. The papal commissioners and the witnesses knew that Provence was once again threatened by extreme levels of mercenary violence. Pope Urban V was forming a league of lords, bishops, and civic representatives to join together to protect against the mercenary companies.[29] He hoped to help these communities withstand the coming attacks of Great Companies entrenched nearby and moving in the region, drawn by the wealth and relative weakness of the Comtat Venaissin and Avignon.[30]

In the longer term, the situation would not improve significantly for Delphine's witnesses and others living in Provence. By the end of the fourteenth century, two more waves of plague would move through the region. Sufferers increasingly turned to saints for healing of the disease, as we see in the pre-inquest for the canonization of Pope Urban V.[31] The spiritual landscape would change dramatically as the Great Schism introduced competing popes, who were increasingly dependent on political rulers for their authority. And continuous warfare in the Iberian and Italian peninsulas and the kingdom of France through the fifteenth century fed the demand for and power of mercenaries. But in 1363, for the witnesses on the curling crest of a wave of changes, theirs was a moment of crisis and transition, and they were adapting the tools they had, in this case saintly intercession and self-transformation, to meet new, overwhelming needs.

Notes

Introduction. Telling Stories of Danger in Fourteenth-Century Provence

1. For the multilingual nature of medieval law and bureaucracy, see Michael Clanchy, *From Memory to Written Record: England, 1066–1307*, 2nd ed. (Oxford: Blackwell, 1993), 206–211. For papal procedures concerning witnesses in canonization inquests, see Christian Krötzl and Sari Katajala-Peltomaa, "Approaching Twelfth- to Fifteenth-Century Miracles: Miracle Registers, Collections, and Canonization Inquest Processes as Source Material," in *Miracles in Medieval Canonization Inquest Processes: Structures, Functions, and Methodologies*, ed. Christian Krötzl and Sari Katajala-Peltomaa, 1–40 (Turnhout: Brepols, 2018), 18–19. For the many ways that notaries shaped canonization inquests and miracle collections, see the essays collected in Raimondo Michetti, ed., *Notai, miracoli e culto dei santi: Pubblicità e autenticazione del sacro tra XII e XV secolo* (Milan: Dott. A. Giuffrè Editore, 2004). See also Jacques Dalarun, *La sainte et la cité: Micheline de Pesaro (1356) Tertiaire Franciscaine* (Rome: École Française de Rome, 1992).

2. For the importance of the timing of Delphine's inquest, see Marthe Dulong, "Les dernières années de sainte Delphine à Apt d'après les procès de canonisation," *Provence Historique* 6, special number (1956): 132–138. This summary is based on her 1928 dissertation at the École des Chartres.

3. For an example of events where stories could be shared, see Michel Hébert, "Du village à l'état: Les assemblées locales en Provence aux XIVe et XVe siècles," in *La société rural et les institutions gouvernementales au Moyen Âge*, ed. John Drendel, (Montréal: Éditions CERES, 1995), 103–116. See also Louis Stouff and Noël Coulet, "Les institutions communales dans les villages de Provence au bas Moyen Âge," *Études rurales* 63 / 64 (1976): 67–81.

4. For an example of this approach, see Robert Bartlett, *The Hanged Man: A Story of Miracle, Memory, and Colonialism in the Middle Ages* (Princeton, NJ: Princeton University Press, 2004).

5. For a broader time span in Avignon, the seat of the papacy for most of the fourteenth century, see Jacques Chiffoleau, *La comptabilité de l'au-dela: Les hommes, la mort et la religion dans la région d'Avignon à la fin du Moyen Âge* (Rome: École Français de Rome, 1980).

6. On a theoretical level, this approach is deeply indebted to Erving Goffman, *Frame Analysis: An Essay on the Organization of Experience* (Boston: Northeastern University Press, 1974; see pages 9–11 for his essential approach. Goffman's concept of frame, similar to what historians often call context, is not static background information

but the dynamic, story- and ritual-based relationships each witness had in their time and place.

7. Jon Arrizabalaga, "Facing the Black Death: Perceptions and Reactions of University Medical Practitioners," in *Practical Medicine from Salerno to the Black Death*, ed. Luis Garcia-Ballester et al. (Cambridge: Cambridge University Press, 1994), 237–239.

8. Monica Green, editor's introduction to "Pandemic Disease in the Medieval World: Rethinking the Black Death," *Medieval Globe* 1 (2014): 9.

9. For reactions to plague in southern Europe, see Geneviève Dumas, *Santé et société à Montpellier à la fin du Moyen Âge* (Leiden: Brill, 2015), 303–329; Arrizabalaga, "Facing the Black Death," 237–288. For plague treatises in southern Europe, see Susan Einbinder, *After the Black Death: Plague and Commemoration among Iberian Jews* (Philadelphia: University of Pennsylvania Press, 2018), 57–87.

10. See the famous account by Gabriele de' Mussis, "Historia de Morbo," in *The Black Death*, ed. Rosemary Horrox (Manchester, UK: Manchester University Press, 1994), 14–26.

11. Ann Carmichael, "Universal and Particular: The Language of Plague, 1348–1500," in *Pestilential Complexities: Understanding Medieval Plague*, ed. Vivian Nutton (London: Wellcome Trust Centre for the History of Medicine, 2008), 17–52; Gabriele Zanella, "La peste del 1348: Italia, Francia, et Germania," in *La Peste Nera: Dati di una realtà et elementi di una interpretazione* (Spoleto: Centro Italiano de Studi sull'alto Medio, 1994), 49–135.

12. Richard Emery, "The Black Death of 1348 in Perpignan," *Speculum* 42 (1967): 611–623.

13. Daniel Lord Smail, "Accommodating Plague in Medieval Marseille," *Continuity and Change* 11 (1996): 11–41; Shona Kelly Wray, *Communities and Crisis: Bologna during the Black Death* (Leiden: Brill, 2009), 45–57.

14. Arrizabalaga, "Facing the Black Death," 237–288; Nicole Archambeau, "Healing Options during the Plague: Survivor Stories from a Fourteenth-Century Canonization Inquest," *Bulletin of the History of Medicine* 85 (2011): 531–59.

15. Philippe Contamine, *La vie quotidienne pendant la Guerre de Cent Ans: France et Angleterre, XIVe siècle* (New York: Hachette, 1978). For a study centering on the interplay of war and plague, see William Caferro, *Petrarch's War: Florence and the Black Death in Context* (Cambridge: Cambridge University Press, 2018), 8.

16. Kelly Devries, "Medieval Mercenaries: Methodology, Definitions, and Problems," in *Mercenaries and Paid Men: The Mercenary Identity in the Middle Ages*, ed. John France (Leiden: Brill, 2008), 43–60.

17. Kenneth Fowler, *Medieval Mercenaries, vol 1, The Great Companies* (Hoboken: Wiley-Blackwell, 2001); Philippe Contamine, "Les companies d'aventure en France pendant la Guerre de Cent Ans," chap. 7 in *La France aux XIVe et XVe siècles: Hommes, mentalités, guerre et paix* (London: Variorum Reprints, 1981).

18. Kenneth Pennington, "Peace and Concord in Medieval Society and Thought," in *Peace and Concord*, ed. Francesco Borghesi (Cambridge: Cambridge University Press, forthcoming).

19. Contamine, *La vie quotidienne*, 42–46.

20. For the complexity of this process, which often reflected long-term processes as well as immediate response to attack, see Gabrielle Démians d'Archimbaud, "Archéologie et villages désertés en Provence résultats desfouilles," in *Village désertés et histoire*

économique, XIe–XVIIIe siècles (Paris: SEVPEN, 1965), 287–301. For the movement of religious communities inside city walls, see Noël Coulet, "Les mendiants à Aix-en-Provence, XIIIe–XVe siècle," *Cahiers de Fanjeaux* 44 (2009): 394–398.

21. Germain Butaud and Vincent Challet, "Guerre et transfert *intra muros* des monastères en Languedoc et en Comtat Venaissin (milieu XIVe–milieu XVe siècle)," *Cahiers de Fanjeaux* 44 (2009): 517–568.

22. For a broad economic view of mercenary impact, see Bruce Campbell, *The Great Transition: Climate, Disease, and Society in the Late-Medieval World* (Cambridge: Cambridge University Press, 2016), 267–277.

23. Katherine Ludwig Jansen, *Peace and Penance in Late Medieval Italy* (Princeton, NJ: Princeton University Press, 2018), 15; Ottavia Niccoli, "Rinuncia, pace, perdono: Rituali di pacificazione della prima età moderna," *Studi Storici* 40 (1999): 219–261.

24. For an overview of this language in penitential literature of the later Middle Ages, see Nicole Bériou, "La confession dans les écrits théologiques et pastoraux du XIIIe siècle: Médication de l'âme ou démarche judiciaire?," in *L'aveu: Antiquité et Moyen Âge*, ed. Jean-Claude Maire Vigueur (Rome: École Française de Rome, 1986), 261–282. See also the collected essays in Leonard Boyle, *Pastoral Care, Clerical Education, and Canon Law, 1200–1400* (London: Variorum Reprints, 1981). For other kinds of literature that use this concept, see Na'ama Cohen-Hanegbi, *Caring for the Living Soul: Emotions, Medicine, and Penance in the Late Medieval Mediterranean* (Leiden: Brill, 2017). For the scholastic shaping of sin, see Eileen Sweeney, "Aquinas on the Seven Deadly Sins: Tradition and Innovation," in *Sin in Medieval and Early Modern Culture: The Tradition of the Seven Deadly Sins*, ed. Richard Newhauser and Susan Ridyard (York: York Medieval Press, 2012), 85–106.

25. For an overview of the importance of peacefulness and health and its spread in Italy via Franciscan preaching, see Jansen, *Peace and Penance*, 3–5, 9–14.

26. Jacme d'Agramont quoted in Arrizabalaga, "Facing the Black Death," 245. According to Arrizabalaga, Gentile of Foligno's treatise shared this view.

27. Roberto Rusconi, "De la prédication à la confession: Transmission et contrôle de modèles de comportement au XIIIe siècle," in *Faire croire: Modalités de la diffusion et de la réception des messages religieux du XIIe au XVe siècle* (Rome: École Française de Rome, 1981), 67–85; Joseph Goering, "The Internal Forum and the Literature of Penance and Confession," *Traditio* 59 (2004): 175–227.

28. For an overview, see Dennis Martin, "Popular and Monastic Pastoral Issues in the Later Middle Ages," *Church History* 56 (1987): 320–332. For the emergence of this expectation of transformation, see Bériou, "La confession dans les écrits théologique et pastoraux," 266. See also Thomas Tentler, *Sin and Confession on the Eve of the Reformation* (Princeton, NJ: Princeton University Press, 1977), 12–13; Anne Thayer, *Penitence, Preaching, and the Coming of the Reformation* (Aldershot: Ashgate, 2002), 1–6.

29. Campbell, *The Great Transition*, 2.

30. For this inquest, see the critical edition by Jacques Cambell, *Enquête pour le procès de canonisation de Dauphine de Puymichel Comtesse d'Ariano* (Turin: Bottega d'Erasmo, 1978). Cambell used two main copies of Delphine's inquest, including the Bibliothèque Méjanes, MS 335 in Aix-en-Provence, France, and what was then St. Leonard College Library, MS 1 in Dayton, Ohio.See Cambell, *Enquête*, xx–xxii. I have used the Bibliothèque Méjanes manuscript to check certain words and phrases used in witness testimonies. Page references in this book will refer to Cambell's critical edition, as

is standard practice for those who use canonization inquest testimony as historical evidence.

31. This anonymous work became a historic monument in 1907. See Sandra Poëzévara and Yann Codou, *Saintetés Aptesiennes: Trésors, architecture et dévotions dans une cité épiscopal* (Apt: Ville d'Apt Éditions, 2019). Photograph taken by Dr. Yann Codou, included here with his permission.

32. See, for example, Sharon Farmer, *Surviving Poverty: Gender, Ideology, and the Daily Lives of the Poor* (Ithaca, NY: Cornell University Press, 2002). She uses miracles collected for King Louis IX to explore the lives of poor men and women in Paris. Didier Lett, *Un procès de canonisation au Moyen Âge: Essai d'histoire sociale, Nicolas de Tolentino, 1325* (Paris: Presses Universitaires de France, 2008), uses the canonization inquest for Nicolas of Tolentino for a similar process. Gérard Veyssière, *Vivre en Provence au XIVe siècle* (Paris: Éditions d'Harmattan, 1998), uses three canonization inquests, including Delphine's, to consider aspects of social and cultural history in Provence.

33. For an example of a similar approach, see Laura Smoller, *The Saint and the Chopped-Up Baby: The Cult of Vincent Ferrer in Medieval and Early Modern Europe* (Ithaca, NY: Cornell University Press, 2014). See also Aviad Kleinberg, *Prophets in Their Own Country: Living Saints and the Making of Sainthood in the Later Middle Ages* (Chicago: University of Chicago Press, 1992), 1–20.

34. The history of this belief goes back almost to the beginning of Christianity. See Peter Brown, *The Cult of the Saints: Its Rise and Function in Latin Christianity* (Chicago: University of Chicago Press, 1981). For a more recent overview, see Robert Bartlett, *Why Can the Dead Do Such Great Things? Saints and Worshippers from the Martyrs to the Reformation* (Princeton, NJ: Princeton University Press, 2013), 3–26.

35. For the great diversity of miracle forms and practices, see Pierre-Andre Sigal, *L'homme et le miracle dans la France médiéval (XIe–XIIe siècle)* (Paris: Les Éditions du CERF, 1985), 32. For adaptation in the longer term, see Chiffoleau, *La comptabilité*, 217–233.

36. The papal curia made significant efforts to assess witness testimony based on their own criteria. For an overview of this process, see Gâbor Klaniczay, "The Inquisition of Miracles in Medieval Canonization Processes," in *Miracles in Medieval Canonization Processes: Structures, Functions, and Methodologies*, ed. Christian Krötzl and Sari Katajala-Peltomaa (Turnhout: Brepols, 2018), 43–73.

37. Elinor Ochs and Lisa Capps, *Living Narrative: Creating Lives in Everyday Storytelling* (Cambridge, MA: Harvard University Press, 2001), 45.

38. For an approach to using witness testimony to understand the moral worldview of witnesses, see Susan Alice McDonough, *Witnesses, Neighbors, and Community in Late Medieval Marseille* (New York: Palgrave Macmillan, 2013), 4–5.

39. Arthur Kleinman, *The Illness Narratives: Suffering, Healing, and the Human Condition* (New York: Basic Books, 1988), 5.

40. John Arnold, "Inside and Outside the Medieval Laity: Some Reflections on the History of Emotions," in *European Religious Cultures: Essays Offered to Christopher Brooke on the Occasion of His Eightieth Birthday*, ed. Miri Rubin (London: Institute of Historical Research, 2008), 123. See also Edward Peters, "*Vir inconstans*: Moral Theology as Paleopsychology," in *In the Garden of Evil: The Vices and Culture in the Middle Ages*, ed. Richard Newhauser (Toronto: Pontifical Institute of Mediaeval Studies, 2005), 59–73. For a recent study, see Damien Boquet and Piroska Nagy, *Medieval*

Sensibilities: A History of Emotions in the Middle Ages (Medford, MA: Polity Press, 2018).

41. The word "emotion" was not used in the fourteenth century, but will be used here to fit my research more clearly into the historical study of emotion. For a discussion of English emotion terms in relation to Romance languages, see Barbara Rosenwein, "Emotion Words," in *Le sujet des émotions au Moyen Âge*, ed. Piroska Nagy and Damien Boquet (Paris: Éditions Beauchesne, 2009), 93–106. For an anthropological exploration of political emotion contextualized in specific situations, see Catherine Lutz and Lila Abu-Lughod, "Introduction: Emotion, Discourse, and the Politics of Everyday Life," in *Language and the Politics of Emotion*, ed. Catherine Lutz and Lila Abu-Lughod (Cambridge: Cambridge University Press, 1990), 1–23.

42. See Frederick Cheyette, *Ermengarde of Narbonne and the World of the Troubadours* (Ithaca, NY: Cornell University Press, 2001). Witnesses had a different perspective than those encountered in other kinds of legal sources. See Richard Barton, "'Zealous Anger' and the Renegotiation of Aristocratic Relationships in Eleventh- and Twelfth-Century France," in *Anger's Past: The Social Uses of an Emotion in the Middle Ages*, ed. Barbara Rosenwein (Ithaca, NY: Cornell University Press, 1998), 153–170; Daniel Lord Smail, "Hatred as a Social Institution in Late-Medieval Society," *Speculum* 76 (2001): 90–126.

43. For an article that looks at a specific historical moment for emotional reaction, see Jeroen Deploige, "Meurtre politique, émotions collectives et catharsis littéraire: Guibert de Nogent et Galbert de Bruges faces aux révolts urbaines de Laon (1111–1112) et de Bruges (1127–1128)," in *Politiques des émotions au Moyen Âge*, ed. Damien Boquet and Piroska Nagy (Florence: Sismel, 2010), 225–254.

44. For an anthropological exploration of difficult emotions, see Byron Good and Arthur Kleinman, eds., *Culture and Depression: Studies in Anthropology and Cross-Cultural Psychiatry of Affect and Disorder* (Berkeley: University of California Press, 1985). For a modern ethnographical approach to emotion, see John Leavitt, "Meaning and Feeling in the Anthropology of Emotions," *American Ethnologist* 23, no. 3 (1996): 514–539.

45. Ruth Harvey, *The Inward Wits: Psychological Theory in the Middle Ages and the Renaissance* (London: Warburg Institute, 1975); Luis Garcia-Ballester, "Changes in the *Regimina Sanitatis*: The Role of the Jewish Physicians," in *Health, Disease, and Healing in Medieval Culture*, ed. Sheila Campbell, Bert Hall, and David Klausner (New York: St. Martin's Press, 1992), 119–131.

46. Goering, "The Internal Forum," 175–227.

47. See Arnold, "Inside and Outside the Medieval Laity," 107–130. See also Jeroen Deploige, "Studying Emotions: The Medievalist as Human Scientist?," in *Emotions in the Heart of the City (14th–16th Century)*, ed. Anne Van Bruaene (Turnhout: Brepols, 2005), 22.

48. Carolyn Walker Bynum, "Did the Twelfth Century Discover the Individual?," *Journal of Ecclesiastical History* 31 (1980): 1–17. For an exploration of the internal self in Wycliffite literature, see Katherine Little, *Confession and Resistance: Defining the Self in Late Medieval England* (South Bend, IN: University of Notre Dame Press, 2006), 49–77.

49. For example, very few artisans testified in this inquest, unlike other inquests in Provence. See for example the witnesses to miracles in the canonization of Louis of Anjou in "Processus Canonizationis et Legendae variae Sancti Ludovici O.F.M.," in *Analecta Franciscana*, vol. 7 (Florence: Ad Claras Aquas, 1951), 122–256.

50. For an overview of some of Delphine's witnesses, see Veyssière, *Vivre en Provence*, 28; Paul Amargier, "Dauphine de Puymichel et son entourage au temps de sa vie Aptésienne (1345–1360)," in *Le peuple des saints: Croyances et dèvotions en Provence et Comtat Venaissin à la fin du Moyen Âge* (Avignon: Institut de Recherches et d'Études du Bas Moyen Âge Avignonnais, 1986), 111–123. See also Pierre-André Sigal, "Les temoins et les temoignages au procès de canonisation de Dauphine de Puimichel (1363)," *Provence Historique* 195–196 (1999): 461–471. See also André Vauchez, "La religion populaire dans la France Méridionale au XIVe siècle d'après les procès de canonisation," in *La religion populaire en Languedoc du XIIIe siècle à la moitié du XIVe siècle* (Toulouse: Édouard Privat, 1976), 91–108. For an overview of Delphine's witnesses and miracles, see Dulong, "Les dernières années de sainte Delphine" 132–138.

51. Countess Delphine has been studied by many scholars, with a sample given here. For her saint's life, see Jacques Cambell, ed., *Vies Occitanes de Saint Auzias et de Sainte Dauphine*, vol. 12 (Rome: Pontificum Athenaeum Antonianum, 1963). For elements of her sanctity, see André Vauchez, "Two Laypersons in Search of Perfection: Elzear de Sabran and Delphine of Puimichel," in *The Laity in the Middle Ages: Religious Beliefs and Devotional Practices*, ed. Daniel Bornstein, trans. Margery Schneider (London: University of Notre Dame Press, 1993), 73–82; André Vauchez, "Aux originies de la 'Fama Sanctitatis' d'Elzear (d. 1323) et de Dauphine de Sabran (d. 1360): Le mariage virginal," in *Le peuple des saints: Croyances et dèvotions en Provence et Comtat Venaissin à la fin du Moyen Âge* (Avignon: Institut de Recherches et d'Études du Bas Moyen Âge Avignonnais, 1986), 153–166; Dyan Elliott, *Proving Woman: Female Spirituality and Inquisitional Culture in the Later Middle Ages* (Princeton, NJ: Princeton University Press, 2004). For her family relationships, see Florian Mazel, *La noblesse et l'Église en Provence, fin Xe–début XIVe siècle: L'exemple des familles d'Agoult-Simiane, de Baux et de Marseille* (Paris: Éditions du CTHS, 2002), 526–527; Georges Passerat, "Douceline, Delphine et les autres ou la sainteté feminine en Occitaine à la fin du Moyen Âge," *Bulletin de littérature ecclésiastique* 98 (1997): 235–250.Marthe Dulong, "Édition critique de la vie provençale de sainte Delphine et l'étude comparée jointe à la vie du procès de canonisation," (Doctoral dissertation, École des Chartres, 1928.)

52. See the collected essays in Noël Coulet and Jean-Michel Matz, eds., *La noblesse dans les territoires Angevins à la fin du Moyen Âge* (Rome: École Française de Rome, 2000). Ultimately Provence was under the control of the Holy Roman Emperors, but they had very little direct influence on Provence. See Jean Dunbabin, *Charles I of Anjou: Power, Kingship, and State-Making in Thirteenth-Century Europe* (London: Routledge, 1998).

53. The Angevin offshoot of the French royal family held a broad, discontiguous kingdom that included the kingdom of Hungary and regions of Greece. David Abulafia, *The Western Mediterranean Kingdoms, 1200–1500: The Struggle for Dominion* (London: Longman, 1997).

54. This phrase was used many times in the inquest. For a particularly dramatic example, see Cambell, *Enquête*, 534.

55. For their chaste marriage, see Rosalynn Voaden, "A Marriage Made for Heaven: The *Vies Occitan* of Elzear of Sabran and Delphine of Puimichel," in *Framing the Family: Narrative and Representation in the Medieval and Early Modern Periods*, ed. Rosalynn Voaden and Diane Wolfthal (Tempe: Arizona Center for Medieval and Renaissance Studies, 2005), 101–116. For Sanxia and Delphine in 1343, see Cristina Andenna, "Women at the Angevin Court between Naples and Provence: Sancia of Majorca,

Delphine of Puimichel, and the 'Struggle' for a Female Franciscan Life," in *Queens, Princesses and Mendicants: Close Relations in a European Perspective*, ed. Nikolas Jaspert and Imke Just (Zurich: LIT Verlag GmbH, 2019), 29–51; Cambell, *Enquête*, 541n2.

56. Michel Hébert, "La cristallisation d'une identité: Les États de Provence, 1347–1360," in *Événement, identité et histoire*, ed. Claire Dolan (Sillery: Les éditions du Septentrion, 1991), 151–164.

57. Gábor Klaniczay, *Holy Rulers and Blessed Princesses: Dynastic Cults in Medieval Central Europe*, trans. Éva Pálmai (Cambridge: Cambridge University Press 2002), 295–393.

58. These are what Goffman refers to as primary frameworks. See Goffman, *Frame Analysis*, 23–39.

59. Ochs and Capps, *Living Narrative*, 19–33. For a different approach to narrative, see Rachel Koopmans, *Wonderful to Relate: Miracle Stories and Miracle Collecting in High Medieval England* (Philadelphia: University of Pennsylvania Press, 2011).

60. For social and political ramifications of friendship and enmity, see Daniel Lord Smail, *The Consumption of Justice: Emotions, Publicity, and Legal Culture in Marseille, 1264–1423* (Ithaca, NY: Cornell University Press, 2003), 90–93.

61. Michael Goodich, "*Mirabilis Deus in sanctis suis*: Social History and Medieval Miracles," in *Signs, Wonders, Miracles: Representations of Divine Power in the Life of the Church*, ed. Kate Cooper and Jeremy Gregory (Woodbridge: Boydell Press, 2005), 135–156. Goodich addresses the issue of hindsight as a distortion of memory, 142.

62. For a discussion of identity and narrative, see K. Little, *Confession and Resistance*, 5–15.

63. For the sale of her goods, see Cambell, *Enquête*, 45–47, Articles 21–23. For an analysis, see Nicole Archambeau, "Remembering Delphine's Books: Reading as a Means to Shape a Holy Woman's Sanctity," in *Writing Medieval Women's Lives*, ed. Amy Livingstone and Charlotte Newman Goldy (New York: Palgrave, 2013), 33–49.

64. André Vauchez, *Sainthood and the Later Middle Ages*, trans. Jean Birrell (Cambridge: Cambridge University Press, 1997), 74–84. For an extensive overview, see Thomas Wetzstein, *Heilige vor Gericht: Das Kanonisationsverfahren im europäischen Spätmittelalter* (Cologne: Böhlau, 2004). For a synthetic overview, see Katajala-Peltomaa and Krötzl, "Approaching Twelfth- to Fifteenth-Century Miracles," 1–39.

65. Krötzl and Katajala-Peltomaa, "Approaching Twelfth- to Fifteenth-Century Miracles," 23.

66. Krötzl and Katajala-Peltomaa, "Approaching Twelfth- to Fifteenth-Century Miracles," 22.

67. For a summary of these different formats, see Krötzl and Katajala-Peltomaa, "Approaching Twelfth- to Fifteenth-Century Miracles," 20. Having the notarial records of the hearings *in partibus*, as we do for Delphine's inquest, means we have the fullest record of what witnesses said that would have been produced at the time.

68. Krötzl and Katajala-Peltomaa, "Approaching Twelfth- to Fifteenth-Century Miracles," 6.

69. Cambell, *Enquête*, 1.

70. Cambell, *Enquête*, 1–30, 102. For the convening of the commissioners in the Franciscan church in Apt, see Cambell, *Enquête*, 14.

71. Abbé Elzear Boze, *Histoire de l'église d'Apt* (Apt: Jh. Trémollière, Imprimeur-Libraire, 1820), 248–250, places the entire inquest in the Franciscan church. But the summary letter of the commissioners' actions while in Apt stated that they heard the

witnesses and then went to the Franciscan church in order to see activity at Delphine's tomb (Cambell, *Enquête*, 109). This suggests that they did not interview witnesses there.

72. Cambell, *Enquête*, 109.

73. For the letter instating Master Nicolau and outlining his duties, see Cambell, *Enquête*, 29–30. For an overview of the training and duties of a fourteenth-century proctor, see James Brundage, *The Medieval Origins of the Legal Profession: Canonists, Civilians, and Courts* (Chicago: University of Chicago Press, 2008), 353–365.

74. See Jacques Cambell, "Le sommaire de l'enquête pour la canonisation de S. Elzear de Sabran, TOF (d. 1323)," *Miscellanea Franciscana* 73 (1973): 438–473.

75. Nicole Archambeau, "'His Whole Heart Changed': Political Uses of a Mercenary's Emotional Transformation," *Micrologus* 34 (2010): 196.

76. This process will be discussed in chapter 3.

77. Krötzl and Katajala-Peltomaa, "Approaching Twelfth- to Fifteenth-Century Miracles," 21.

78. "Processus Canonizationis et Legendae variae Sancti Ludovici O.F.M.," in *Analecta Franciscana*, vol. 7 (Florence: Ad Claras Aquas, 1951), xliii.

79. Of the sixty-eight witnesses, forty were described as hearing the articles and testifying in the vulgar tongue, their *lingua materna*, or *romansio*. The terms are at times used together. For example, Monna Beesa is described as speaking "lingua materna expositio ac vulgarisato in romansio." See Cambell, *Enquête*, 456.

80. See for example the testimony of Margarita Sicard, Cambell, *Enquête*, 503–504.

81. Laura Smoller, "Miracle, Memory, and Meaning in the Canonization of Vincent Ferrer, 1453–1454," *Speculum* 73 (1998): 429–454.

82. For the credibility of miracles and testimony, see Michael Goodich, "Reason or Revelation? The Criteria for the Proof and Credibility of Miracles in Canonization Inquest Processes," in *Procès de canonisation au Moyen Âge: Aspects juridiques et religieux*, ed. Gábor Klaniczay (Rome: École Française de Rome, 2004), 181–197.

83. This is not to say that the testimonies leave the narrative structures familiar to miracle stories, but instead that they described miracles that were not included in the official articles of interrogation. For miracle story structure, see, among others, Koopmans, *Wonderful to Relate*, 1–8.

84. See Cambell, *Enquête*, 29. Commissioners asked these questions of both eyewitnesses and witnesses who heard about events from others. For those who heard about events, they were asked where and when they heard and who was present when they heard. For the standard questioning procedure in a canonization inquest, see Krötzl and Katajala-Peltomaa, "Approaches to Twelfth- to Fifteenth-Century Miracles," 22.

85. As we will see in later chapters, this did not seem to be a hostile tactic, but a reassuring one. Several witnesses, including Catherine de Pui who told such engaging stories to the commissioners, reveal significantly more information after being urged with questions. See Cambell, *Enquête*, 386–410, for examples from Catherine de Pui's testimony.

86. Cambell, *Enquête*, 29: "Et series testimonii et verba testis cuiuslibet plene et distincte fideliter redigantur in scriptis."

87. I did not include in this number witnesses who spoke to either Article 1 or Article 35 because these witnesses tended to speak about many different issues under the umbrella of these general articles.

88. Cambell, *Enquête*, 467.

89. Cambell, *Enquête*, 478.

90. See Cambell, *Enquête*, 421–424.

91. For Francisca Bot's testimony, see Cambell, *Enquête*, 425–428. For Ysoarda Laugier's testimony, see Cambell, *Enquête*, 428.

92. For Alazays Mesellano's testimony, see Cambell, *Enquête*, 429–442.

93. The information that follows is a summary of Cambell, *Enquête*, 131–134.

94. Cambell, *Enquête*, 132: Lord Peire Audenque,* canon and *precentor*; Durand Andree* and Peire de Sancta Maria, canons; Lord Aycard Bot,* Giraud de Fonte, *beneficiati*, and other chaplains and beneficed clerics of the bishop's church and others making their personal residence there; and religious men, brother Jacme Bot, *vicarious* and brother Arnau Garnier, *lector*; Bertran Nicolau et Raymon Fresquet, in the house of the order of Minors in Apt; the noble and *circumspectis* man, Lord Peire de Montilio, legal professional, bailie, and judge in the curia of Apt; Johan Autrici, syndic of the city of Apt; Raybaud St. Mitri,* Raymon Olerii, Uguo de Salice, magister Johan Gale,* Guilhem de Mediolano, Iacob Cariloci, Raybaud Pinholi, councilors of the city; other nobles Theobald Bot, Franses Bassauna, Laugier de Gorda, et Savaric Bot,* and others of the city; and indeed so many clerics and lay people, men and women, of the city of Apt and surroundings, that the crowd seemed to number four thousand or more (asterisks indicate witnesses in the inquest).

95. This would have been Raymon Savini, bishop from 1362 to 1382. Joseph-Hyancinth Albanés, *Gallia Christiana Novissima: Histoire des archevèchés, évèchés, et abbayes de France*, vol. 1 (Montbéliard: Société Anonyme d'Imprimerie Montbéliardaise, 1899), columns 255–256.

96. Cambell, *Enquête*, 133.

97. Cambell, *Enquête*, 134: "pro maiori parte manus elevaverunt et extenderunt versus altare dicte ecclesie." It is unclear why some people chose not to participate, but it may reveal potential disagreement within the community or simply that some people had not heard of Delphine.

98. Cambell, *Enquête*, 14–16, 546–548.

99. This was typical procedure by the fourteenth century. See Vauchez, *Sainthood*, 45–46.

100. My understanding is influenced here by the dimensional approach to narrative in Ochs and Capps, *Living Narrative*, 18–19.

101. For the original study of the "danger of death story," see William Labov, "The Transformation of Experience in Narrative Syntax," in *Language in the Inner City: Studies in the Black English Vernacular* (Philadelphia: University of Pennsylvania Press, 1972), 354–396.

102. Elinor Ochs and Lisa Capps, "Narrating the Self," *Annual Review of Anthropology* 25 (1996): 19–43.

103. Ochs and Capps, *Living Narrative*, 45–54.

104. This approach is inspired by Barbara Rosenwein, *Emotional Communities in the Early Middle Ages* (Ithaca, NY: Cornell University Press, 2006), 25–26.

105. For a well-known presentation of the fourteenth century as an irrational moment, see Johan Huizinga, *The Autumn of the Middle Ages*, trans. Rodney J. Payton and Ulrich Mammitzsch, (Chicago: University of Chicago Press, 1996).

1. Bertranda Bertomieua and the Death of King Robert of Naples

1. Noël Coulet, *Aix-en-Provence: Espace et relations d'une capitale (milieu XIVe s.–milieu XVe s.)* (Aix-en-Provence: Publications de l'Université de Provence, 1988), 60–78.

2. André Vauchez, "The Virginal Marriage of Elzear and Delphine," in *The Laity in the Middle Ages: Religious Beliefs and Devotional Practices*, ed. Daniel Bornstein, trans. Margery Schneider (London: University of Notre Dame Press, 1993), 191–203; Dyan Elliott, *Spiritual Marriage: Sexual Abstinence in Medieval Wedlock* (Princeton, NJ: Princeton University Press, 1993), 219.

3. R. Voaden, "A Marriage Made for Heaven," especially 104–106. See Cambell, *Vies Occitan*.

4. Lady Catherine de Pui is the only witness who calls her Lady Bertranda. For example, see Cambell, *Enquête*, 396. Friar Giraud Raybaud identifies her as coming from Puimichel; Cambell, *Enquête*, 174.

5. Theresa Earenfight, *Queenship in Medieval Europe* (London: Palgrave Macmillan, 2013).

6. Goodich, "*Mirabilis Deus in Sanctis Suis*," 135–156, 143–144; Smoller, "Miracle, Memory, and Meaning," 429–454.

7. Klaniczay, *Holy Rulers and Blessed Princesses*, 297.

8. Elizabeth Casteen, *From She-Wolf to Martyr: The Reign and Disputed Reputation of Johanna of Naples* (Ithaca, NY: Cornell University Press, 2015), 156–195.

9. The questions took many forms, but were common to inquest procedure. See Brundage, *The Medieval Origins of the Legal Profession*, 365–370.

10. For inquest questions, see Jacques Paul, "Expression et perception du temps d'après l'enquête sur le miracles de Louis d'Anjou," in *Temps, memoire, tradition au Moyen Âge*, ed. Bernard Guillemain (Aix-en-Provence: Université de Provence, 1983), 19–42.

11. For an analysis of how Bertranda and others used the phrase "first mortality," see Nicole Archambeau, "The 'First Mortality' as a Time Marker in 14th-Century Provence," in *Viral Networks: Connecting Digital Humanities and Medical History*, ed. E. Thomas Ewing and Katherine Randall (Blacksburg, VA: VT Publishing, 2018), 157–184.

12. Leif Søndergaard, "Imagining Plague: The Black Death in Medieval Mentalities," in *Living with the Black Death*, ed. Lars Bisgaard (Gylling: University of Southern Denmark, 2009), 207–233.

13. Cambell, *Enquête*, 306–307.

14. Cambell, *Enquête*, 326–327.

15. For an overview of political changes at this moment, see Charles M. de la Roncière, "L'état Angevin 1265–1340: Pouvoirs et sociétés dans le Royaume et le Comté, Bilan d'un colloque," in *L'état Angevin: Pouvoir, culture, et société entre XIIIe et XIVe siècle* (Rome: École Française de Rome, 1998), 661–664. For a sense that 1343 was a moment of change, see Gérard Giordanengo, "*Arma legesque colo*: L'état et le droit en Provence (1246–1343)," in *La noblesse dans les territoires Angevins à la fin du Moyen Âge*, ed. Noël Coulet and Jean-Michel Matz (Rome: École Français de Rome, 2000), 35–80. For changes before King Robert's death, see, in the same volume, Florian Mazel, "La

noblesse Provençal face à la justice souveraine (1245–1320): L'âge du pragmatism," 343–370.

16. John Watts, *The Making of Polities, 1300–1500* (Cambridge: Cambridge University Press, 2009). For fourteenth-century Provence, see Justine Firnhaber-Baker, "Techniques of Seigneurial War in the Fourteenth Century," *Journal of Medieval History* 36 (2010): 90–103. For an earlier time period, see Cheyette, *Ermengard of Narbonne*, 199–220.

17. Others in Provence marked King Robert's death as a moment of change. For example, see the anonymous poem "Glorios Dieus don totz ben ha creysensa," in *Poesie Provenzali storiche relative all'Italia*, vol. 2, ed. Vincenzo de Bartholomaeis (Rome: Botega d'Erasmo, 1931), 316–317. For an analysis of this poem, see Jean-Paul Boyer and Thierry Pécout, introduction to *La Provence et Fréjus sous la première maison d'Anjou (1246–1382)*, ed. Boyer and Pécout (Aix-en-Provence: Publications de l'Université de Provence, 2010), 11–12.

18. Hébert, "La cristallisation d'une identité," 151–164; John Drendel, "The Institutions of Village Government in Later Medieval Provence and the Origins of the Council of Trets," *Historical Reflections/Réflexions Historiques* 19 (1993): 249–266.

19. For a family tree, see Mazel, *La nobless et l'Église*, 615.

20. Other options certainly existed, especially among his daughters and their children, who included Margaret (married to Charles of Valois), Blanche (queen consort to James II of Aragon), and Eleanor (queen consort to Frederick III of Sicily).

21. This was his son Charles, who married Marie of Valois (a sister of King Philip VI of France). See Casteen, *From She-Wolf to Martyr*, 2–6.

22. See Samantha Kelly, *The New Solomon: Robert of Naples (1309–1343) and Fourteenth-Century Kingship* (Leiden: Brill 2003), 281–283.

23. For perceptions of King Robert of Naples, see Kelly, *The New Solomon*. Not all chroniclers agreed, however. For another view of this moment of transition, see Casteen, *From She-Wolf to Martyr*, 30–35. Other historians also see the cultural transition as less abrupt; see Isabelle Heullant-Donat, "Quelques réflexions autour de la cour angevine comme milieu culturel au XIVe siècle," in Roncière, *L'état Angevin*, 173–191.

24. Émile-Guillaume Léonard, *Histoire de Jeanne 1re, reine de Naples, comtesse de Provence (1343–1382)*, 3 vols. (Monaco: Imprimerie de Monaco, 1936), 1:214–215. For a brief overview of Cabassole's life, see Victor Saxer, "Philippe Cabassole et son *Libellus hystorialis Marie beatissime Magdalene," in L'état Angevin: Pouvoir, culture, et société entre XIIIe et XIVe siècles*, (Rome: École de Française de Rome, 1998) 193–204. By 1363, Philippe Cabassole would be a cardinal and the titular patriarch of Jerusalem.

25. See Léonard, *Histoire*, 1:220–224.

26. Norman Zacour, "Talleyrand: The Cardinal of Périgord (1301–1364)," *Transactions of the American Philosophical Society* 50 (1960): 31–42; Albano Sorbelli, ed., *Domenico de Gravina, notarii, Chronicon de rebus in Apulia gestis (aa. 1333–1350)* (Città de Castello: Tipi dell'Editore S. Lapi, 1903), 10, "agniculus inter lupos."

27. Cardinal Talleyrand of Périgord was close to the papacy and a diplomat during the Hundred Years War. Zacour, "Talleyrand," 43–63.

28. Émile-Guillaume Léonard, *Les Angevins de Naples* (Paris: Presses Universitaires de France, 1954), 342–345.

29. Klaniczay, *Holy Rulers and Blessed Princesses*, 333–335.

30. Catherine of Valois was the titular Empress of Constantinople, a half-sister of Philip VI of France, and the regent of her son, Robert of Taranto, in the Principality of Achaea (which included parts of what is now Greece).

31. Johanna's grandmother was Robert's first wife, Yolanda of Aragon, who died in 1302. See Casteen, *From She-Wolf to Martyr*, xii.

32. Caroline Bruzelius, "Queen Sancia of Mallorca and the Convent Church of Sta. Chiara in Naples," *Memoirs of the American Academy in Rome* 40 (1995): 69–100. See pages 72–78 for Sanxia's role in its founding. For Robert's tomb, see Darleen Pryds, *The King Embodies the Word: Robert d'Anjou and the Politics of Preaching* (Leiden: Brill, 2000), 32.

33. For the impact of the bombing and responses of historians, see Roncière, "L'état Angevin 1265–1340," 650.

34. For an in-depth assessment of depictions of Queen Johanna in chronicles and other sources at this time, see Casteen, *From She-Wolf to Martyr*, 37–66. For an assessment of evidence from chronicles and sources that emphasized Provençal interests, see Léonard, *Angevins*, 347–349. They both provide a thoughtful statement about their approach to the many chronicle accounts.

35. Léonard, *Angevins*, 346. For an overview of chronicle accounts, see Léonard, *Histoire*, 1:470–473. Léonard built this account primarily from the chronicle of Domenico of Gravina. Perhaps the best known account for modern scholars is that of the famous Florentine chronicler, Giovanni Villani, who claimed to have spoken to Andrew's bailiff, who accused Queen Johanna of being part of the assassination. See Rala I. Diakité and Matthew Sneider, eds. *The Final Book of Giovanni Villani's New Chronicle* (Kalamazoo: Medieval Institute Publications, 2016), 97–100. A lesser known account from Provence appears in the chronicle of the venerable abbey of S. Victor in Marseille. Interestingly, this account did not record the death of King Robert in 1343, but did record the assassination of Andrew of Hungary in 1345. The anonymous chronicler did not speculate about the perpetrators, saying only that Andrew was killed "per suos in Aversa civitate." See George Pertz, ed., *Annales S. Victoris Massiliensis*, MGH SS 23 (Hannover, 1924), 6.

36. Léonard, *Histoire*, 1:479, remarks on the strange tone of the official letter that appears to partially blame Andrew for his own murder.

37. Casteen, *From She-Wolf to Martyr*, 47.

38. For a deeper analysis of this event, see Casteen, *From She-Wolf to Martyr*, 29–66.

39. Although her older son, Robert, who was ruling the Principality of Achaea at this time, also wished to marry Johanna, Catherine supported her younger son, Louis. See Léonard, *Angevins*, 347. Robert soon after married an heiress of Bohemia and no longer opposed Louis.

40. The initial investigation was mainly carried out by Charles of Artus, King Robert's bastard son and Count of Saint Agata. See Léonard, *Angevins*, 335.

41. Léonard, *Histoire*, 2:1–5.

42. Léonard, *Histoire*, 1:514, "que salutem animarum ipsorum respiciunt." For the beginning of the pope's inquest, see Léonard, *Histoire*, 1:533–534.

43. Uguo de Baux was well connected to the court of Naples, and his family was linked to the royal line. See Mazel, *La noblesse et l'Église*, 55, 280, 628–629. See also

Jean-Paul Boyer, "Les Baux et le modèle royal: Une oraison funèbre de Jean Regina de Naples (1334)," *Provence Historique* 181 (1995): 447–450.

44. Casteen, *From She-Wolf to Martyr*, 52.

45. Léonard, *Histoire*, 1:680–682. Louis's older brother, Robert, at first a rival for Johanna's hand, became a support after he negotiated a favorable marriage.

46. Léonard, *Histoire*, 1:645–649.

47. Léonard, *Histoire*, 1:680–682.

48. Cambell, *Enquête*, 304: "iurataque ad sancta Dei ewangelia puram, meram, et plenam dicere et deponere veritatem quam sciverit super articulis infrascriptis."

49. Cambell, *Enquête*, 304: "Et primo, super primo articulo . . . eidem testi loquenti lecto et de verbo ad verbum exposito et vulgarizato lingua materna."

50. Some of the local words and phrases did not translate well and were left in Provençal.

51. Cambell, *Enquête*, 304: "Interrogata quomodo scit quod fuerit reputacio et publica vox et fama, etc., ut in articulo continentur et prout deposuit."

52. For a discussion of narrative genres surrounding sainthood, see Gábor Klaniczay, "Hagiography and Historical Narrative," in *Chronicon: Medieval Narrative Sources*, ed. Janos Bak and Ivan Jurkovic (Leiden: Brepols, 2013), 111–118. See also Koopmans, *Wonderful to Relate*, 1–8.

53. For a description of the process, see Anders Frömark, "Telling the Miracle: The Meeting between Pilgrim and Scribe as Reflected in Swedish Miracle Collections," in *Miracles in Medieval Canonization Processes*, ed. Christian Krötzl and Sari Katajala-Peltomaa (Turnhout: Brepols, 2018), 131–155.

54. Michael Goodich, introduction to *Voices from the Bench: The Narratives of Lesser Folk in Medieval Trials*, ed. Michael Goodich (New York: Palgrave Macmillan, 2006), 1–13. For a comparison of canonization inquest testimony with other kinds of testimony, see Elliott, *Proving Woman*, 119–179.

55. Michael Richter, "The Search for Spoken Language in Medieval Texts: Mission Impossible? The Case of Italy in the Ninth Century," in *La fabrique du signe: Linguistique de l'émergence entre micro- et macro-structures*, ed. Michel Banniard and Dennis Philps (Toulouse: Presses Universitaires du Mirail, 2010), 106–113.

56. For an overview of narrative qualities, see Ochs and Capps, *Living Narrative*, 2–6.

57. For example, Robert and Sanxia were with Delphine in Avignon when Elzear died in Paris, while negotiating Robert's son's marriage. The royal couple witnessed Delphine's wondrous knowledge that Elzear had died and helped her through her year of grieving. Cambell, *Enquête*, 42–43. For Elzear's death, see Cambell, *Vies Occitan*, 179–183.

58. Cambell, *Enquête*, 307: "dominam Iohannam de Meleto, familiarem et servitricem domine regine Sanxie, gravi infirmitate febris detentam, ita quod, ut dici audivit, non sperabatur de vita ipsius uixta relacionem medicorum. Et dicta domina Dalphina visitavit et tetigit ipsam cum manu sua; et eadem nocte dimisit eam febris, et post, infra tres dies, ivit ad palacium sana et incolumis, ut ab eadem Iohanna audivit dici post aliquod tempus. Et eciam audivit dici a quadam, vocata Almodia, familiari dicte domine regine, idem, videlicet quod post tactum et visitacionem dicte domine Dalphine predicta domina Iohanna curata fuerat; et iverat ad palacium regium predictum."

59. Cambell, *Enquête*, 308: "Interrogata unde erat dicta Iohanna oriunda, dixit quod de Meleto, ducatus Calabrie."

60. Cambell, *Enquête*, 326: "Vidit eciam in civitate Neapolitana quadam vice quod, dum dicta domina Dalphina incederet per carrerias, quidam iuvenes—erant tunc de capella ducis Calabrie—derisiones intulerunt et fecerunt dicte domine Dalphine, audientes ipsam esse comitissam; et unus illorum interrogavit et dixit: 'que est ista bizoca?' et audiens que erat dicta domina comitissa, elevavit digitum, deridendo eam in comtemptum eius."

61. Cambell, *Enquête*, 327: "Interrogata de tempore, dixit quod illa que vidit in Neapoli, vidit sunt bene XX anni elapsi vel circa, ante obitum regis Roberti."

62. Andrée Courtemanche, "La rumeur de Manosque: Femmes et honneur au XIVe siècle," in *Normes et pouvoir à la fin du Moyen Âge*, ed. Marie-Claude Déprez-Masson (Montreal: CERES, 1989), 127.

63. Chris Wickham, "*Fama* and the Law in Twelfth-Century Tuscany," in *Fama: The Politics of Talk and Reputation in Medieval Europe*, ed. Thelma Fenster and Daniel Lord Smail (Ithaca, NY: Cornell University Press, 2003), 19. For the workings of *fama*, see also Steven Bednarski, *Curia: A Social History of a Provençal Criminal Court in the Fourteenth Century* (Montpellier: Presses Universitaire de la Méditerranée, 2013), 35.

64. In Bertranda's testimony, as in most others, this reads "quod de eis fuit et est commune dictum, communis opinion, assercio et reputacio ac publica vox et fama in partibus regni Sicilie et Provincie et in civitate Avinionis."

65. For the definition of *bizoca*, see Cambell, *Enquête*, 223n2. This is from the testimony of Friar Bertran Jusbert, one of Delphine's confessors in the last ten years of her life. He heard the story from Bertranda Bertomieua and verified it with Delphine in confession.

66. Cambell, *Enquête*, 56: "ipsa domina comitissa magnam familiaritatem haberet cum serenissima domina Sanxia, Ierusalem et Sicilie regina."

67. Cambell, *Enquête*, 532.

68. Margaret Toynbee, *S. Louis of Toulouse and the Process of Canonisation in the Fourteenth Century* (Manchester, UK: Manchester University Press, 1929), 161.

2. Bishop Philippe Cabassole and the "War of the Seneschals"

1. For the use of this term and a brief overview of the events and their implications, see Martin Aurell, Jean-Paul Boyer, and Noël Coulet, *La Provence au Moyen Âge* (Aix-en-Provence: Publications de l'Université de Provence, 2005), 278. See also Coulet, *Aix-en-Provence*, 59–67.

2. For the political centrality of Aix-en-Provence to Angevin governance, see Noël Coulet, "Aix, capitale de la Provence Angevine," in *L'état Angevin: Pouvoir, culture et société entre XIIIe et XIVe siècle* (Rome: École Française de Rome, 1998), 317–338.

3. Cambell, *Enquête*, 541: "nisi fecisset, fuisset, ut credit, magna divisio in Provincia et magna scandala et guerra."

4. For Enric's involvement, see Léon-Honoré Labande, ed., *Inventaire sommaire des archives communales antérieures à 1790*, Série BB, vol. 1 (Marseille: Imprimerie Moullot, 1909), p. 69, col. 1, Département des Bouches-du-Rhône, Ville de Marseille.

5. For Enric's history in law in Provence, see Fernand Cortez, *Les Grands Officiers Royaux de Provence au Moyen Âge* (Aix-en-Provence: Société d'Études Provençales, 1921), 240–241. For background on the *juge mage* of Provence, see Jean-Luc Bonnaud, "Les

juges mages du comté de Provence et de Forcalquier à la fin du Moyen Âge (XIIIe-XVe siècle)" in Riccardo Rao, ed. *Les grands officiers dans les territoires Angevins: I grandi ufficiali nei territori angioini,* (Rome: École Française de Rome, 2017), 189–206. See also Cortez, *Grands Officiers*, xii–xiii. Noël Coulet, "Un fragment de registre de la cour du juge mage de Provence à la fin du XIIIe siècle," in *La justice temporelle dans les territoires Angevins aux XIIIe et XVe siècles*, ed. Jean-Paul Boyer, Anne Mailloux, and Laure Verdon (Rome: École Française de Rome, 2005), 187–189.

6. See Alessandro Barbero, "Letteratura e politica fra Provenza e Napoli," in *L'état Angevin: Pouvoir, culture et société entre XIIIe et XIVe siècle* (Rome: École Française de Rome, 1998), 168–172.

7. I have estimated his age based on the events in which he participated. He did not state his age in his testimony.

8. Cambell, *Enquête*, 137.

9. Victor Saxer, "Philippe Cabassole et son *Libellus hystorialis Marie beatissime Magdalene*: Préliminaires à une édition du *Libellus*," in *L'état Angevin*, 193–194; Cortez, *Grands Officiers*, 211–212.

10. For an overview, see C. F. H. Barjavel's *Dictionnaire historique, biographique et bibliographique de Département de Vaucluse*, vol. 1 (Carpentras: de l. Devillario, 1841), 311–316. See also Ulysse Chevalier, *Réportoire des sources historiques de Moyen Âge: Bio-Bibliographie* (Paris: Librairie de la Société Bibliographique, 1877), vol. 1, col. 740; Cortez, *Grands Officiers*, 205–209. For Jean's role as a proctor for Louis of Anjou's canonization, see "Processus Canonizationis et Legendae variae Sancti Ludovici O.F.M.," 7:20.Toynbee does not mention him in her discussion of the proctors, however. See Toynbee, *S. Louis of Toulouse*, 157–158.

11. Germain Butaud, "Aperçus sur la coseigneurie en Comtat Venaissin (XIIe–XVe siècles)," *Mélanges de l'École française de Rome* 122 (2010): 63–87.

12. Cortez, *Grands Officiers*, 211; Saxer, "Philippe Cabassole et son *Libellus*," 193–194.

13. Before Cabassole's death in 1372, he would be named bishop of Marseille and made a cardinal by Pope Urban V. Although his final title was cardinal, I shall refer to him as bishop, since that is the title he held in 1363 when he testified. See Cortez, *Grands Officiers*, 112–113, 156–16, 205–212.

14. For a list of letters, see Ernest Wilkins, "Philippe de Cabassoles on Petrarch," *Speculum* 35 (1960): 69.

15. For example, see André Longpré, ed., *Pétrarque: Lettres familières*, vol. 4 (Paris: Les Belles Lettres, 2004), 56–59.

16. For Petrarch's friendship with Louis Heyligen, see Paul Amargier, "Pétrarque et ses amis au temps de la verte feuillée," *Cahier de Fanjeaux* 26 (1991): 127–140. See also, Jan Papy, "Creating an 'Italian' Friendship: From Petrarch's Ideal Literary Critic 'Socrates' to the Historical Reader Ludovicus Sanctus of Beringen," in Karl A. E. Enenkel and Jan Papy, eds. *Petrarch and His Readers in the Renaissance* (Leiden: Brill, 2006), 13–30. For letters between Petrarch and Talleyrand, at least one of which Cabassole delivered, see Zacour, *Talleyrand*, 28. Talleyrand's sister, Agnes of Pèrigord, died from poison, with Catherine de Valois (Louis of Taranto's mother) as his most likely suspect. Talleyrand wrote angry letters, especially after Louis of Taranto married Johanna.

17. See Saxer, "Philippe Cabassole et son *Libellus*," 193–204; Katherine Jansen, *Making of the Magdalen: Preaching and Popular Devotion in the Later Middle Ages* (Princeton,

NJ: Princeton University Press, 2000), 325–327; Barjavel, *Dictionnaire*, 314; Neal Clemens, "The Establishment of the Cult of Mary Magdalene in Provence, 1279–1543," PhD diss., Columbia University, 1997, 100–102, 257–258. The book also put Philippe in famous company. Vincent of Beauvais, Salimbene de Adam, and Bernard Gui (among others) wrote histories of King Charles II of Naples's discovery of Mary Magdalene's relics. See Clemens, "Cult of Mary Magdalene," 86–109.

18. Other histories were written by Bernard Gui, Vincent of Beauvais, and Salimbene de Adam, among others. See Clemens, "Cult of Mary Magdalene," 86–100.

19. As we will see in chapter 6, Mary Magdalene was thought to be the original evangelist of Provence.

20. Cambell, *Enquête*, 55: "Article 38: Item, quod commune dictum, communis opinio et communis assercio, publica vox et fama in partibus Provincie et alibi fuit et est quod dicta domina Dalphina, quamdiu in humanis agebat, fuit et erat magno amoris et caritatis in Deum et proximum fervore repleta; et quod summe gaudebat et cupiebat animas hominum salvas fieri; et propterea labores magnos et sollicitudines magnas sustentare non formidabat. Et quod, cum aliorum dissensiones et discordias audiebat, pro ipsorum concordia affectuosissime laborabat et ad loca eciam longinqua, dum sperabat sedare scandala, se propterea transferebat, licet nec equitare nec peditare posset propter senectutis et infirmitatum suarum impedimenta. Et se propterea in lectica vili et humili per homines cum magno sui corporis labore et detrimento portari faciebat. Quodque ipsa, dum et quando gravia peccata, quibus Deus graviter offendebatur, committi aut christianos infidelibus aliqualiter subici audiebat, ipsa domina magnas lacrimas effundebat et corpus suum affligebat, adeo quod frequenter propterea infirmitas febris fortiter in ea invalescebat."

21. Cheyette, *Ermengarde of Narbonne*, 202. See chapter 10 for a further discussion of emotion in the language of oaths. Some lordly anger could be useful to point out untenable political situations; see Barton, "'Zealous Anger,'" 152–170. For an overview, see Boquet and Nagy, *Medieval Sensibilities*, 222–223.

22. Smail, "Hatred as a Social Institution," 90–91.

23. For a discussion of this, see Caroline Walker Bynum, "The Female Body and Religious Practice," in *Fragmentation and Redemption: Essays on Gender and the Human Body in Medieval Religion*, ed. Caroline Walker Bynum (New York: Zone Books, 1992), 181–238; and Esther Cohen, "Animated Pain of the Body," *American Historical Review* 105 (2000): 61–62. For the theological complexity of voluntary suffering for sin, see Donald Mowbray, *Pain and Suffering in Medieval Theology* (Suffolk: Boydell Press, 2009), 61–80. For the specific act of weeping, see Piroska Nagy, *Le don des larmes au Moyen Âge* (Paris: Albin Michel, 2000).

24. Testimony linked to the third part of the article concerned the treatment of Christians by the king of Armenia, Leo V, in 1333. Only two witnesses mentioned this event, however, and only one had specific details, so it did not appear to be a moment of danger for this community. For the fullest testimony to this event, see Cambell, *Enquête*, 338.

25. For an overview of cultural understandings of anger, see Stephen D. White, "The Politics of Anger," in *Anger's Past: The Social Uses of and Emotion in the Middle Ages*, ed. Barbara Rosenwein (Ithaca, NY: Cornell University Press, 1998), 127–152. For hatred in legal settings, see Smail, "Hatred as a Social Institution," 90–92.

26. For an overview, see Nicole Archambeau, "Medical and Scientific Understandings," in *A Cultural History of the Emotions in the Medieval Age*, ed. Juanita Feros Ruys and Clare Monagle (London: Bloomsbury, 2019), 17–30. For an in-depth study, see Cohen-Hanegbi, *Caring for the Living Soul*, 18–67.

27. For the workings of the brain, see Harvey, *The Inward Wits*; Nancy G. Siraisi, *Taddeo Alderotti and His Pupils: Two Generations of Italian Medical Learning* (Princeton, NJ: Princeton University Press, 1981), 203–236; and Mary Carruthers, *The Book of Memory: A Study of Memory in Medieval Culture* (Cambridge: Cambridge University Press, 1990), 46–79. For a contemporary description of the physical and spiritual impact of anger in political dispute, see Longpré, *Pétrarque*, 4:83. The letter, written to Giovanni Barrili, is from volume 12, letter 14.

28. Cohen-Hanegbi, *Caring for the Living Soul*, 119–133; Bériou, "La confession dans les écrits théologiques et pastoraux," 261–282.

29. For the Agoult and Baux families in Provençal politics in the early to mid-fourteenth century, see Mazel, *La noblesse et l'Église*, 591–596.

30. Casteen, *From She-Wolf to Martyr*, 79–92.

31. Andrew's mother and others made the legal argument that Andrew of Hungary, as Johanna's husband, should also have stood as God to his wife, giving him the right to rule. See Casteen, *From She-Wolf to Martyr*, 52–53.

32. Guido Guerri dall'Oro, "Les mercenaires dans les campagnes Napolitaines de Louis le Grand, Roi de Hongrie, 1347–1350," in *Mercenaries and Paid Men: The Mercenary Identity in the Middle Ages*, ed. John France (Leiden: Brill, 2008), 61–88.

33. Dall'Oro, "Les mercenaires," 61–63; Léonard, *Histoire*, 2:1–5. For mercenaries in the Italian peninsula, see William Caferro, *Mercenary Companies and the Decline of Siena* (Baltimore: Johns Hopkins University Press, 1998), 1–14 and 25–35. For a contemporary chronicle account of King Louis of Hungary's advance, see Diakité and Sneider, eds., *The Final Book of Giovanni Villani's New Chronicle*, 161–175.

34. Ole Benedictow, *The Black Death, 1346–1353: The Complete History* (Woodbridge, UK: Boydell Press, 2004), 97.

35. Benedictow, *The Black Death*, 72–73. Benedictow indicates that there is some debate about when plague entered Provence. He ultimately places it in Marseille in late 1347. The chronicle of the abbey of St. Victor in Marseille, indicated it emerged there in November. See *Annales S. Victoris Massiliensis*, MGH SS 23, 6. For a recent analysis of when plague spread in the Mediterranean, see Hannah Barker, "Laying the Corpses to Rest: Grain, Embargoes, and Yersinia pestis in the Black Sea, 1346–1348," Forthcoming in Speculum, January 2021. For an overview of French sources on plague, see Pierre Toubert, "La Peste Noire dans les Abruzzes (1348–1350)," *Le Moyen Âge* 120 (2014): 11–26.

36. For an overview of these events in Marseille, see François Otchakovsky-Laurens, *La vie politique à Marseille sous la domination Angevine (1348–1385)* (Rome: École de Français de Rome, 2017), 201–227. See also Thierry Pécout, "Marseille et la reine Jeanne," in Thierry Pécout, ed. *Marseille au Moyen Âge, entre Provence et Méditerranée: Les horizons d'une ville portuaire* (Paris: Éditions Désiris, 2009), 215–224.

37. See Samantha Kelly, "Noblesse de robe et noblesse d'esprit à la cour de Robert de Naples: La question d''Italianisation,'" in *La noblesse dans les territoires Angevins à la fin du Moyen Âge*, ed. Noël Coulet and Jean-Michel Matz (Rome: École Française

de Rome, 2000), 347–361. For more on Bishop Philippe Cabassole, see Léonard, *Histoire*, 2:69–70.

38. For the early 1340s as a moment of change, see Roncière, "L'état Angevin 1265–1340," 649–664. For background to this change, see Jean Dunbabin, *The French in the Kingdom of Sicily, 1266–1305* (Cambridge: Cambridge University Press, 2011), 68–73. For the changes in the political status of Provençal lords under different rulers, see Gérard Giordanengo, "Droit nobiliaire en Provence Angevin," in *La noblesse dans les territoires Angevins à la fin du Moyen Âge*, ed. Noël Coulet and Jean-Michel Matz (Rome: École Française de Rome, 2000), 261–301.

39. Léonard, *Histoire*, 2:71. For the participants, see Michel Hébert, *Regeste des états de Provence, 1347–1480* (Paris: CTHS, 2007), 5–8.

40. Aurell, Boyer, and Coulet, *La Provence au Moyen Âge*, 278; Michel Hébert, "La noblesse Provençale et les états de Provence," in *La noblesse dans les territoires Angevins à la fin du Moyen Âge*, ed. Noël Coulet and Jean-Michel Matz (Rome: École Française de Rome, 2000), 327–345.

41. Léonard, *Histoire*, 2:74.

42. This had also been a stipulation in King Robert's last will. See Léonard, *Histoire*, 2:223.

43. For an overview of Clement VI's relationship to Johanna, see Guillaume Mollat, *The Popes at Avignon, 1305–1378*, trans. Janet Love (London: Thomas Nelson and Sons, 1963), 175–185.

44. The kingdom of Naples was, in part, a papal fief in return for which the rulers protected the Papal States on the Italian peninsula. At the same time, the rulers of Naples were counts of Provence, which meant they owned Avignon and the Comtat Venaissin, the papal lands surrounding Avignon. Dunbabin, *The French in the Kingdom of Sicily*, 73; Henri Dubled, *Histoire du Comtat Venaissin* (Villelaure: CREDEL, 1982), 56–57.

45. He was accompanied by Nicola Acciaiuoli, his highly effective grand seneschal. Léonard, *Histoire*, 2:75.

46. The pope while living in Avignon was technically Queen Johanna's vassal in her position as Countess of Provence. Léonard, *Histoire*, 2:91.

47. Benedictow, *The Black Death*, 93–95. See also George Christakos et al., "Recent Results on the Spatiotemporal Modeling and Comparative Analysis of Black Death and Bubonic Plague Epidemics," *Public Health* 121 (2007): 700–720.

48. Cortez, *Grands Officiers*, 66–67.

49. Although Johanna had promised the Estates that no part of Provence would be sold, there were few protests to the sale, though there was some confusion as to whether the people of Avignon were still part of the Estates of Provence.

50. Léonard, *Histoire*, 2:91.

51. For Queen Johanna's relationship with Pope Clement VI, see Casteen, *From She-Wolf to Martyr*, 72.

52. If any of the lords of Provence were uncomfortable with Johanna's sale of Avignon to Pope Clement VI—a sale of a Provençal region to an outside party, which she had promised not to do—they did not say.

53. Émile-Guillaume Léonard, "Un ami de Petrarque, senechal de Provence: Giovanni Barrili," *Études Italiennes* 9 (1927): 109–142.

54. Justine Firnhaber-Baker, "Seigneurial War and Royal Power in Later Medieval Southern France," *Past and Present* 208 (2010): 37–76.

55. For a documentary history of this complex moment, see Otchakovsky-Laurens, *La vie politique à Marseille*, 41–48, 142–143, 216–218.

56. For the long-term importance of this moment, see Hébert, "La cristallisation d'une identité," 151–164.

57. For the relations between Naples and Florence, see Kelly, *The New Solomon*, 227–235; Léonard, "Un ami de Petrarque," 128–129.

58. Léonard, "Un ami de Petrarque," 128–129; Otchakovsky-Laurens, *La vie politique à Marseille*, 210–211. Christian Maurel, "Pouvoir royal et pouvoir municipal (XIVe—XVe siècle)," in Thierry Pécout, ed. *Marseille au Moyen Âge, entre Provence et Méditerranée: Les horizons d'une ville portuaire* (Paris: Éditions Désiris, 2009), 225–231. For warfare between lords, see Firnhaber-Baker, "Techniques of Seigneurial War," 93.

59. For a list of letters between Petrarch and Cabassole, see Wilkins, "Philippe de Cabassoles on Petrarch," 69. For Petrarch's attitude toward Cabassole, see Longpré, *Pétrarque*, 4:56–59.

60. Léonard, *Histoire*, 2:148–162.

61. Léonard, *Histoire*, 2:174–180. Louis of Taranto had some ties to the Agoult family, especially Fulk d'Agoult, Raymon's son. For relations between Johanna and Louis at this time, see Casteen, *From She-Wolf to Martyr*, 81–85.

62. Léonard, "Un ami de Petrarque," 130.

63. Léonard, "Un ami de Petrarque," 131–132.

64. For this translation and others, I have been guided by Aldo Bernardo's translations. See Francis Petrarch, *Letters on Familiar Matters, Rerum familiarum libri, IX–XVII*, trans. Aldo Bernardo (Baltimore: Johns Hopkins University Press, 1982). This quotation is from book 12, letter 14, pp. 162–163. The Latin edition is Longpré, *Pétrarque*, 4:83: "Is ergo cum distinctis receptaculis 'iram in pectore,' concupiscentiam 'subter precordia collocasset, rationem' in vertice velut 'in arce' constituit, ut moderatricem illam ac dominam passionum vel ipse situs ostenderet; quod nec poetas nostros ignorasse crediderim, quamvis eam rem, ut solent, secretius exequantur. . . . Illud tibi brevissime quod nemo doctus ignorat, inculcandum reor: ubi passiones habitant, nubilum esse teterrimum et horrendas anime tenebras, ac rationis, ut proprie dixerim, eclipsim; quod cum de omnibus tum de ira convenientissime dici arbitror. . . . Oportet igitur, si felices esse volumus, ea felicitate quam recipit vita mortalis, etsi per hanc ad aliam aspiramus, oportet, inquam, illam etheree mentis altissimam esse particulam, ut quod de supremo dicitur Olimpi iugo, nulla eam passionum nubes possit attingere."

65. See Siraisi, *Taddeo Alderotti and His Pupils*, 203–236; and Carruthers, *The Book of Memory*, 46–79.

66. Luke Demaitre, *Medieval Medicine: The Art of Healing from Head to Toe* (Santa Barbara: Praeger, 2013), 129–140.

67. Cambell, *Enquête*, 531. As we saw in chapter 1, Agnes of Pèrigord was Cardinal Talleyrand's sister, who may have been poisoned in 1345 in the court of Naples.

68. Cambell, *Enquête*, 541: "ut retulit ipsa domina Dalphina sibi testi loquenti, ivit ad partes Neapolitanas vocata per dominam Sanxia reginam tunc infirmam, ut eam consolaretur."

69. Cambell, *Enquête*, 541: "nisi fecisset, fuisset, ut credit, magna divisio in Provincia et magna scandala et guerra."

70. All six were important witnesses in the inquest. See, among others, Amargier, "Dauphine de Puymichel et son entourage," 111–123.

71. Cambell, *Enquête*, 233: "propter controversiam et dissensiones periculosas."

72. Campell, *Enquête*, 233: "et post osculum pacis ut amici recesserunt."

73. See Kiril Petkov, *The Kiss of Peace: Ritual, Self, and Society in the High and Late Medieval West* (Leiden: Brill, 2003). By the fourteenth century the kiss of peace may have been losing its legal meaning, but it was still commonly described in negotiations and in literary and art representations of negotiation. The weakness of the central authorities in this moment may have led to the use of an old tactic for producing peace—the use of relics; see Patrick Geary, *Furta Sacra: Thefts of Relics in the Central Middle Ages*, (Princeton: Princeton University Press, 2011), 26; Herbert Cowdrey, "The Peace and Truce of God in the Eleventh Century," *Past and Present* 46 (1970): 42–67.

74. See Thomas Head and Richard Landes, eds., *The Peace of God: Social Violence and Religious Response in France around the Year 1000* (Ithaca, NY: Cornell University Press, 1992), 2, 14.

75. For the miracle at St. Louis's church in Marseille, see Article 51, the first in the miracle series; Cambell, *Enquête*, 64–65. At least two witnesses referred to it, including Bertran Jusbert and Peire Clodi, who gave the date as 1338. Cambell, *Enquête*, 240–241 and 149, respectively. For the holy light, see Article 40, Cambell, *Enquête*, 56–57. The article includes reference to the first mortality. Five people testified about the holy light, including Friar Giraud Raybaud (p. 188), Bertran Jusbert (p. 235), and Durand Andree (p. 270), who heard about it; and Raybaud St. Mitri (p. 382) and Pons Rostang (p. 546).

76. Daniel Callahan, "The Peace of God and the Cult of Saints in Aquitaine in the Tenth and Eleventh Centuries," in Head and Landes, *The Peace of God*, 174.

77. Geoffrey Koziol, "Monks, Feuds, and the Making of Peace in Eleventh-Century Flanders," in Head and Landes, *The Peace of God*, 246–253.

78. Koziol, "Monks, Feuds, and the Making of Peace," 245.

79. For the ability of noblewomen to negotiate peace, see Angus Kennedy, "Christine de Pizan's *Epistre a la reine*: A Woman's Perspective on War and Peace?," in Albrecht Classen and Nadia Margolis, eds. *War and Peace: Critical Issues in European Societies and Literature, 800–1800* (Berlin: De Gruyter, 2011), 395–423. For an analysis of the function of negotiators, see Jenny Benham, *Peacemaking in the Middle Ages: Principles and Practices* (Manchester, UK: Manchester University Press, 2011), 117–142.

80. Raymon d'Agoult was Delphine's uncle by marriage. See Mazel, *La noblesse et l'Église*, 526.

81. Jacques Cambell, "Le sommaire de l'enquête pour la canonisation de S. Elzear de Sabran, T.O.F. (1323)," *Miscellanea Francescana* 73 (1973): 439.

82. Mazel, *La noblesse et l'Église*, 534.

83. Mazel, *La noblesse et l'Église*, 534.

84. Holy noblewomen could have significant influence in political disputes. See Gábor Klaniczay, "Legends as Life Strategies for Aspirant Saints in the Later Middle Ages," *Journal of Folklore Research* 26 (1989): 151–171. See especially page 160.

85. Voluntary poverty of the elite had a spiritual valence that poverty caused by circumstances did not. See Kenneth Baxter Wolf, *The Poverty of Riches: St. Francis of Assisi Reconsidered* (Oxford: Oxford University Press, 2003). For virginity in marriage, see Elliott, *Spiritual Marriage*.

86. Inquest commissioners frequently asked witnesses about the *publica fama* of the events they spoke of. As in other medieval inquests, organizers were interested in where and from whom non-eyewitnesses had learned about the events. See Michael Goodich, "Canonization and the Hagiographical Text," in *Miracles and Wonders: The Development of the Concept of Miracle, 1150–1350* (Aldershot: Ashgate, 2007), 88.

87. Cambell, *Enquête*, 155–190.

88. Cambell, *Enquête*, 187: "loca ubi sperabat ponere concordiam inter discordes."

89. Cambell, *Enquête*: "Interrogatus, dixit quod fuit et est de eis que supra deposuit commune dictum, communis opinio et communis assercio, et publica vox et fama in civitatibus Avinionis et Aptensi."

90. Cambell, *Enquête*, 337: "dixit quod post primam mortalitatem."

91. Cambell, *Enquête*, 236. Since Friar Bertran met Delphine in 1348, he used "the first mortality" to date many events in the inquest. Overall he used the phrase sixteen times to date various events.

92. Arrizabalaga, "Facing the Black Death," 237–288.

93. Baratier, *Demographie*, 5.

94. Baratier, *Demographie*, 65–66. While hearths are probably the best demographic marker that survive from the time, it is not easy to estimate the number of people from the number of hearths. As Baratier points out on pages 14–15, a hearth was a legal taxation term originally referring to a household, but not limited to a household by the fourteenth century. The term could mean a house, outbuildings, and all the people and animals within. But it could also include more. For an analysis of taxation and studies of it in Provence, see Noël Coulet, "Les villages Provençaux, la queste et le cadastre," in *La société rurale et les institutions gouvernementales au Moyen Âge*, ed. John Drendel (Montreal: Éditions CERES, 1995), 117–129.

95. Baratier, *Demographie*, 65–66. Baratier refers to these cities as *vigeuries*, but that term did not become common until after the fourteenth century.

96. Thierry Pécout, "Le destin heuristique d'une histoire de la panique: La crise en Provence au Moyen Âge finissant; Jalons historiographiques pour le XIVe siècle," in *Crisis in the Later Middle Ages: Beyond the Postan-Duby Paradigm* (Turnhout: Brepols, 2015), 225–250; Baratier, *Demographie*, 80.

97. Fernand Sauve, *Les épidémies de pest à Apt, notamment en 1588 et 1720–1721* (Aix: Typographie et Lithographie B. Niel, 1905), 5–8; Monique Zerner, "Une crise de mortalité au XVe siècle a travers les testaments et les rôles d'imposition," *Annales, Histoire, Science Sociales*, 34e Année (1979): 566–589. In 1359, Queen Johanna I of Naples and King Louis of Taranto visited Apt to assess the damages done by plague, war, and brigandage. They gave a ten-year remittance of twelve deniers per hearth to the city. For a translation, see Fernand Sauve, "La vie Aptésienne d'autrefois," *Mercure Aptésien*, July 21, 1907.

98. Baratier, *Demographie*, 80–85. For a visual representation, see Édouard Baratier, Georges Duby, and Ernest Hildersheimer, *Atlas historique: Provence, Comtat Venaissin, Principaute de Monaco, Princepaute d'Orange, Comte de Nice* (Paris: Librairie Armand Colin, 1969). See maps 93–96. For a close analysis of the nearby region surrounding Nice, see Jean-Paul Boyer, "Contribution à la demographie de la Provence Savoyarde au XIVe siècle," *Provence Historique* 135 (1984): 36–53; Augustin A. Roux, *Apt: Quelques aspects de son histoire* (Apt: Imprimerie Reboulin, 1967), 48.

99. Claude Faure, *Étude sur l'administration et l'histoire du Comtat Venaissin du XIIIe au XVe siècle (1229–1417)* (Paris: Honoré Champion, 1909), 145–147. For areas in Languedoc under French control at the time, see John Henneman Jr., "The Black Death and Royal Taxation in France, 1347–1351," *Speculum* 43 (1968): 410–416.

100. Smail, "Accommodating Plague in Medieval Marseille," 11–41.

101. Records from other regions of Mediterranean Europe show the economic difficulties of this time. For example, see Melanie Shirk, "The Black Death in Aragon, 1348–1351," *Journal of Medieval History* 7 (1981): 357–367; Wray, *Communities and Crisis*. The annual *compte de clavaire* in Provence, however, showed few changes even during the plague. See Jean-Luc Bonnaud, "L'origine géographique de clavaires et notaires de cour de l'administration comtale locale en Provence au XIVe siècle," in *La société rurale et les institutions gouvernementales au Moyen Âge*, ed. John Drendel (Montréal: Éditions CERES, 1995), 133.

102. Louis Stouff, "Une enquête économique en Provence au XIVe siècle," *Le Moyen Âge* 3–4 (1968): 522–523.

103. Stouff, "Une enquête économique," 527. These types of records are explored in more detail in chapter 4.

104. Francine Michaud, "La peste, la peur et l'espoir. Le pèlerinage jubilaire de romeux marseillais en 1350," *La Moyen Âge* 104 (1998), 399–434.

105. For a will from Apt in 1348, see Apt Municipal Archive GG23, written by the notary Master Nicolau Nicholay.

106. Chiffoleau, *La comptabilité.*

107. Chiffoleau, *La comptabilité*, 174. Cabassole's tomb was located in the Chartreux of Bonpas, which no longer exists; see Jean Schopfer, "Description analytique des documents relatifs à l'histoire de l'art contenus dans les manuscrits N.-C. Fabri de Peiresc, conservés à la bibliothèque de la ville de Carpentras," *Bulletin archéologique du Comité des travaux historiques et scientifiques* (1899), 365.

108. Hugh Willmott et al., "A Black Death Mass Grave at Thornton Abbey, Lincolnshire: The Discovery and Examination of a 14th-Century Rural Catastrophe," *Antiquity* 94 (2020), 179–196.

109. Cambell, *Enquête*, 281. She mentions the fever in her main story, but only mentions the buboes in later questioning. See Cambell, *Enquête*, 283. Lord Giraud de Simiana also testified in Delphine's inquest, though he did not mention this miraculous healing.

110. Cambell, *Enquête*, 281: "sperantes de convalescencia sua."

111. Cambell, *Enquête*, 282.

112. For funeral preparations in later medieval Provence, see Louis Stouff, "Les Provençaux et la mort dans les testaments (XIIIe–XVe siècle)," *Cahiers de Fanjeaux* 33 (1998): 199–222. For general expectations in the fourteenth century, see Roger S. Wieck, "The Death Desired: Books of Hours and the Medieval Funeral," in *Death and Dying in the Middle Ages*, ed. Edelgard Dubruck and Barbara Gusick (New York: Peter Lang, 1999), 431–476.

113. For a careful approach to literary sources, see Shona Kelly Wray, "Boccaccio and the Doctors: Medicine and Compassion in the Face of Plague," *Journal of Medieval History* 30 (2004): 301–322. For an overview of medical and municipal reactions to multiple waves of plague in a southern French city, see Dumas, *Santé et société*, 306–329.

114. That the three men knew each other well we can see from Petrarch, *Letters on Familiar Matters*, trans. Aldo Bernardo, book 6, letter 9, 330.

115. See Benedictow, *The Black Death*, 72–73.

116. Petrarch returned to Italy later in the year and over the years revised these letters into a collection and dedicated them to Socrates, the name he used for Louis Heyligen. Ursmer Berlière, *Un ami de Pétrarque: Louis Heyligen de Beeringen* (Rome: Institute Historique Belge, 1905). Heyligen is also referred to as Louis Sanctus in modern scholarship.

117. Petrarch, *Letters on Familiar Matters*, book 8, letter 7, 416–417. "qui non solum nos amicis, sed mundum omnem gentibus spoliavit; cui siquid defuit, sequens ecce annus illius reliquias demetit, et quicquid illi procelle superfuerat, mortifera falce persequitur. . . . quando unquam tale aliquid visum aut fando auditum? quibus hoc unquam in annalibus lectum est, vacuas domos, derelictas urbes, squalida rura, arva cadaveribus angusta, horrendam vastamque toto orbe solitudinem?" For the latin, see Longpré, *Pétrarch: Lettres Familières*, 3:81.

118. Petrarch, *Letters on Familiar Matters*, book 8, letter 7, 418. "Vel ergo pessimi omnium vere sumus, quod negare velim potius quam ausim, vel ad futura bona presentibus malis exercitatiores purgatioresque servamur, vel omnino aliquid est quod nec cogitare sufficimus." For the latin, see Longpré, *Pétrarch: Lettres Familières*, 3:85. Carmichael, "Universal and Particular," 25.

119. This was not a unique response but an example of a long-term trend. See Carol Lansing, *Passion and Order: Restraint of Grief in Medieval Italian Communes* (Ithaca, NY: Cornell University Press, 2008).

120. For Louis Heyligen's letter, which survives because it was copied into a chronicle by its recipients, see J.-J. de Smet, ed., "Breve Chronicon Clerici Anonymi," in *Recueil des Chroniques de Flandre*, vol. 3 (Brussels: Commission Royale Histoire, 1856), 14–18. The first part of the letter is paraphrased by an anonymous chronicler. Heyligen's language in both the paraphrased and quoted material reflected many chronicle reports—see Carmichael, "Universal and Particular," 17–52, and Zanella, "La peste del 1348," 49–135.

121. Anna Montgomery Campbell, *The Black Death and Men of Learning* (New York: AMS Press, 1996.) Melissa Chase, "Fevers, Poisons, and Apostemes: Authority and Experience in Montpellier Plague Treatises," *Annals of the New York Academy of Sciences* 441 (1985): 153–170.

122. These were common ways of presenting the first mortality. People used the well-known medical theory of the six nonnaturals to understand how so many people could become sick at once. See Arrizabalaga, "Facing the Black Death," 237–288, and Zanella, "La peste del 1348," 49–135.

123. Chiffoleau, *La comptabilité*, 207, uses the letter to highlight the deaths of the poor, especially rural workers coming to Avignon to work with the dead and dying.

124. Faure, *Étude sur l'administration*, 146–147.

125. See Mollat, *Popes at Avignon*, 40, and Jean-Noël Biraben, *Les hommes et la peste en France et dans les pays européens et méditerranéens*, vol. 2, (Paris: Mouton, 1975–1976), 62–69.

126. Otto Gescer, "Doctors and Preachers against the Plague: Attitudes toward Disease in Late Medieval Plague Tracts and Plague Sermons," in *The Sacred and the*

Secular in Medieval Healing: Sites, Objects, and Texts, eds. Barbara Bowers and Linda Keyser (London: Routledge, 2016), 78–102.

127. Andries Welkenhuysen, "La peste en Avignon (1348) décrite par un témoin oculaire, Louis Sanctus de Beringen (Édition critique, traduction, élements de commentaire)," in *Pascua Mediaevalia: Studies voor Prof. Dr. J. M. de Smet* (Leuven: Universitaire pers Leuven, 1983), 468–469.

128. For an early sense of the concept of Sicut Judaeis, see Jeremy Cohen, *Living Letters of the Law: Ideas of the Jew in Medieval Christianity* (Berkeley: University of California Press, 1999), 73–94. For papal treatment of the Jews in Provence, see Valérie Theis, "Jean XXII et l'expulsion des juifs du Comtat Venaissin," *Annales. Histoire, Sciences Sociales*, 67 (2012): 41–77.

129. Simonsohn, *Apostolic See*, 1:375.

130. For an example of violence against Jewish communities, see Anna Colet et al., "The Black Death and Its Consequences for the Jewish Community in Tàrrega: Lessons from History and Archaeology," *Medieval Globe* 1 (2014): 63–97. For an overview, see Noël Coulet, "Les Juifs en Provence au bas Moyen-Âge: Les limites d'une marginalite?," in *Minorités et marginaux en France méridionale et dans la péninsule ibérique, VIIe–XVIIIe siècles* (Paris: Presses du CNRS, 1986), 203–219; Joseph Shatzmiller, "Les Juifs de Provence pendant la Peste Noire," *Revue des Études Juives* 133 (1974): 457–480. He particularly analyzes the violence in Toulon, but Jews in Apt faced significant violence. Delphine's witnesses do not mention it, but evidence of a violent attack in Apt appears in an official copy of a letter from the seneschal, Lord Raymon d'Agoult, dated 1349. The text describes the rejection of an appeal by several lords of Apt against accusations that they attacked and killed Jewish men and women in Apt and stole their goods in 1348. The letter ordered these lords to pay 800 gold florins. As of 2009 when I photographed this document, it was an unnumbered manuscript in Series FF in the Apt Municipal Archive.

131. Ann Carmichael, *Plague and the Poor in Renaissance Florence* (Cambridge: Cambridge University Press, 1986), 108–110; Dumas, *Santé et société*, 320–329.

132. "Quis finis vel quod principium, Deus scit; quidam tamen timent quod pro morte Andree regis, qui ita trucidatus fuit, Deus his malis mundum flagellat," (Smet, *Recueil de Chroniques de Flandres*, 3:17); Welkenhuysen, "La peste en Avignon (1348), 468–469, also states that Louis Heyligen could easily have observed Queen Johanna in Avignon. For other literary works that linked Johanna's actions to the plague, see Léonard, *Histoire*, 2:20. For other works that accused Johanna and Louis of Andrew's murder, see Léonard, *Histoire*, 2:29.

133. Alessandro Barbero, "Letteratura e politica fra Provenza e Napoli," 170–171.

134. Faure, *Étude sur l'administration*, 134–135. See especially note 4 on page 135.

135. Cambell, *Enquête*, 541.

136. This moment had parallels to Delphine's wondrous awareness of Elzear's death in 1323, when she was living with King Robert and Queen Sanxia in Avignon. She knew about her husband's death before messengers arrived from Paris and had already begun to mourn him. See Article 18, Cambell, *Enquête*, 42–43.

137. Cambell, *Enquête*, 58–60.

138. There is some indication that Johanna may have agreed to the marriage in return for Uguo's help. See Léonard, *Histoire*, 2:281. For the royal aspirations of the Baux family, see Boyer, "Les Baux et le modèle royal," 431–432, and Zacour, "Talleyrand," 36.

139. Louis Barthélémy, *Histoire d'Aubagne, chef-lieu de Baronnie: depuis son origine jusqu'en 1789* (Marseille: Barlatier et Barthelet, 1889), 111–112.

140. Barthélémy, *Histoire d'Aubagne*, 112. Louis Barthélémy, *Inventaire chronologique et analytique des chartes de la maison de Baux* (Marseille: Barlatier-Feissat, 1882), 375–376.

141. Casteen, *From She-Wolf to Martyr*, 95.

3. Master Nicolau Laurens and the Mercenary Invasion

1. For an overview of these events, see Coulet, *Aix-en-Provence*, 67–72.

2. The anonymous author of the chronicle of the abbey of St. Victor in Marseille also saw this as a highly political moment. See *Annales S. Victoris Massiliensis*, MGH SS 23, 6.

3. The lords of Baux and Charles of Durazzo had been rebelling against Philippe of Taranto, the vicar-general of the king and queen of Naples in Provence, and brother of Louis of Taranto, since 1355. Boyer and Pécout, introduction to *La Provence et Fréjus*, 10–16. See also Faure, *Étude sur l'administration*, 147–148; Cortez, *Grands Officiers*, 74. For an overview, see Zacour, "Talleyrand," 37–40.

4. Firnhaber-Baker, *Violence and the State in Languedoc*, 117.

5. For an analysis of mercenary warfare, see Contamine, "Les compagnies d'aventure," chap. 7; Jonathan Sumption, *Trial by Fire*, vol. 2 of *The Hundred Years War* (Philadelphia: University of Pennsylvania Press, 1999), 359–365; Hébert, "La cristallisation d'une identité," 156–159; and Michel Hébert, "Guerre, finance et adminstration: Les états de Provence de novembre 1359," *Revue d'Histoire de Philologie: Le Moyen Âge* 83 (1977): 103–130.

6. Italians in the papal court such as Francis Petrarch would have been more familiar with mercenary violence like this, which had been conducted for decades in the peninsula. See Daniel Waley, "Condotte and Condottieri in the Thirteenth Century," *Proceedings of the British Academy* 61 (1975): 337–371.

7. Firnhaber-Baker, *Violence and the State in Languedoc*, 115–152. For the perceived danger of a somewhat later attack in Provence, see McDonough, *Witnesses, Neighbors, and Community*, 123–149.

8. Cambell, *Enquête*, 29–30.

9. Sigal, "Les temoins et les temoignages au procès de canonisation," 461–471. Nicolau's name appears several times in the notarial register of Jourdan Manent of Apt in relation to the convent of St. Catherine in 1360, the year Delphine died. See ADV 3 E 33 MS 1.

10. See Archambeau, "Remembering Delphine's Books," 33–49.

11. Brundage, *The Medieval Origins of the Legal Profession*, 353.

12. Brundage, *The Medieval Origins of the Legal Profession*, 353–364.

13. Inquest witnesses were not bound by the articles, however, and they could have very different versions of events. See Smoller, "Miracle, Memory, and Meaning," 429–454.

14. For Laurens's active construction of the articles, see Archambeau, "'His Whole Heart Changed,'" 169–190.

15. Although including testimony from those who could not be questioned by the papal commissioners was not overly common in canonization inquests, an inquest

proctor was expected to gather witnesses and testimony even from distant places. See Brundage, *The Medieval Origins of the Legal Profession*, 353.

16. For changing violence and peace in western France, see Firnhaber-Baker, *Violence and the State in Languedoc*, 115–149.

17. Albert Rigaudière, "Le financement des fortifications urbaines en France du milieu du XIVe siècle à la fin du XVe siècle," *Revue Historique* 273 (1985): 19–95. For an economic study of mercenary activity in the Italian peninsula, see Caferro, *Petrarch's War*, 84–112. For a broad economic study, see Campbell, *The Great Transition*, 267–277. For a more regional economic study, see especially the work of Edouard Perroy, "At the Origin of a Contracted Economy: The Crises of the 14th Century," in *Essays in French Economic History*, eds. Rondo Cameron, Franklin Mendels, and Judith Ward (Homewood, IL: Richard D. Irwin, 1970), 91–105.

18. For an overview of the changes in warfare and the mercenary groups, see Norman Housley, "The Mercenary Companies, the Papacy, and the Crusades, 1356–1378," *Traditio: Studies in Ancient and Medieval History, Thought, and Religion* 38 (1982): 253–255. For an overview of this process in France, see Firnhaber-Baker, *Violence and the State in Languedoc*. For the mercenaries, see Fowler, *Medieval Mercenaries*; Philippe Contamine, *War in the Middle Ages*, trans. Michael Jones (Oxford: Basil Blackwell, 1984), 65–165; Maurice Hugh Keen, *Nobles, Knights, and Men-at-Arms in the Middle Ages* (London: Hambledon Press, 1996).

19. Petrarch, *Letters on Familiar Matters*, trans. Aldo Bernardo, book 8, letter 10, 430.

20. DeVries, "Medieval Mercenaries," 43–60; Sumption, *Trial by Fire*, 214–215.

21. Housley, "Mercenary Companies," 254.

22. Henri Denifle, La *désolation des églises, monastères et hopitaux en France pendant la Guerre de Cent Ans, vol. 2 La Guerre de Cent Ans jusqu'a la mort de Charles V (Paris: Alphonse Picard et Fils, 1899)*, 200–201n5. The letter was written August 3, 1357. See Léonard, *Histoire*, 3:290.

23. Caferro, *Petrarch's War*, 49–83.

24. Sumption, *Trial by Fire*, 360.

25. For an example of a mercenary leader, see William Caferro, *John Hawkwood: An English Mercenary in Fourteenth-Century Italy* (Baltimore: Johns Hopkins University Press, 2006).

26. Maurice Hugh Keen, *The Laws of War in the Middle Ages* (London: Routledge, 1965).

27. Frederick Cheyette, "Some Reflections on Violence, Reconciliation, and 'The Feudal Revolution,'" in *Conflict in Medieval Europe: Changing Perspectives on Society and Culture*, ed. Warren Brown and Piotr Górecki (Aldershot: Ashgate, 2003), 243–264.

28. For an overview of the war subsidy and repeated fiscal crises in France, see John Bell Henneman, *Royal Taxation in Fourteenth-Century France* (Princeton, NJ: Princeton University Press, 1971).

29. Philippe Contamine, "En guise de conclusion: Les villes de Languedoc et la chevauchée d'Édouard, prince de Galles (12 octobre–28 novembre 1355)," in *Défendre la ville dans les pays de la Méditerranée Occidentale au Moyen Âge*, ed. Daniel Le Blévec (Montpellier: Centre historique de recherches et d'études sur la Méditerranée médiévale occidentale 2002), 194–210; Robert-André Michel, "La défense d'Avignon sous Urbain

V et Grégroire XI," *Mélanges d'archéologie et d'histoire* 30 (1910): 129–154. For examples, see Sumption, *Trial by Fire*, 211–213, 352–356.

30. Denifle, *La désolation des églises*, 2:205. See also Noël Coulet, "La désolation des églises de Provence à la fin du Moyen Age," *Provence Historique* 23 (1956): 34–53. In 1359, the consuls of the city of Apt were given the right to destroy buildings and other possessions as needed for public safety. See Archives Civiles, ADBR B, MS1690, f. Clxxiiiv (numbering in a later hand). For an overview of these issues, see Kathryn Reyerson, "Medieval walled space: Urban development vs. defense," in James D. Tracy, ed. *City Walls: The Urban Enceinte in Global Perspective* (Cambridge: Cambridge University Press, 2000), 88–116.

31. For an example, see Coulet, *Aix-en-Provence*, 69.

32. Firnhaber-Baker, *Violence and the State in Languedoc*, 118–132.

33. Norman Housley, *The Italian Crusades: The Papal-Angevin Alliance and the Crusades against Christian Lay Powers, 1254–1343* (Oxford: Clarendon Press, 1982).

34. See Innocent VI's 1357 issuing of the papal bull *Ad reprimendas insolentias* in Denifle, *La désolation des églises*, 2:182.

35. Elisabeth Vodola, *Excommunication in the Middle Ages* (Berkeley: University of California Press, 1986), 67–69.

36. This idea appears even more clearly in Urban V's letter to the bishop of Rouen, written in 1365, in Paul Lecacheux, ed., *Lettres secrètes et curiales de Pape Urbain V (1362–1370)* (Paris: Ancienne Librarie Thorin et Fils, 1902), letter 1747, pp. 300–301. Philippe Contamine, "L'idée de guerre à la fin du Moyen Âge: Aspects juridiques et éthiques," in *La France au XIVe et VXe siècles: Hommes, mentalités, guerre et paix* (London: Variorum Reprints, 1981), chap, 13, 82–83.

37. Sumption, *Trial by Fire*, 244–282; Nigel Bryant, ed., *The True Chronicles of Jean le Bel, 1290–1360* (Woodbridge, UK: Boydell Press, 2011), 225–235, 242–247.

38. According to Chérest, Cervole was a significant fief, though it would not place Cervole in the high nobility of the region. Aimé Chérest, *L'archiprêtre: Épisodes de la Guerre de Cent Ans au XIVe siècle* (Paris: A. Claudin, 1879), 5–6.

39. Denifle, *La désolation des églises*, 2:188–190; Coulet, *Aix-en-Provence*, 67–72.

40. Firnhaber-Baker, *Violence and the State in Languedoc*, 121–122.

41. Émile-Guillaume Léonard, "Niccolò Acciaiuoli victime de Boccace," in *Mélanges de philologie, d'histoire, et littérature offerts à Henri Hauvette* (Paris: Presses Françaises, 1934), 139–148.

42. Faure, *Étude sur l'administration*, 148–149.

43. Cortez, *Grands Officiers*, 74.

44. Léonard, *Histoire*, 2:27–31.

45. Odile Maufras, "Le castrum des Baux-de-Provence: Histoire d'un site fortifié médiéval," *Provence Historique* 159 (1990): 79–95. See especially pages 80–81.

46. Barthélémy, *Histoire d'Aubagne*, 115.

47. Léonard, *Histoire*, 3:280. See also Chérest, *L'archipretre*, 5, and Denifle, La *désolation des églises*, 2:188.

48. A letter from the queen of Aragon stated the situation explicitly: "The dauphin of Vienne, son of the king of France, went against the king of Naples with 4000 glaives." See Léonard, *Histoire*, 3:289. See also Sumption, *Trial by Fire*, 358–359; and Denifle, *La désolation des églises*, 2:192–193.

49. Léonard, *Histoire*, 3:277–278. King Jean also had strong ties to the Durazzo branch of the family. Lord Robert of Durazzo died fighting for him in the battle of Poitiers.

50. Anne-Marie Hayez, "La défense d'Avignon au temps des papes," in *Défendre la ville dans les pays de la Méditerranée occidentale au Moyen Âge*, ed. Daniel le Blévec (Montpellier: Université Paul-Valéry, 2002), 63–101

51. Léonard, *Histoire*, 3:284–288.

52. Stouff, "Une enquête économique," 511; Coulet, *Aix-en-Provence*, 68; Léonard, *Histoire*, 3:287, 302–303.

53. Barthéléme, *Histoire d'Aubagne*, 116–117.

54. Léonard, *Histoire*, 3:288–289.

55. Hayez, "La défense d'Avignon," 66–67.

56. Léonard, *Histoire*, 3:285, and Sumption, *Trial by Fire*, 195–215; Firnhaber-Baker, *Violence and the State in Languedoc*, 125–132.

57. Léonard, *Histoire*, 3:284.

58. Hayez, "La défense d'Avignon," 66–67; Denifle, *La désolation des églises*, 2:196–198; and Léonard, *Histoire*, 3:287.

59. Hayez, "La défense d'Avignon," 72–75.

60. Denifle, *La désolation des églises*, 2:195; Anthony Luttrell, "Juan Fernandez de Heredia at Avignon: 1351–1367," in *El Cardenal Albornoz y el Colegio de España*, ed. E. Verdera y Tuells (Bologna: Publicaciones de real Colegio de España, 1972), 1:289–316.

61. For an overview of these events, see Coulet, *Aix-en-Provence*, 67–72.

62. Léonard, *Histoire*, 3:289; see note 3.

63. Léonard, *Histoire*, 3:289. Barthélémy, *Histoire d'Aubagne*, 116–117.

64. Stouff, "Une enquête économique," 510.

65. Coulet, *Aix-en-Provence*, 68–69.

66. Coulet, *Aix-en-Provence*, 72.

67. For an overview of city leaders' decision making during this time, see Labande, *Inventaire sommaire des Archives communales*, Série BB, vol. 1, 68–82. For an example of property abandoned in the suburbs, see Daniel Lord Smail, *Imaginary Cartographies: Possession and Identity in Late Medieval Marseille* (Ithaca, NY: Cornell University Press, 1999), 14n30.

68. Léonard, *Histoire*, 3:298–300. Sending crossbowmen to Aix was not a purely selfless act. Both of those cities were between the main body of Arnau de Cervole's troops and Marseille. If they held, they protected Marseille.

69. Hayez, "La défense d'Avignon," 73–80.

70. Hayez, "La défense d'Avignon," 85–87.

71. Barthélémy, *Histoire d'Aubagne*, 118.

72. Aubagne was seen by some at the time as a stronghold for the rebelling Baux. Léonard, *Histoire*, 3:291–300; Coulet, *Aix-en-Provence*, 68.

73. Léonard, *Histoire*, 3:307. On October 21, King Louis of Naples sent a letter to the lords of Marseille, urging them to stay strong, resist the invaders, and wait for his great offensive action. He promised reinforcements, including three hundred troops.

74. Léonard, *Histoire*, 3:302–306.

75. Coulet, *Aix-en-Provence*, 69.

76. For the difficulties of feeding a besieged port city, see S. J. Burley, "The Victualling of Calais, 1347–1365," *Bulletin of the Institute of Historical Research* 31 (1958): 49–57.

77. Léonard, *Histoire*, 3:313.

78. Coulet, *Aix-en-Provence*, 69.

79. Léonard, *Histoire*, 3:313–315.

80. Stouff, "Une enquête économique," 508–512, discusses the economic instability and the inability to collect taxes because of plague, mercenary invasion, and the difficulties of Queen Johanna's early reign in the region. For many defense expenses just in Avignon, see Hayez, "La défense d'Avignon," 63–101. For a study of the expenses of warfare like this, see Caferro, *Petrarch's War*, 84–112.

81. Léonard, *Histoire*, 3:626: "si istud fieret, posset esse tocius patrie salus."

82. Hébert, "Le cristallisation d'une identité," 151–164.

83. Léonard, *Histoire*, 3:318–320.

84. Denifle, *La désolation des églises*, 2:203–206, and Léonard, *Histoire*, 3:315–316. For grain price fluctuation, see Stouff, "Une enquête economique," 530–542.

85. Léonard, *Histoire*, 3:320, 334–335.

86. Aurell, Boyer, and Coulet, *La Provence au Moyen Âge*, 279; Léonard, *Histoire*, 3:321–326. King Louis of Naples's promised reinforcements had never come.

87. Léonard, *Histoire*, 3:335.

88. Denifle, *La désolation des églises*, 2:200.

89. Butaud and Challet, "Guerre et transfert *intra muros*," 517–568.

90. Turning to saints during warfare was an accepted method of protection and healing. See Michael Goodich, *Violence and Miracle in the Fourteenth Century: Private Grief and Public Salvation* (Chicago: University of Chicago Press, 1995), 121–146.

91. Cambell, *Enquête*, 389: "anno videlicet quo Vascones erant in Provincia."

92. Cambell, *Enquête*, 389–390.

93. Cambell, *Enquête*, 398–390.

94. Faure, *Étude sur l'administration*, 148.

95. Cambell, *Enquête*, 389–390.

96. Cambell, *Enquête*, 390: "Tunc dicta domina, iunctis et erectis manibus ad celum, dixit hec verba, 'O Domine Deus, habeas pietatem de isto paupere populo!' subiungens, 'Adiuro te per Deum vivum, per Deum sanctum et per Deum omnipotentem,' que verba ipsa loquens audivit." This is the language of exorcism; see Nancy Caciola, *Discerning Spirits: Divine and Demonic Possession in the Middle Ages* (Ithaca NY: Cornell University Press, 2003), 242–243, 256–268.

97. Cambell, *Enquête*, 389–390.

98. For the process of stories as a place to understand and control unexpected events, see Ochs and Capps, *Living Narrative*, 156.

99. Denifle, *La désolation des églises*, 2:208. For the difficulty of retaking towns from the mercenaries, see Coulet, *Aix-en-Provence*, 70–73.

100. Cambell, *Enquête*, 67: "videntes se dampnificari cotidie per gentes predicti loci de Ansoysio." For another analysis, see Veyssière, *Vivre en Provence*, 180.

101. Cambell, *Enquête*, 67, Article 54.

102. Cambell, *Enquête*, 67, Article 54.

103. For a discussion of mercenaries in Provençal canonization inquests, see Veyssière, *Vivre en Provence*, 181–187. He specifically mentions Gailhardo on page 182. For recognition of Delphine's help during this and later mercenary invasions, see Hébert, *Regeste des états de Provence*, 66–67.

104. Cambell, *Enquête*, 351. Cambell states in a footnote that this was 1357.

105. Neither of these men appear in the table of mercenary captains in Fowler, *Medieval Mercenaries*, 1:323–328. Neither are they likely to have been the same Gailhardo de Bazaran who was an important captain under Arnau de Cervole. See *Léonard, Histoire*, 3:312–313.

106. Cambell, *Enquête*, 351–352: "nec erant in dicto castro nisi tres parvi roncini, qui non fuissent sufficientes ad equitandum pro aliquo homine armato."

107. Cambell, *Enquête*, 444.

108. For an exploration of the religious values of thirteenth- and fourteenth-century mercenaries in the kingdom of Aragon, see Hussain Fancy, *The Mercenary Mediterranean: Sovereignty, Religion, and Violence in the Medieval Crown of Aragon* (Chicago: University of Chicago Press, 2016), 90–94. Fancy also provides an overview of cultural historians' approaches to religion on pages 67–74. For a contrasting view, see Brian Catlos, "'Mahomet Abenadalill': A Muslim Mercenary in the Service of the Kings of Aragon, 1290–1291," in *Jews, Muslims and Christians in and around the Crown of Aragon: Studies in Honour of Professor Elena Lourie*, ed. Harvey Hames (Leiden: Brill, 2003), 257–302.

109. Housley, "Mercenary Companies," 278–279.

110. For Enric's political background, see Cortez, *Grands Officiers*, 240–241.

111. Cambell, *Enquête*, 372–373: "et hoc contigisse dicebatur ad terrorem inimicorum, ne invaderent dictum castrum de Ansoysio."

112. For Johan de Revest's letter, see Léonard, *La jeunesse de Jeanne Ire: Reine de Naples, Comtesse de Provence* (Paris: Librairie Auguste Picard, 1932), 3:626.

113. For a further exploration of this miracle, see Nicole Archambeau, "Miraculous Healing for the Warrior Soul: Transforming Fear, Violence, and Shame in the Canonization Inquest for Delphine de Puimichel, 1363," *Historical Reflections/Réflexions Historiques* 41 (2015): 14–27.

114. Cambell, *Enquête*, 69: "ut non remaneret vituperatus et ad pusillanimitatem sive verecundiam non ascriberetur sibi."

115. Cambell, *Enquête*, 69: "promitti fecit sibi quod neminem occideret et quod pro eo Deum eadem domina deprecaretur."

116. Cambell, *Enquête*, 69: "recommendavit se in corde suo dicte domine comitisse."

117. Cambell, *Enquête*, 299–301.

118. Cambell, *Enquête*, 300.

119. Cambell, *Enquête*, 300.

120. Catherine de Pui did not mention this in her testimony.

121. Cambell, *Enquête*, 301. None of the men he named testified in the inquest.

122. Cambell, *Enquête*, 301: "processisset et ivisset contra dictos inimicos."

123. Contamine, *War in the Middle Ages*, 253.

124. Thelma Fenster and Daniel Lord Smail, introduction to *Fama: The Politics of Talk and Reputation in Medieval Europe* (Ithaca, NY: Cornell University Press, 2003), 1–11; Sumption, *Trial by Fire*, 216–217.

125. Contamine, *War in the Middle Ages*, 253.

126. Contamine, *War in the Middle Ages*, 253–259.

127. For more on the complexity of pacifism in the Middle Ages, see Contamine, *War in the Middle Ages*, 292–296.

128. Andrew Taylor, "Chivalric Conversation and the Denial of Male Fear," in *Conflicted Identities and Multiple Masculinities*, ed. Jacqueline Murray (New York: Garland Publishing, 1999), 169–188.

129. Contamine, "Les compagnies d'aventure," 382–383.

130. Although Delphine was never canonized, this miracle may have been the signature miracle around which her cult could be built. For an exploration of the uses and transformations of a signature miracle, see Smoller, *The Saint and the Chopped Up Baby*.

131. For a seventeenth-century image of this event, see Poëzévara and Codou, *Saintetés Aptésiennes*, 38.

132. Cambell, *Enquête*, Article 56, 70: "totis cordis affectibus se convertit, supplicans sibi in corde suo, et eciam tacita voce exprimens, ut ipsa eum in tanto periculo deberet adiuvare, maxime quia, si mortem evaderet, ad eam veniret, quecumque preciperet impleturus."

133. For Durand Arnau's full testimony, see Cambell, *Enquête*, 116–119. For an overview of this event, see Veyssière, *Vivre en Provence*, 182. It was not uncommon for either soldiers or those condemned to death to pray to saints. See Goodich, *Violence and Miracle in the Fourteenth Century*, 51–57.

134. Cambell, *Enquête*, 116–120.

135. This letter is reproduced in Denifle, *La désolation des églises*, 2:182. See Housley, "Mercenary Companies," 257–259.

136. Cambell, *Enquête*, 234: "blasphemabant beatam virginem Mariam, appellando eam meretricem."

137. Cambell, *Enquête*, 233–234.

138. Housley, "Mercenary Companies," 255–256.

139. Edmund Martene and Ursini Durand, eds., *Thesaurus novus anecdotorum*, vol. 2 (Paris, 1717), column 853: "feverioris rigorem judicis."

140. *Thesaurus novus anecdotorum*, vol. 2, column 853: "Illius tamen sequendo vestigia, qui quos vocat ad poenitentiam patienter exspectat; ac pii more patris, qui non quaerit mortem filiorum aberrantium, sed salutem, eosdem nostris monitis & mandatis praeveniendos duximus." The letter comes from 1361 and is discussed further in chapter 4. For a discussion of later portions of this letter, which offer limited indulgences for people fighting against the mercenaries, see Housley, "Mercenary Companies," 253–280.

141. For further analysis of Article 57, see Archambeau, "'His Whole Heart Changed,'" 187–190.

142. Cambell, *Enquête*, 72: "Que quidem domina comitissa . . . et salubrem de recognicione gracie per Dei misericordiam sibi facte, cor ipsius contritum intelligens et humiliatum in consideracione beneficii tam immensi."

143. See Pierre Michaud-Quantin, *Sommes de casuistique et manuels de confession au Moyen Âge (XII–XVI Siècles)* (Louvain: Edit. Nauwelaerts, 1962), 20.

144. Cambell, *Enquête*, 72: "Vade et noli amplius peccare. Et antequam similia mala que comisisti hactenus in futurum committeres, elige prius mori, quoniam multas temptaciones et instigaciones demonum provide sustinebis."

145. Cambell, *Enquête*, 72.

146. Archambeau, "'His Whole Heart Changed,'" 186–189.

4. Lady Andrea Raymon and the Great Companies

1. This date is based on the testimony of Friar Bertran Jusbert and Catherine de Pui. Master Durand Andree placed it three days before the feast of St. Catherine; Cambell, *Enquête*, 272.

2. Cambell, *Enquête*, 63–64.

3. Cambell, *Enquête*, 64; Donald Weinstein and Rudolph Bell, *Saints and Society: The Two Worlds of Western Christendom, 1000–1700* (Chicago: University of Chicago Press, 1982), 149–150.

4. The prostitute's kiss is depicted in the anonymous painting of Delphine's vigil. See figure 1.

5. Sumption, *Trial by Fire*, 445–447; Fowler, *Medieval Mercenaries*, 2–5.

6. Fowler, *Medieval Mercenaries*, 4, 27.

7. Fowler, *Medieval Mercenaries*, 24–30.

8. Guy de Chauliac, *Inventarium sive chirurgia magna*, ed. Michael McVaugh (Leiden: Brill 1997), 1:119. For an analysis of this passage, see Carmichael, "Universal and Particular," 37–38. See also Jean Glénisson, "La seconde peste: L'épidémie de 1360–1362 en France et en Europe," *Annuaire-Bulletin de la Société de l'Histoire de France* (1969): 27–38, especially p. 31. For another contemporary association of war and plague, see Diakité and Sneider, eds., *The Final Book*, 173.

9. Fowler, *Medieval Mercenaries*, 4. According to Fowler, chroniclers at the time discerned three main groups of mercenaries: those who went home, those who went to fight for Charles of Navarre, and those who made war on their own account. See also Mollat, *Popes at Avignon*, 50–51.

10. Fowler, *Medieval Mercenaries*, 2–8.

11. For estimates of the numbers of mercenaries assembled after the Treaty of Bretigny, see Fowler, *Medieval Mercenaries*, 5. He quotes Bascot de Mauléon in an estimate of twelve thousand men. Fowler's appendix C, "The Numerical Strength of the Great Companies," 329–332, has a broader analysis, though of later battles.

12. Contamine, "Les compagnies d'aventure," 365–386.

13. Léon-Honoré Labande, "L'occupation de Pont-Saint-Esprit par les Grandes Compagnies," *Revue Historique de Provence* (1901): part 1, 79–95, and part 2, 146–164. See page 82.

14. Labande, "L'occupation," 80.

15. Fowler, *Medieval Mercenaries*, 28.

16. Fowler, *Medieval Mercenaries*, 32; Labande, "L'occupation," 82.

17. Fowler, *Medieval Mercenaries*, 33.

18. A. Hayez, "La défense d'Avignon," 75–76.

19. Reyerson, "Medieval Walled Space," 109–112. *Le Petit Thalamus de Montpellier* (Montpellier: Jean Martel Ainé, 1811), 357–360.

20. Butaud and Challet, "Guerre et transfert *intra muros*," 520–521; Fowler, *Medieval Mercenaries*, 30–32; Labande, "L'occupation," 81–82; A. Hayez, "La défense d'Avignon," 79.

21. Labande, "L'occupation," 84.

22. A. Hayez, "La défense d'Avignon," 80–81.

23. Fowler, *Medieval Mercenaries*, 32.

24. Fowler, *Medieval Mercenaries*, 3–4.

25. After the loss of King Jean's ransom, there were rumors that the mercenaries planned to capture Innocent VI and hold him for ransom. See Labande, "L'occupation," 80.

26. See Fowler, *Medieval Mercenaries*, 30; Caferro, *John Hawkwood*, 43–45. The unlikely mercenary Giannino Guccio also found himself at Pont-Saint-Esprit; see Tommaso di Carpegna Falconieri, *The Man Who Believed He Was the King of France: A True Medieval Tale*, trans. William McCuaig (Chicago: University of Chicago Press, 2008), 80–91.

27. Coulet, *Aix-en-Provence*, 72–73.

28. Labande, "L'occupation," 147.

29. Fowler, *Medieval Mercenaries*, 35; Luttrell, "Juan Fernandez de Heredia at Avignon," 298.

30. Léonard, *Histoire*, 3:447–449.

31. Housley, "Mercenary Companies," 262.

32. Housley, "Mercenary Companies," 262.

33. Fowler, *Medieval Mercenaries*, 34–35; Mollat, *Popes of Avignon*, 50–51; Sumption, *The Hundred Years War*, 2:466–469.

34. Labande, "L'occupation," 147–149. According to Froissart, they followed John Hawkwood.

35. Léonard, *La jeunesse*, 3:449–450.

36. Fowler, *Medieval Mercenaries*, 36–39, and Labande, "L'occupation," 149.

37. Labande, "L'occupation," 150.

38. Martene and Durand, *Thesaurus novus anecdotorum*, 2:852–854.

39. Martene and Durand, *Thesaurus novus anecdotorum*, 2:852: "nonnulli iniquitatis filii, quos de diversis nationibus in societatem, imo perversitatem unam congregavit impietas ad turbationem communis commodi et tranquillitatis & pacis Christi fidelium temerariis ausibus intendentes."

40. Martene and Durand, *Thesaurus novus anecdotorum*, 2:853: "alioquin contra eos spiritualiter et temporaliter procedere curaremus."

41. Martene and Durand, *Thesaurus novus anecdotorum*, 2:853: "feverioris rigorem judicis."

42. Martene and Durand, *Thesaurus novus anecdotorum*, 2:853: "ac pii more patris, qui non quaerit mortem filiorum aberrantium, sed salutem."

43. Lester Little, "Pride Goes before Avarice: Social Change and the Vices in Latin Christendom," *American Historical Review* 76 (1971): 23.

44. Cambell, *Enquête*, 233–234.

45. Though popes continued to consider it possible for mercenaries to redeem themselves by going on crusade. See Contamine, "Les companies d'aventure," 382–383.

46. See Housley, "Mercenary Companies," 262–263.

47. Robert Shaffern, *The Penitents' Treasury: Indulgences in Latin Christendom, 1175–1375 (Scranton: University of Scranton Press, 2007)*, 131–132.

48. Martene and Durand, *Thesaurus novus anecdotorum*, 2:853: "per quem mercimonia ac victualia plurima eidem curiae necessaria ac opportuna etiam deferuntur."

49. Contamine, "Les compagnies d'aventure," 369–378.

50. Cambell, *Enquête*, 449–453.

51. Cambell, *Enquête*, 450.

52. Cambell, *Enquête*, 450.

53. Cambell, *Enquête*, 451: "per spacium unius longe lancee sive glavii."

54. Cambell, *Enquête*, 451: "Vade in mala hora!" Et ipsa testis loquens resondit: "Et vos remaneatis in mala hora!"

55. See Cambell, *Enquête*, 85–86, for the article, and 485–486 for Ayselena's testimony.

56. For the companies of Spain, Ayselena may be referring to the company under the exiled Enrique of Trastámara. See Fowler, *Medieval Mercenaries*, 5.

57. Cambell, *Enquête*, 86: "Ac si essent rationis participes."

58. For a general view of the impact on Church lands, see C. T. Allmand, "The War and the Non-combatant," in *The Hundred Years War*, ed. Kenneth Fowler (London: Macmillan, 1971), 172; Caferro, *John Hawkwood*, 45.

59. Stouff, "Une enquête économique," 528.

60. Chauliac, *Inventarium*, 1:119; Carmichael, "Universal and Particular," 37–38; Glénisson, "La seconde peste," 31.

61. Microbes moving from one region to another in their human hosts can have a significant impact. Nükhet Varlik, *Plague and Empire in the Early Modern Mediterranean World: The Ottoman Experience, 1347–1600* (Cambridge: Cambridge University Press, 2015), 44–45. For just one modern example, see Chen-Shan Chin et al., "The Origin of the Haitian Cholera Outbreak Strain," *New England Journal of Medicine* 364 (2011): 33–42.

62. Glénisson, "La seconde peste," 36. See Chauliac, *Inventarium*, 1:119. See also Denifle, *La désolation des églises*, 2:401.

63. John W. I. Lee, *A Greek Army on the March: Soldiers and Survival in Xenophon's "Anabasis"* (Cambridge: Cambridge University Press, 2007), 236. No similar studies have been undertaken for the Great Companies, whose numbers are difficult to estimate.

64. For human average waste production, see Richard Hoffmann, "Footprint Metaphor and Metabolic Realities: Environmental Impacts of Medieval European Cities," in *Nature's Past: The Environment and Human History*, ed. Paolo Squatriti (Ann Arbor: University of Michigan Press, 2006), 309.

65. Contamine, *La vie quotidienne*, 117–132. For an overview of city sanitation concerns, see Guy Geltner, *Roads to Health: Infrastructure and Urban Wellbeing in Later Medieval Italy* (Philadelphia: University of Pennsylvania Press, 2019), 20–41. Hoffmann, "Footprint Metaphor and Metabolic Realities," 309–312.

66. Guy Geltner, "The Path to Pistoia: Urban Hygiene before the Black Death," *Past and Present* 246 (2020), 10.

67. Hoffmann, "Footprint Metaphor," 309.

68. See also Carole Rawcliffe, *Urban Bodies: Communal Health in Late Medieval English Towns and Cities* (Woodbridge, UK: Boydell Press, 2013), 127–131.

69. Hoffmann, "Footprint Metaphor," 310.

70. Michael Wolfe, "Siege Warfare and the *Bonnes Villes* of France during the Hundred Years War," in *The Medieval City under Siege*, ed. Ivy Corfis and Michael Wolfe (Woodbridge: Boydell Press, 1995), 49–66.

71. Piers Mitchell, *Medicine in the Crusades: Warfare, Wounds, and the Medieval Surgeon* (Cambridge: Cambridge University Press, 2004), 1–2, 56–57.

72. Michael McVaugh, "Arnald of Villanova's *Regimen Almarie (Regimen Castra Sequentum)* and Medieval Military Medicine," *Viator* 23 (1992): 201–214. For an overview

of this topic, see Guy Geltner, "In Camp and on the March: Military Manuals as Sources for Studying Premodern Public Health," *Medical History* 63 (2019): 44–60.

73. For an overview of life within city walls in fourteenth-century Montpellier, see Reyerson, "Medieval Walled Space," 88–116. For disease in the city environment, see Carole Rawcliffe, *Urban Bodies: Communal Health in Late Medieval English Towns and Cities*, (Woodbridge: The Boydell Press, 2013), 62–78.

74. Denifle, *La désolation des églises*, 1:680.

75. For the notarial record of Laurent Laurent, a notary of Apt, 1346–1375, ADV, Avignon, France, 3 E 4 MS2, f50v–53v. These notarial entries suggest that the convent was negotiating for property inside the city walls in 1360.

76. Boze, *Histoire de l'eglise d'Apt*, 138–139.

77. ADV 3 E 4 MS 2, f.47r–48r.

78. Boze, *Histoire de l'église d'Apt*, 160.

79. ADV 3 E 33 MS 1, f.16v–16r.

80. Constance Hoffman Berman, "Medieval Agriculture, the Southern French Countryside, and the Early Cistercians: A Study of Forty-Three Monasteries," *Transactions of the American Philosophical Society*, New Series, 76 (1986): 1–179. Although focusing on an earlier time period, this study provides a varied discussion of food production.

81. William Caferro, "Warfare and Economy in Renaissance Italy, 1350–1450," *Journal of Interdisciplinary History* 39 (2008): 167–209; Yuval Noah Harari, "Strategy and Supply in Fourteenth-Century Western European Invasions," *Journal of Military History* 64 (2000): 301–303.

82. For aspects of grain production, harvest, and storage, see Carola Small, "Grain for the Countess: The 'Hidden' Costs of Cereal Production in Fourteenth-Century Artois," in *Proceedings of the Annual Meeting of the Western Society for French History*, ed. Gordon Bond (Auburn, IN: Western Society for French History, 1990), 56–63.

83. Denifle, *La désolation des églises*, 1:398.

84. Martene and Durand, *Thesaurus novus anecdotorum*, 2:853.

85. Louis Stouff, "Alimentation et démographie en Provence aux XIVe et XVe siècles," *Annales de démographie historique* (1976): 61–69.

86. Ian Kershaw, "The Great Famine and Agrarian Crisis in England, 1315–1322," *Past and Present* 59 (1973): 3–50; Mavis Mate, "High Prices in Early Fourteenth-Century England: Causes and Consequences," *Economic History Review* 28 (1975): 1–16. Although these examples are from England, they give a sense of the multiple impacts of the loss of cattle.

87. Butaud and Challet, "Guerre et transfert," 517–568.

88. Meat was limited to Sundays and feast days, and even poultry consumption was limited, sometimes to those who were sick or for guests. Stouff, "Alimentation et démographie en Provence," 67.

89. Stouff, "Alimentation et démographie en Provence," 67–68. Stouff built his picture of daily food consumption from town fiscal documents, institutional documents, notarial records of alimony left to widows, and records from a papal *studium* in Arles.

90. The witness does not give a specific date, but it likely occurred in early December, after her vigil.

91. Cambell, *Enquête*, 381–382.

92. The uses of wood and woodlands were, of course, more diverse than the example of firewood. See John Drendel, "Note sur l'exploitation de la terre gaste dans le finage de Brignoles au XIVe siècle," *Provence Historique* 256 (2014): 371–379.

93. Hoffmann, "Footprint Metaphor," 305–308.

94. J. L. Bolton, "Looking for *Yersinia Pestis*: Scientists, Historians and the Black Death," in *The Fifteenth Century XII: Society in an Age of Plague*, ed. Linda Clark and Carole Rawcliffe (Woodbridge, UK: Boydell and Brewer, 2013), 24.

95. Kenneth Gage and Michael Kosoy, "Natural History of Plague: Perspectives from More Than a Century of Research," *Annual Review of Entomology* 50 (2005): 505–528; Rebecca J. Eisen and Kenneth L. Gage, "Adaptive Strategies of *Yersinia pestis* to Persist during Inter-epizootic and Epizootic Periods," *Veterinary Research* 40 (2009): doi:10.1051/vetres:2008039.

96. This reflects the findings of Arrizabalaga, "Facing the Black Death," 237–288.

97. For a more medical approach to these testimonies, see Archambeau, "Healing Options during the Plague," 531–559. For reactions to the 1382 plague in Avignon, see Susan Einbinder, *No Place of Rest: Jewish Literature, Expulsion, and the Memory of Medieval France* (Philadelphia: University of Pennsylvania Press, 2009), 112–136.

98. Cambell, *Enquête*, 360.

99. This appears to be a local term for the plague. See Veyssière, *Vivre en Provence*, 150.

100. Cambell, *Enquête*, 371.

101. Luis Garcia-Ballester, "On the Origins of the 'Six Non-natural Things' in Galen," in *Galen and Galenism: Theory and Medical Practice from Antiquity to the European Renaissance*, eds. Luis Garcia-Ballester and Jon Arrizabalaga (Aldershot: Ashgate, 2002), chap. 4, 105–115.

102. For a discussion of the nonnaturals in the regimens of health, see Michael McVaugh, *Medicine before the Plague: Practitioners and Their Patients in the Crown of Aragon, 1285–1345* (Cambridge: Cambridge University Press, 1993), 144–150. See also Pedro Gil Sotres, "The Regimens of Health," in *Western Medical Thought from Antiquity to the Middle Ages*, ed. Mirko Grmek (Cambridge, MA: Harvard University Press, 1998), 313–314. See also Siraisi, *Taddeo Alderotti and His Pupils*, 226–236; Luis Garcia-Ballester, "Changes in the *Regimina Sanitatis*, 119–131.

103. For Raymon's testimony, see Cambell, *Enquête*, 515–517. Raymon spoke to Article 77, which is on page 85.

104. Cambell, *Enquête*, 516: "Totis affectibus ac toto corde et mente sua invocabat."

105. Cambell, *Enquête*, 517.

106. His experience incorporates what historian Mary Carruthers describes as the "somatic psychology" expressed by medieval scholars like Thomas Aquinas and Hugh of St. Victor. See Carruthers, *The Book of Memory*, 51–54.

107. Carruthers, *The Book of Memory*, 54.

108. Siraisi, *Taddeo Alderotti and His Pupils*, 209–216.

109. For the knowledge of plague among the clergy, see Gescer, "Doctors and Preachers against the Plague," 78–102.

110. Arrizabalaga, "Facing the Black Death," 245.

111. Jacme d'Agramont, "Regiment de Preservacio a Epidemia o Pestilencia e Mortaldats Epistola de Maestre Jacme d'Agramont als honrats e discrets seynnors pa-

hers e conseyll di la Ciutat de Leyda, 1348," trans. M. L. Duran-Reynals and C.-E. A. Winslow, *Bulletin of the History of Medicine* 23 (1949): 57–89, quotation on 84.

112. For an analysis of this text, see Arrizabalaga, "Facing the Black Death," 237–288.

113. Cambell, *Enquête*, 516.

114. Sara Ritchey, "Illness and Imagination: The Healing Miracles of Clare of Montefalco," in *The World of St. Francis: Essays in Honor of William R. Cook*, ed. Bradley Franco and Beth Mulvaney (Leiden: Brill, 2014), 113–143.

115. Cambell, *Enquête*, 145.

116. Cambell, *Enquête*, 82. The article of interrogation states, "Item, quod Anthonetus . . . graviter infirmus de febre continua, et bossam et carbunculum habuit supra bossam." No one identified this as the present mortality or *lo cat*, but it did happen at the time when the illness was in the region.

117. Cambell, *Enquête*, 143, 82. For signs of death in canonization inquests, see Leigh Ann Craig, "Describing Death and Resurrection: Medicine and the Humors in Two Late Medieval Miracles," in *The Sacred and the Secular in Medieval Healing: Sites, Objects, and Texts*, ed. Barbara Bowers and Linda Keyser (London: Routlege, 2016), 103–115.

118. Cambell, *Enquête*, 82–83.

119. Cambell, *Enquête*, 146.

120. Cambell, *Enquête*, 434.

121. Cambell, *Enquête*, 435.

122. Cambell, *Enquête*, 434–435.

123. Cambell, *Enquête*, 436

124. Cambell, *Enquête*, 436. Although she does not specify, she likely meant that she hastened to Delphine in her heart, as the noble Lady Andrea Raymon did when she saw the mercenaries.

125. Cambell, *Enquête*, 81, 448–449.

126. Cambell, *Enquête*, 452.

127. Labande, "L'occupation," 87–95.

128. Labande, "L'occupation," 86.

5. Master Durand Andree and the Sacrament of Penance

1. For an overview of debates surrounding the intellectual history of the efficacy of confession, see Martin, "Popular and Monastic Pastoral Issues," 320–332.

2. For an overview of understandings of confession and its practice, see the collected essays in *L'aveu, antiquité et Moyen Âge*, ed. Jean-Claude Maire Vigueur (Rome: École Français de Rome, 1986).

3. Thayer, *Penitence, Preaching, and the Coming of the Reformation*, 1–12.

4. Peregrine Horden, "Ritual and Public Health in the Early Medieval City," in *Histories of Urban Public Health*, ed. Sally Sheard and Helen Power (Aldershot: Ashgate, 2000), 17–40.

5. Cambell, *Enquête*, 207.

6. Louis Stouff, "Les Provençaux et la mort," 200–201. This synthetic article brings together the work of Jacques Chiffoleau, Noël Coulet, and others. See also Michaud, "La peste, la peur et l'espoir: 399–443.

7. Stouff, "Les Provençaux et la mort," 204–216.

8. For more on Durand as a medical doctor, see Joseph Ziegler, "Practitioners and Saints: Medical Men in Canonization Processes in the Thirteenth to Fifteenth Centuries," *Social History of Medicine* 12 (1999): 191–225. Master Durand also appears in Amargier, "Dauphine de Puymichel et son entourage," 117, and in Sigal, "Les temoins et les temoignages au procèes de canonisation," 470–471.

9. ADV 3 E 33 MS 1 fol. 25v-26v. This was a donation involving the Holy Cross convent in 1361. Nicolau Laurens, the proctor of Delphine's inquest, appeared in this document as well, receiving the donation documents. When Master Durand Andree died in 1377, he was buried in the convent of the Holy Cross in Apt. See Albanés, *Gallia Christiana Novissima*, 1:300–301.

10. ADV 2MI 193. This microfilm contains ADV 1G 9, "Comtes de recettes et dépenses de l'évêché d'Avignon, 1363–1368." Master Durand also interacted with the papal court in his attempt in 1360 to be considered for a vacant office. See ADV 3E 4 MS 2, fol. 58v. In 1373, he followed Pope Gregory XI to Rome and acted as his almoner until his death in 1377. See Albanés, *Gallia Christiana Novissima*, 1:300–301.

11. For the local workings of Lenten confession in the region around Avignon, see Clément Lenoble, *L'exercice de la pauvreté: Économie et religion chez les franciscains d'Avignon (XIIIe–XVe siècles)* (Rennes: Presses Universitaires de Rennes, 2013).

12. Cohen-Hanegbi, *Caring for the Living Soul*, 18–66.

13. Rusconi, "De la prédication," 67–85; Siegfried Wenzel, "Preaching the Seven Deadly Sins," in *In the Garden of Evil*, ed. Richard Newhauser, 145–169; Carolyn Muessig, "Sermon, Preacher and Society in Middle Ages," *Journal of Medieval History* 28 (2012): 73–91. For Dominican preaching in Provence, see Jacques Paul, "Les frères Prêcheurs de la province de Provence," *Cahiers de Fanjeaux* 36 (2001): 19–59.

14. Tentler, *Sin and Confession*, 104.

15. William J. Courtenay, "Curers of Body and Soul: Medical Doctors as Theologians," in *Religion and Medicine in the Middle Ages*, ed. Peter Biller and Joseph Ziegler (York: York Medieval Press, 2001), 69–75.

16. Cambell, *Enquête*, 267: "movebantur corda audiencium et predictorum fuerunt mutata ad penitenciam, contricionem, compunctionem, lacrimarum effusionem et de offensis quas in Deum commiserant dolorem, eo quod peccatorum omnium vite sue recordabantur et eis reducebantur ad memoriam, ac si omnia illa in scriptis haberent cum summo desiderio confitendi."

17. Pierre Payer, *Sex and the New Medieval Literature of Confession, 1150–1300* (Toronto: Pontifical Institute of Medieval Studies, 2009), 50–58.

18. For the importance of tears in contrition, see Mary Carruthers, "On Affliction and Reading, Weeping and Argument: Chaucer's Lachrymose Troilus in Context," *Representations* 93 (2006): 1–21. For tears in Delphine's inquest, see Archambeau, "Remembering Countess Delphine's Books," 33–49.

19. See Silvana Vecchio, "Peccatum Cordis," *Micrologus* 11 (2003): 332–333. She points out the importance of *compunctio* to Augustine, Isidore of Seville, Bernard of Clairvaux, and Guglielmo Alvernia. For Gregory the Great, *compunctio* could be caused by both fear and love, and Isidore defined it as "humility of the mind, accompanied by tears, that is born from the memory of sin and the fear of judgement." (Conpunctio cordis est humilitas mentis cum lacrimis, exoriens de recordatione

peccati et timore iudicii." From Isidore of Seville, *Sententia* vol. 2, book 12 PL 83, 613–614.)

20. Bertranda placed the events about twenty years before the inquest, making it 1343. Cambell, *Enquête*, 338–339.

21. The ladies were two of Queen Sanxia's *familiares*, Francesca de Mari and Iohanna de Meleto. See Cambell, *Enquête*, 339.

22. Cambell, *Enquête*, 56: "domine nobiles et magnifice socie."

23. Cambell, *Enquête*, 56: "ab ore dicte domine comitisse scintille ignee processerunt."

24. Cambell, *Enquête*, 56: "ex cuius visionis, miraculo ammirantes dicte due nobiles domine et compuncte intrinsecus, confiteri statim, sine intervallo alio, voluerunt; et confesse fuerunt peccata earum."

25. Virginia Reinburg, "Hearing Lay People's Prayer," in *Culture and Identity in Early Modern Europe (1500–1800)*, ed. Barbara Diefendorf and Carla Hesse (Ann Arbor: University of Michigan Press, 1993), 19–39.

26. Gérard Jacquin, "Éducation et culture de la noblesse en Anjou au XIVe siècle," in *La noblesse dans les territoires Angevins à la fin du Moyen Âge*, ed. Noël Coulet and Jean-Michel Matz, 677–688 (Rome: École Française de Rome, 2000). For the general popularity of books of vices and virtues, see Richard Newhauser, introduction to *In the Garden of Evil*, vii–xix. For analyses of poetry, see the essays collected in Herman Braet and Verner Verbeke, eds., *Death in the Middle Ages* (Leuven: Leuven University Press, 1983). For confession in particular, see Rusconi, "De la prédication," 67–85. For an overview of the spread of Franciscan ideas about the works of mercy in frescoes and other art forms, see Federico Botana, *The Works of Mercy in Italian Medieval Art (c. 1050–1400)* (Leiden: Brepols, 2011), 49–81. For a study of the complexity of education and change before the Reformation, see Thayer, *Penitence, Preaching, and the Reformation*, 2–3.

27. For women's education, see Anne Marie de Gendt, *L'art d'éduquer les nobles damoiselles: Le livre de chevalier de la Tour Landry* (Paris: Honoré Champion, 2003); Pierre Boisard, "La vie intellectuelle de la noblesse Angevine à la fin du XIVe siècle d'après *Le Chevalier de la Tour Landry*," in *La littérature Angevine médiévale* (Paris: Honoré Champion, 1981), 135–154; Susan Groag Bell, "Medieval Women Book Owners: Arbiters of Lay Piety and Ambassadors of Culture," *Signs* 7 (1982): 742–768. For an early fourteenth-century Occitan prayer book, see Geneviève Hasenohr, "Un donat de dévotion en Langue d'oc du XIIIe siècle: Le *Liber divini amoris*," *Cahier de Fanjeaux* 35 (2000): 219–243.

28. A fourteenth-century copy of Jacobus Voragine's *Golden Legend*, found in Forqualquier and written in Occitan, suggests a lay readership of saints' lives in Provence. Paul Meyer, "La traduction Provençale de la Légende Dorée," *Romania* 27 (1898): 93–137.

29. In a list of liturgical manuscripts of Apt compiled by the Ministère de la Culture, de la Communication, des Grands Travaux et du Bicentenaire, this book is identified as #19, Livres d'heures, dit "de sainte Delphine" XIVe. When I accessed this book in 2008, it was held in the Musée Trésor de la Cathédrale Sainte-Anne in Apt, Provence. The book is poetically described in Abbé Henri Théolas, *Le vitrail d'Apt et le retour de la papauté d'Avignon à Rome* (Avignon: Imprimerie D. Seguin, 1924), 37–41. The book is briefly described in Abbé Joseph Sautel, "Catalogue descriptif des manuscrits liturgiques de l'église d'Apt," *Annales d'Avignon et du Comtat Venaissin* (1919): 104. The

Archives Départmentales de Vaucluse owns a rather difficult to read microfilm of the document, 1 Mi 435. The list of liturgical manuscripts also includes one other book of hours, five breviaries, and two books of sermons, all from the fourteenth century, among its far more famous musical documents, all of which are described by Joseph Sautel. I sincerely thank Marie-Claude Leonelli, Jean-Laurent Rosenthal, Mike Osborne, and Mme. Pion for help in gaining access to the physical document.

30. *Le breviari d'amor de Matfre Ermengaud*, ed. Peter T. Ricketts, with collaboration of Cyril P. Hershon, vols. 2–4 (Turnhout: Brepols, 1989–2004). An earlier edition is Matfre Ermengaud, *Le breviari d'amor*, ed. Gabriel Azaïs (Paris: Librairie A. Frank, 1862).

31. Thirty-two manuscripts and fragments of the text have been identified. All fourteen of the complete manuscripts include at least two hundred miniatures. See Federico Botana, "Virtuous and Sinful Uses of Temporal Wealth in the *Breviari d'Amor* of Matfre Ermengaud (MS BL Royal 19.C.I.)," *Journal of the Warburg and Courtauld Institutes* 67 (2004): 50.

32. Botana, "Virtuous and Sinful Uses of Temporal Wealth," 58.

33. Botana, "Virtuous and Sinful Uses of Temporal Wealth," 50.

34. For example, Master Durand Andree, who came to Apt from a town outside Bèziers. See the notarial register of Laurent Laurent, ADV, 3E 4 MS 2, 61v–62v.

35. Michelle Bolduc, "The *Breviari d'Amor*: Rhetoric and Preaching in Thirteenth-Century Languedoc," *Rhetorica* 24 (2006): 403–425.

36. Bolduc, "*Breviari*," 418.

37. Wenzel, "Preaching the Seven Deadly Sins," 145–169.

38. For example, Katherine Jansen described sermons as dialogical, since they could incorporate revisions based on reactions to earlier versions. See Jansen, *The Making of the Magdalen*, 7.

39. Cambell, *Enquête*, 441: "sed ex tunc portavit vestes humiles et vitam suam mutavit in melius; et ad inductionem dicte domine Dalphine pluries ipsa testis loquens confessionem fecit generaliter de omnibus peccatis suis."

40. For metaphors of illness and health, see Bolduc, "*Breviari*," 416–418.

41. Cambell, *Enquête*, 482–483: "ipsa testis loquens et plures alie de dicto monasterio moniales dimiserunt vestes nimis curiosas et maioris precii et anulos ac taccas et coclearia argentea, Agnus Dei de argento et plura alia iocalia que habebant vendiderunt, et pecunias seu precia pauperibus erogaverunt."

42. See Janzen, *The Making of the Magdalen*, 161–162.

43. Cambell, *Enquête*, 474–475: "audivit semel ipsam dominam Dalphinam dicentem quod, quando Deus fecit alicui persone graciam et consolacionem in confessione, debet attribuere totum Deo et humiliare seipsam. Et ipsa testis loquens ex dictis verbis perpendit quod dicta domina Dalphina tetigit interiora cordis sui, quia, quandoque ipsa testis loquens, dum vacaverat oracioni et devote oraverat, dabat sibi vanam gloriam et attribuebat sibi totum et non attribuebat Deo cum humilitate, a quo totum procedebat. Et propter dicta verba et tunc, quantum Deus dedit sibi graciam, emendavit se de predictis et Deo attribuit."

44. See Archambeau, "Remembering Countess Delphine's Books," 42–44.

45. Cambell, *Enquête*, 252: "O quam vane et perverse visiones que non deducunt animam, nisi ad noxios mundi honores, famam, et favores!"

46. Cambell, *Enquête*, 252.

47. Cambell, *Enquête*, 252: "tangentibus salutem anime."

48. Cambell, *Enquête*, 252.

49. Tentler, *Sin and Confession*, 109–111. The quote is on page 109.

50. For the importance of memory and for preparing for confession by trying to recall sins, see Tentler, *Sin and Confession*, 109–113.

51. See Anne Thayer and Katharine Lualdi *Handbook for Curates: A Late Medieval Manual on Pastoral Ministry*, trans. Anne Thayer (Washington, DC: Catholic University of America Press, 2011), xiii. There are roughly 250 surviving manuscript copies of this text, suggesting its popularity.

52. Guido de Monte Rochen, *Manipulus curatorum* (Rome: Per magistrum Steffanum Plank de Patavia, 1490), f. lxiii r.: "debet enim hoc probabiliter homo credere quod in multis offendit deum quorum non recordatur. Et si sub ista extimatione doleat: sicut si certus esset contritus esset et penitens." Translation from Thayer, *Handbook for Curates*, 175.

53. Thayer, *Handbook for Curates*, 87.

54. Guido of Monte Rochen, *Manipulus curatorum*, Thayer trans., 184.

55. Etiquette or courtesy books, often referred to as mirrors, for women became more popular in the thirteenth century. See Diane Bornstein, *The Lady in the Tower: Medieval Courtesy Literature for Women* (Hamden, CT: Archon Books, 1983), 133–134. Versions and translations of mirrors for princes, especially *Le somme le roi*, written in the vernacular in 1279 for Philippe III of France, were also read by and adapted for women. For an overview, see Roy Harris, "The Occitan Translations of John XII and XIII–XVIII from a Fourteenth-Century Franciscan Codex (Assisi, Chisea Nuova MS. 9)," *Transactions of the American Philosophical Society* 75 (1985): 15–18. For an example of the mirror's incorporation into other texts, see Ellen Kosmer, "Gardens of Virtue in the Middle Ages," *Journal of the Warburg and Courtauld Institutes* 41 (1987): 303.

56. Cohen-Hanegbi, *Caring for the Living Soul*, 120–121.

57. Cambell, *Enquête*, 522: "Interrogata in quo sensiit in corde suo quod dicta domina Dalphina sciret interiora consciencie sue." Rossolina d'Agoult was a relative of the seneschal Raymon d'Agoult involved in the so-called war of the seneschals discussed in chapter 2.

58. Cambell, *Enquête*, 522: "esset anxia in mente sua de quodam peccato suo quod confiteri volebat, spectans confessorem cui confiteretur ibidem, nec propter anxietatem predictam adverteret bene ad verba dicte domine Dalphine."

59. The requirement to speak aloud to a priest was considered by some unnecessary and problematic, but Delphine's witnesses do not speak of it that way, even when they describe it as difficult. For the Wycliffite view that the priest was not necessary to confession, see K. Little, *Confession and Resistance*, 49–77.

60. Cambell, *Enquête*, 263: "ac si colligeret florum manipulos diversorum."

61. Cambell, *Enquête*, 263: "Qualis confessor estis vos, quod non reprehendatis me de iniquitatibus meis, quas vobis confessa sum!"

62. Cambell, *Enquête*, 263.

63. Peter Biller and A. J. Minnis, eds., *Handling Sin: Confession in the Middle Ages* (York: University of York Press, 1998).

64. Quoted in Tentler, *Sin and Confession*, 242.

65. Michelle Armstrong-Partida, "Conflict in the Parish: Antagonistic Relations between Clerics and Parishioners," in *A Companion to Pastoral Care in the Late Middle Ages (1200–1500)*, ed. Ronald Stansbury (Leiden: Brill, 2010), 173–212.

66. Guido of Monte Rochen, *Manipulus curatorum*, tract 2, chaps. 1–7. For an overview of thirteenth- and fourteenth-century attitudes, see Tentler, *Sin and Confession*, 235–236.

67. Cambell, *Enquête*, 401: "Vis servire Deo, et eris filia mea?" Et dicta Huga respondit ita: "Libenter!" Et tunc dicta domina Dalphina dixit dicte Hugue: "Removeas dictos pilos, qui impediunt animam tuam!"

68. Cambell, *Enquête*, 402: "mutavit animum quem habebat primo de pilis."

69. Cambell, *Enquête*, 402. For another analysis of this encounter, see Amargier, "Dauphine de Puymichel et son entourage," 119.

70. Katherine Jansen, "Mary Magdalen and the Mendicants: The Preaching of Penance in the Late Middle Ages," *Journal of Medieval History* 21 (1995): 1–25.

71. Mazel, *La noblesse et l'Église*, 526–527.

72. Cambell, *Enquête*, 507, 523.

73. ADV 3 E 33 MS 1 fol. 24r-24v. This register includes a document that lists the nuns of St. Catherine's convent, which includes Jordana de Viens.

74. Since both Rossolina and Tiburga agreed to the details as written in Article 61 rather than telling the story in their testimonies, I use the language of Article 61 here.

75. Cambell, *Enquête*, 73, Article 61.

76. Susan Snyder, "The Left Hand of God: Despair in Medieval and Renaissance Tradition," *Studies in the Renaissance* 12 (1965): 19–21.

77. Cambell, *Enquête*, 73–74, Article 61.

78. Cambell, *Enquête*, 74–75, Article 62.

79. Cambell, *Enquête*, 74, Article 61: "statim a dicta temptacione liberata fuit penitus et omnino, et in tantum quod, eciam si voluisset, non poterat postea cogitare, nec potuit res de quibus temptacionem huiusmodi sustinebat tam gravem."

80. It is not clear from the article if her aversion to food was a spiritual expression linked to her renouncing of worldly things that she testified to in Article 35, but it does suggest the complex relationship with food many women experienced in the later Middle Ages. See Caroline Walker Bynum, *Holy Feast and Holy Fast: The Religious Significance of Food to Medieval Women* (Berkeley: University of California Press, 1987).

81. Cambell, *Enquête*, 58: "Cumque nec modum nec formam perfecte confessionis faciende in seipsa inveniret, neque haberet de peccatis memoriam sicut vellet, tristabatur, quia dubitabat dampnari."

82. Tentler, "The Conduct of Confession," in *Sin and Confession*, 82–95. For comparison to another geographical region, see Eljenholm Nichols, "The Etiquette of Pre-Reformation Confession in East Anglia," *Sixteenth Century Journal* 17 (1986): 145–163.

83. Cambell, *Enquête*, 58: "puram et humilem et veram confessionem, Dei indignacio tollebatur et anima reconciliabatur Creatori suo." This is consistent with theological views from the fourteenth century. See Martin, "Popular and Monastic Pastoral Issues," 320–332.

84. Cambell, *Enquête*, 58: "ac si tunc eadem peccata commisisset et si in uno libro videret eadem peccata descripta." This language, especially Maria's reference to a book, reflects the influence of the literature of confession. See Tentler, *Sin and Confession*, 110.

85. Cambell, *Enquête*, 58.

86. Cambell, *Enquête*, 58: "ad portas mortis."

87. Cambell, *Enquête*, 288: "dixit contenta in articulo esse vera."

88. Cambell, *Enquête*, 288.

89. For an analysis of conflicting statements, see Smoller, "Miracle, Memory, and Meaning," 429–454.

90. Cambell, *Enquête*, 400: "magna tristicia propter peccata sua, quod timebat non habere tempus sufficiens ad agendam penitenciam de peccatis, et ex hoc posset dampnari."

91. Cambell *Enquête*, 401: "dedit sibi exemplum de duabus mollis: una superiori, alia inferiori; et quod per superiorem mollam intelligebatur confidencia Dei, et per inferiorem mollam, cognicio suorum peccatorum."

92. Cambell, *Enquête*, 401: "Et dicebat sic: "Cum consideras mollam inferiorem, que est cognicio peccatorum, et non consideras mollam superiorem, que est confidencia Dei, et sicut molla inferior sine alia superiori non potest molere bladum, sic de te. Modo considera illam mollam superiorem et habeas confidenciam in Deo, et sic eris consolata ab huiusmodi tristicia!"

93. Payer, *Sex*, 66–67.

94. For an overview of changes, see Payer, *Sex*, 68–73. For theological debates on penance, see Tentler, *Sin and Confession*, 318–340. As Tentler points out, the *Raymundina*, a summa for confessors written by Raymon of Penyafort, at least seven years of penance for serious sins like adultery, perjury, fornication, and homicide. See especially pages 320–322.

95. A subtly different millstone metaphor appears in the *Manipulus curatorum*. In this metaphor, the top millstone is fear of penalty for sin, and the bottom millstone is hope of divine mercy. Thayer, *Handbook for Curates*, 165.

96. Tentler, *Sin and Confession*, 22–27.

97. Payer, *Sex*, 66–71.

98. Our modern word "sadness" does not capture the complexity of this emotion in the fourteenth century. See Rosenwein, "Emotion Words," 93–106. For an exploration of this term, and the idea of affective piety, see Boquet and Nagy, *Medieval Sensibilities*, 183–185.

99. This evokes the theological debate about doing one's best. See Martin, "Popular and Monastic Pastoral Issues," 322–325.

6. Sister Resens de Insula and the Desire for Certainty

1. A local notarial record lists her among the nuns of the Holy Cross convent in 1362. See ADV 3 E 4 MS2 fol. 47r.

2. The convent moved inside the walls permanently by 1375. See Denifle, *La désolation des églises*, 2:680.

3. Cambell, *Enquête*, 490. When the papal commissioners asked Resens about when this happened, she said that about twelve years had elapsed: "Interrogata de tempore, dixit quod sunt bene XII anni elapsi vel circa."

4. Cambell, *Enquête*, 490: "Item, dixit quod, cum esset in quadam tristicia et dolore cordis propter quoddam dubium consciencie sue, quod quidem dubium non poterat a se removere, licet pluries fuisset confessa."

5. Cambell, *Enquête*, 490: "Dalphina dixit sibi bona vera et consolatoria, propter que ipsa testis loquens fuit consolata, et ex tunc ipsa testis loquens dictam tristiciam non habuit."

6. Greg Peters, "Religious Orders and Pastoral Care in the Late Middle Ages," in *A Companion to Pastoral Care in the Late Middle Ages (1200–1500)*, ed. Ronald Stansbury (Leiden: Brill, 2010), 263–284; Payer, *Sex*, 22–24. The language of law could also appear in pastoral care manuals; Bériou, "La confession dans les écrits théologiques et pastoraux," 261–282.

7. Tentler, *Sin and Confession*, 347.

8. Guido of Monte Rochen, *Manipulus curatorum*, part 2, tract 3, chap. 6: "licet enim dolore debeat propter peccata que commisit debet tamen gaudere propter vitam quam recuperavit." Translation from Thayer, *Handbook for Curates*, 211.

9. Didactic literature for confessors dealt more directly with this, but still struggled to answer basic questions about how confessees should know they had experienced the right kind and/or amount of contrition. See Tentler, *Sin and Confession*, 236–238.

10. Cambell, *Enquête*, 53–54: "Item, quod commune dictum, communis opinio, communis assercio et reputacio ac publica vox et fama in partibus Provincie et alibi notorium fuit et est quod ipsa domina Dalphina, ex magna eius devocione et spiritus fervore erga Deum, ut plurimum et quasi continue verba de Deo ex ore suo proferebat. Et quod per verba ipsius persone audientes ad vite earum mutacionem et penitenciam agendam sepissime et mirabiliter movebantur. Et dicebant se nunquam audivisse verba ad mutacionem vite et penitenciam et emendacionem de peccatis tantum inducencia et allicencia sicut erant verba dicte domine. Quodque dictam dominam Dalphinam Deus in hoc mirabiliter et singulariter predotaverat et ei graciam dederat quod quicumque, eam videns et verba eius audiens, dicebat et senciebat quod ipsa particularia et interiora consciencie et status et vite cuiuslibet ipsorum eandem videncium et audiencium sciebat et tangebat. Et quelibet persona, ipsam audiens et documenta eius precipere cupiens, reddebatur in sua mente et animo consolata et de sue consciencie dubiis certificata, licet eadem dubia per personam aliquam eidem domine non fuissent patefacta; ymmo, quod mirabilius erat, in una eademque locucione seu collacione loquendo de Deo multas personas circumstantes et eam simul audientes, verbis suis spiritualiter reficiebat et edificabat, quamvis audientes, eandem diversas consideraciones et voluntates et varias consciencias et dubitaciones haberent. Et unaquaque persona audiencium quod sibi opus erat ex verbis ipsius domine reportabat. Et quod propterea multe et multe persone, mares et femine, tam seculares quam regulares et religiose, eciam iuvenes, de vita seculari pomposa, lasciva et lubrica fuerunt ad vitam bonam, sanctam et honestam et ad humilem statum et penitenciam mirabiliter commutate, converse et translate."

11. Caroline Walker Bynum, *Christian Materiality: An Essay on Religion in Late Medieval Europe* (Cambridge, MA: MIT Press, 2015), 130–138.

12. Voice and touch were common ways that people described miracles. See Sigal, *L'homme et le miracle*, 68.

13. For other approaches to widows in the years after the plague, see Smail, "Accommodating Plague in Medieval Marseille," 11–41; Mavis Mate, *Daughters, Wives and Widows after the Black Death: Women in Sussex, 1350–1535* (Woodbridge, UK: Boydell Press, 1998); Christiane Klapisch-Zuber, "Plague and Family Life," in *The New Cambridge Medieval History* (Cambridge: Cambridge University Press, 2000), 6:124–154.

14. Sister Resens briefly described Lauduna's transformation, but gave more information about the transformation of a woman identified as Barrassa d'Apt, whose husband may have died the year before the first mortality. Cambell, *Enquête*, 488–489. Resens also described several other women who did not become nuns, but did give up their worldly lifestyles after hearing Delphine speak. She remembered this occurring in the year before the first mortality.

15. Lauduna d'Apt appeared in the notarial record of Apt in 1362 giving up her right to certain properties at the marriage of her relative, Raymon d'Apt. See ADV 3 E 4 MS2 fol. 47v.

16. Cambell, *Enquête*, 484: "cum aliis pluribus viduis mulieribus in hac civitate Aptensi."

17. Cambell, *Enquête*, 484.

18. Cambell, *Enquête*, 385: "ad desperacionem inducebatur."

19. Cambell *Enquête*, 385: "staret perplexa nec haberet aliquam leticiam sed in tristicia magno maneret et dolore."

20. Cambell, *Enquête*, 385: "Et omnis tristicia recessit a corde suo, et eciam omnis prava cogitacio; et temptaciones varias et diversas quas prius habuerat non senciit, sed leta et firma in suo voto permansit, sicut adhuc permanet."

21. Welkenhuysen, "La peste en Avignon (1348)," 468: "cum luctibus et fletibus incendentes et capillos trahentes, cum acerrimis flagellis usque effusionem sanguinis se percutiebant."

22. For an overview of the relationship between mind and body in later medieval medicine, see Siraisi, *Taddeo Alderotti and His Pupils*, 203–236.

23. For how nuns and others should consider Christ, see Rachel Fulton, *From Judgment to Passion: Devotion to Christ and the Virgin Mary, 800–1200* (New York: Columbia University Press, 2002), 142–192.

24. Cambell, *Enquête*, 267.

25. Cambell, *Enquête*, 267: "desiderantes de eorumdem conscienciis informari et de dubiis conscienciarum ipsorum certificari cum eadem."

26. Cambell, *Enquête*, 267.

27. Cambell, *Enquête*, 267.

28. Weinstein and Bell, *Saints and Society*, 149–151.

29. Fifteenth-century authors wrote more directly about this issue for lay readers. See Martin, "Popular and Monastic Pastoral Issues," 321–323.

30. For the anxiety about sin and separation from the Christian community, see Tentler, *Sin and Confession*, 234–235.

31. For a discussion of doubt in Augustine's Sermon 393, "De poenitentibus," PL 39, 1713–1715, see Tentler, *Sin and Confession*, 8–9.

32. For an overview of the Franciscan practices of Delphine and her husband Elzear, see Lenoble, *L'exercice de la pauvreté*, 61–63.

33. St. Bonaventure, "Legenda Sancti Francisci," in *Doctoris Seraphici S. Bonaventurae, S. R. Episcopi Cardinalis, Opera Omnia* (Florence: Typographia Collegii S. Bonaventurae, 1898), 511: "certificatus est de remissione plenaria omnium delictorum." For a version of this event in Provençal, see *La vida del glorios Sant Frances: Version Provençale de la legenda maior Sancti Francisci de Saint Bonaventure*, ed. Ingrid Arthur (Uppsala: Almqvist & Wiksells Boktryckeri AB, 1955), 157–158. I sincerely thank Mary Carruthers for pointing out this usage of *certificare*.

34. Heiko Oberman, *The Harvest of Medieval Theology: Gabriel Biel and Late Medieval Nominalism* (Cambridge, MA: Harvard University Press, 1963), 146–160.

35. For an overview, see Martin, "Popular and Monastic Pastoral Issues," 323–324. For the dangers of thinking too much about sin, see Tentler, *Sin and Confession*, 113–116.

36. Lawrence G. Duggan, "Fear and Confession on the Eve of the Reformation," *Archiv für Reformationsgeschichte* 75 (1984): 153–157.

37. Some transformations were described elsewhere. For example, the woman who repented prostitution at Delphine's vigil was considered in testimonies about the vigil, not as an internal transformation.

38. See the testimonies of Catherine de Pui, Bertranda Bertomieua, and Catherine Giraud.

39. Cambell, *Enquête*, 402.

40. Cambell, *Enquête*, 442. In Delphine's saint's life, Bartholomeo de Pertuis was called a usurer, but that accusation does not appear in the inquest. See Cambell, *Vies Occitan*, 208–209.

41. Cambell, *Enquête*, 481–482.

42. For preaching in monastic settings, see Muessig, "What Is Medieval Monastic Preaching?," in *Medieval Monastic Preaching*, ed. Carolyn Muessig (Leiden: Brill, 1998), 3–8. For more formal sermons in the cloister, see Gabriella Zarri, "Places and Gestures of Women's Preaching in Quattro- and Cinquecentro Italy," in *Charisma and Religious Authority: Jewish, Christian, and Muslim Preaching, 1200–1500*, ed. Katherine Jansen and Miri Rubin (Turnhout: Brepols, 2010), 177–196.

43. For women educating others in the convent, see Carolyn Muessig, "Prophecy and Song: Teaching and Preaching by Medieval Women," in *Women Preachers and Prophets through Two Millennia of Christianity*, ed. Beverly Mayne Kienzle and Pamela J. Walker (Berkeley: University of California Press, 1998), 146–158.

44. Cambell, *Enquête*, 482.

45. See Vauchez, *Sainthood*, 394–395.

46. Cambell, *Enquête*, 483: "Dixit eciam interrogata quod nunquam audivit, dum vixit, aliquam personam per cuius verba sive documenta aliquis sive aliqua persona melius induceretur ad mutacionem vite sue et ad peragendum penitenciam sicut per verba antedicte domine."

47. Cambell, *Enquête*, 52. For an overview of the *ars praedicandi*, see Roberts, "The *Ars Praedicandi* and the Medieval Sermon," in *Preacher, Sermon, and Audience in the Middle Ages*, ed. Carolyn Muessig (Leiden: Brill, 2002), 41–62.

48. Cambell, *Enquête*, 52. For the nuances of the phrase "word of God" in women's public speaking, see Claire M. Waters, *Angels and Earthly Creatures: Preaching, Performance, and Gender in the Later Middle Ages (Philadelphia: University of Pennsylvania Press, 2004)*, 121–123. See also Timothy Johnson, introduction to *Franciscans and Preaching: Every Miracle from the Beginning of the World Came about through Words*, ed. Timothy Johnson (Leiden: Brill, 2012), 1–8.

49. Alcuin Blamires, "Women and Preaching in Medieval Orthodoxy, Heresy, and Saints' Lives," *Viator* 26 (1995): 135–152.

50. Nicole Bériou, "The Right of Women to Give Religious Instruction in the Thirteenth Century," in *Women Preachers and Prophets through Two Millennia of Chris-*

tianity, ed. Beverly Mayne and Pamela J. Walker Kienzle (Berkeley: University of California Press, 1998), 134–145.

51. Clemens, "Cult of Mary Magdalene"; Saxer, *Le culte de Marie Madaleine en Occident* (Auxerre: Publications de la Société des Fouilles Archéologiques et des Monuments Historiques de l'Yonne, 1959), 228–249; Jansen, *The Making of the Magdalen*, 324–327.

52. Cambell, *Enquête*, 540. For Philippe Cabassole's interest in Mary Magdalene, see Saxer, "Philippe Cabassole et son *Libellus*," 193–204. For an excerpt of the *Libellus*, see Étienne M. Faillon, *Monuments inédit sur l'apostolat de Sainte Marie-Madeleine en Provence*, vol. 2 (Paris: J.P. Migne, 1865), columns 789–796.

53. The palm frond was one of the ways Charles II was able to identify the remains as Mary Magdalene's. See Jansen, *Making of the Magdalen*, 62–82.

54. Clemens, "Cult of Mary Magdalene," 216–221.

55. For Francis Meyronne at King Robert I's court in Naples, see Kelly, *The New Solomon*, 41–42. Francis Meyronne was also important in Delphine's life as the person who heard her husband Elzear's last confession in Paris in 1323. See Mazel, *La noblesse et l'Église*, 528. Meyronne would have been at Elzear's inquest in Apt in 1351.

56. See Mazel, *La noblesse et l'Église*, 12–13.

57. Hébert, "La noblesse Provençale," 327–345.

58. Cambell, *Enquête*, 542–543.

59. Cambell, *Enquête*, 543: "ab infusione Spiritus sancti." It is important to reiterate that Delphine's words do not come from a vision, but her clarity comes from divine influence.

60. Some papal audiences reading these testimonies might have understood this to reflect the idea that women's ability to speak of God came not from intelligence or education but from an outside gift. See Muessig, "Prophecy and Song," 146–148.

61. Cambell, *Enquête*, 54–55: "fuerunt eis reddita clara, lucida et decisa."

62. Philippe Cabassole used the phrase "*magnos clericos litteratos*" to describe the people Delphine spoke to. Cambell, *Enquête*, 540–541. Perhaps Francis Meyronne's name was included here not just for his well-known theological presence and links to the kings of Naples, but also because of his support for the preaching and erudition of Mary Magdalene, which may have made him a natural supporter of learned, eloquent women. See Jansen, *The Making of the Magdalen*, 73.

63. Cambell, *Enquête*, 232: "ante mortalitatem primam." For an analysis of this figure, see Sylvain Piron, "Les studia Franciscains de Provence et d'Aquitaine (1275–1335)," in *Philosophy and Theology in the Studia of the Religious Orders at the Papal and Royal Courts. Acts of the XVth International Colloquium of the Société Internationale pour l'Étude de la Philosophie Médiévale*, University of Notre Dame, 8–10 October, 2008 (2012): 303–358.

64. Cambell, *Enquête*, 232.

65. Cambell, *Enquête*, 233: "quod de tribus dubiis magnis in sacra pagina factis." The commissioners asked Friar Bertran what those doubts were, but he did not know.

66. Cambell, *Enquête*, 268: "Qui habitat in adiutorio Altissimi." This is Psalm 90 in the Vulgate.

67. Cambell, *Enquête*, 540–541.

68. Cambell, *Enquête*, 540–541: "videlicet quomodo in incarnatione Verbi Dei concurrerunt virtus innata, virtus infusa et virtus increata, ut simul fuerit unus homo."

69. For a witness who was initially suspicious of Delphine's speaking, see Cambell, *Enquête*, 298–299.

Conclusion. Lord Giraud de Simiana and the Health of Body and Soul

1. Jean-Luc Bonnaud, *Un état en Provence. Les officiers locaux du comte de Provence au XIVe siècle (1309–1382)* (Rennes: Presses Universitaires de Rennes, 2007), annexe S, 12.

2. Cortez, *Grands Officiers*, 82–83.

3. Cambell, *Enquête*, 544. Interestingly, Giraud testified to different words that Delphine spoke than were included in the article, though they have the same general meaning. I present Giraud's words here: "Videas, fili, quomodo mundus satisfacit nobis. Tu vides in quo statu ego sum. Tu fuisti in magnis periculis et in infirmitatibus, quas ego vidi et de quibus non erat spes quod curareris ab illis; et non sis ingratus Deo de graciis quas fecit tibi; quia, cum velles fecisse plura bona quando eris in fine dierum tuorum!"

4. Cambell, *Enquête*, 544.

5. Cambell, *Enquête*, 544: "et placuit sibi plus multum stare tunc iuxta ipsam dominam Dalphinam quam primo." Giraud's testimony also differs from the article here. In the article, he was described as making a general confession in two or three sessions over several days. See Cambell, *Enquête*, 61–62.

6. Cambell, *Enquête*, 544: "propter verba dicte domine Dalphine et sanctitatem ipsius."

7. Cambell, *Enquête*, 544. Lord Giraud's wife, Lady Maria d'Evenos, also remarked on Lord Giraud's transformation. See Cambell, *Enquête*, 289.

8. Conrad Rawski, ed., *Petrarch's Remedies for Fortune Fair and Foul: Book II, Remedies for Adversity* (Bloomington: Indiana University Press, 1991).

9. Rawski, *Petrarch's Remedies for Adversity*, 322. For more on Petrarch's Stoic responses to emotional distress in the fourteenth century, see Lansing, *Passion and Order*, 187–216.

10. Rawski, *Petrarch's Remedies for Adversity*, 322–323. These reasons for delaying confession appeared in confession literature as well. See Tentler, *Sin and Confession*, 72.

11. For the importance of externalization of internal experience, see Arnold, "Inside and Outside the Medieval Laity," 107–130.

12. Cambell, *Enquête*, 184–185.

13. Cambell, *Enquête*, 348–350.

14. Cambell, *Enquête*, 375–376.

15. Cambell, *Enquête*, 480–485.

16. Cambell, *Enquête*, 385.

17. Cambell, *Enquête*, 231. For the resignation, see ADV 3E 4, MS 2. fol. 51v–52v. We should be cautious with this resignation of a benefice, however, since Master Durand may not have done this out of contrition, but in hopes of being able to take a more lucrative office in the papal court.

18. See, among many others, Carmichael, *Plague and the Poor*, 108–126.

19. David C. Lindberg, "Medieval Science and Its Religious Context," *Osiris*, 2nd ser., 10 (1995): 67.

20. Monica Green, "Integrative Medicine: Incorporating Medicine and Health into the Canon of Medieval European History," *History Compass* 7 (2009): 1218–1245.

21. Katharine Park, "The Criminal and the Saintly Body: Autopsy and Dissection in Renaissance Italy," *Renaissance Quarterly* 47 (1994): 1–33.

22. Ziegler, "Practitioners and Saints," 191–225.

23. Sara Ritchey, "Health, Healing, and Salvation: Hagiography as a Source for Medieval Healthcare," In *Hagiography and the History of Latin Christendom, 500–1500*, ed. Samantha Herrick (Leiden: Brill, 2019), 417–436.

24. Jacalyn Duffin, *Medical Miracles: Doctors, Saints and Healing in the Modern World* (Oxford: Oxford University Press, 2009).

25. Sari Katala-Peltomaa, *Gender, Miracles, and Daily Life: The Evidence of Fourteenth-Century Canonization Processes* (Turnhout: Brepols, 2009); Sharon Farmer, *Surviving Poverty in Medieval Paris: Gender, Ideology, and the Daily Lives of the Poor* (Ithaca, NY: Cornell University Press, 2002).

26. See Cheyette, *Ermengarde of Narbonne*. Witnesses had a different perspective than those encountered in other kinds of legal sources. See Barton, "'Zealous Anger,'" 153–170; Smail, "Hatred as a Social Institution," 90–126.

27. For an article that looks at a specific historical moment for emotional reaction, see Deploige, "Meurtre politique," 225–254.

28. For an anthropological exploration of difficult emotions, see Good and Kleinman, *Culture and Depression*. For a modern ethnographical approach to emotion, see Leavitt, "Meaning and Feeling," 514–539.

29. Denifle, *La désolation des églises*, 2:441–442.

30. Housley, "Mercenary Companies," 272.

31. Goodich, *Violence and Miracle in the Fourteenth Century*, 117–120.

Bibliography

Manuscript Sources

Archives Civiles, Archives Départmentales des Bouches-du-Rhône, Marseille and Aix-en-Provence, France, Série B, MS1690.

Archives Départmentales de Vaucluse, Avignon, France. 3E, 33, MS 1. Notarial register of Jourdan Manent, 1360.

Archives Départmentales de Vaucluse, Avignon, France. 3E 4 MS 2. Notarial Register of Laurent Laurent, 1346–1375.

Comptes de recettes et dépenses de l'évêché d'Avignon, 1363–1368. Archives Départmentales de Vaucluse, Avignon, France. G 1, MS 9.

Gordon, Bernard de. *Practica, seu Lilium Medicinae*, 1419. National Library of Medicine, History of Medicine Division. Bethesda, Maryland. Early Western Manuscripts, Microfilm, 63–14; 48–105.

Grand prieure de Saint-Gilles des Hospitaliers de Saint-John de Jerusalem. Archives Départmentales de Bouches-du-Rhône, Marseille and Aix-en-Provence, France. H 56.

Livres d'heures, dit "de sainte Delphine," XIVe siècle, Musée Trésor de la Cathédrale Sainte-Anne. Apt, France. Manuscrits Liturgiques d'Apt, MS 19.

Processus, Delphine de Sabran. Bibliothèque Méjanes, Fonds Anciennes. Aix-en-Provence, France. Microfilm, MS. 335.

Printed Primary Sources

Anonymous. "Glorios Dieus don totz ben ha creysensa." *Poesie Provenzali storiche relative all'Italia*, vol. II, edited by Vincenzo de Bartholomaeis. Rome: Botega d'Erasmo, 1931, 316–317.

Agramont, Jacme d'. "Regiment de Preservacio a Epidimia o Pestilencia e Mortaldats." Translated by M. L. Duran-Reynals and C.-E. A. Winslow. *Bulletin of the History of Medicine* 23 (1949): 57–89.

Albanés, J. H., and U. Chevalier, eds. *Actes anciens et documents concernant le Bienheureux Pape Urbain V*. Vol. 1 (Paris, 1897).

Augustine. *Soliloquies and Immortality of the Soul*. Edited and translated by Gerard Watson. Warminster, UK: Aris & Phillips, 1990.

Bonaventure. "Legenda Sancti Francisci." In *Doctoris Seraphici S. Bonaventurae, S. R. Episcopi Cardinalis, Opera Omnia*. Florence: Typographia Collegii S. Bonaventurae, 1898.

Cambell, Jacques. *Enquête pour le procès de Dauphine de Puimichel Comtesse d'Ariano (d. 26—XI—1360): (Apt et Avignon: 14 Mai—30 Octobre 1363)*. Turin: Bottega d'Erasmo, 1978.

——. *Vies Occitanes de Saint Auzias et de Sainte Dauphine*. Rome: Pontificium Athenaeum Antonianum, 1963.

Chauliac, Guy de. *Inventarium sive chirurgia magna*, vol. 1 Text. Edited by Michael McVaugh. Leiden: Brill, 1997.

Diakité, Rala I. and Matthew Sneider, eds. *The Final Book of Giovanni Villani's New Chronicle*. Kalamazoo: Medieval Institute Publications, 2016.

Ermengaud, Matfre. *Le breviari d'amor*. Edited by Gabriel Azaïs. Paris: Librairie A. Frank, 1862.

Faillon, Étienne M. ed. An excerpt of the *Libellus hystorialis Marie beatissime Magdalene,* by Cardinal Philippe Cabassoles. In *Monuments inédits sur l'apostolat de Sainte-Marie-Madeleine en Provence*, volume 2, columns 789–796. Paris: J.P. Migne, 1865

Hayez, Anne-Marie. *Le terrier Avignonnais de l'évêque Anglic Grimoard (1366–1368)*. Paris: CTHS, 1993.

Hébert, Michel, ed. *Regeste des états de Provence 1347–1480*. Paris: CTHS, 2007.

Jurkovic, I., and Janos Bak, eds. *Chronicon: Medieval Narrative Sources; A Chronological Guide with Introductory Essays*. Turnhout: Brepols, 2013.

Krueger, Haven C. *Avicenna's Poem on Medicine*. Springfield, IL: Charles C Thomas, 1963.

Labande, Léon-Honoré, ed. *Inventaire sommaire des Archives communales antérieurs à 1790*, ville de Marseille, Série BB, Vol. 1. Marseille: Imprimerie Moullot, 1909.

Le Petit Thalamus de Montpellier. Montpellier: Jean Martel Ainé, 1811.

Lecacheux, Paul, ed. *Lettres secrètes et curiales de Pape Urbain V (1362–1370)*. Paris: Ancienne Librarie Thorin et Fils, 1902.

Longpré, André, ed. *Pétrarque: Lettres familières*. Vol. 2–4. Paris: Les Belles Lettres, 2004.

Martene, Edmund, and Ursini Durand, eds. *Thesaurus novus anecdotorum*. Vol. 2. Paris, 1717.

McVaugh, Michael, ed. Armengaud Blaise's Translation of Galen, *De Cognitione*. In "Armengaud Blaise as a Translator of Galen." In *Texts and Contexts in Ancient and Medieval Science: Studies on the Occasion of John E. Murdoch's Seventieth Birthday*, edited by Edith Sylla and Michael McVaugh. Leiden: Brill, 1997.

Monte Rochen, Guido de. *Manipulus curatorum*. Rome: Per magistrum Steffanum Plank de Patavia, 1490. Available at Bibliothèque nationale de France, Italian Books before 1601, 519.5.

Mussis, Gabriele de. "Historia de Morbo." In *The Black Death*, edited by Rosemary Horrox, 14–26. Manchester, UK: Manchester University Press, 1994.

Petrarch, Francis. *Letters on Familiar Matters. Rerum familiarum libri*. Vols 1–3. Edited and translated by Aldo Bernardo. Baltimore: Johns Hopkins University Press, 1982.

"Processus Canonizationis et Legendae variae Sancti Ludovici O.F.M." In *Analecta Franciscana*, vol. 7. Florence: Ad Claras Aquas, 1951.

Rawski, Conrad, ed. *Petrarch's Remedies for Fortune Fair and Foul*. Book 2, *Remedies for Adversity*. Bloomington: Indiana University Press, 1991.

Raymond of Penyafort. *Summa de paenitentia*. Edited by Xaverio Ochoa and Aloisio Diez. Rome: Commentarium pro religiosis, 1976.

Reit, S. Van, ed. *Liber de Anima seu Sextus de Naturalibus, IV–V*. Leiden: Brill, 1968.
Reyerson, Kathryn, and Debra Salata, eds. and trans. *Medieval Notaries and Their Acts: The 1327–1328 Register of Jean Holanie*. Kalamazoo, MI: Medieval Institute Publications, 2004.
Ricketts, P. T., ed. *Le breviari d'amor de Matfre Ermengaud*. Vols. 2–4. Turnhout: Brepols, 1989–2004.
Rollo-koster, Joelle. *The People of Curial Avignon: A Critical Edition of the Liber Divisionis and the Lists of Matriculation of the Confraternity of Notre Dame La Majour*. Lewiston, NY: Edwin Mellen Press, 2009.
Pertz, George, ed. *Annales S. Victoris Massiliensis*. MGH SS 23 Hannover, 1924, 1–8.
Sauve, Fernand, ed. "Anciens privilèges d'Apt," in "La vie Aptésienne d'autrefois," *Le Mercure Aptésien*, Sunday, March 24–Sunday, June 30.
Smet, Joseph Jean de, ed. "Breve Chronicon Clerici Anonymi." In *Recueil des Chroniques de Flandre*, Vol. 3. Brussels: Commission Royale Histoire, 1856.
Sorbelli, Albano, ed. *Domenico de Gravina, notarii, Chronicon de rebus in Apulia gestis (aa. 1333–1350)*. Città de Castello: Tipi dell'Editore S. Lapi, 1903.
Stouff, Louis, and Noël Coulet, "Les institutions communales dans les villages de Provence au bas Moyen Âge," *Études rurales* No. 63 / 64 (1976): 67–81.
Welkenhuysen, Andries. "La peste en Avignon (1348) décrite par un témoin oculaire, Louis Sanctus de Beringen (Édition critique, traduction, élements de commentaire)." In *Pascua Mediaevalia: Studies voor Prof. Dr. J. M. de Smet*, 452–492. Leuven: Universitaire pers Leuven, 1983.
Wenzel, Sigfried, ed. *Fasciculus Morum: A Fourteenth-Century Preacher's Handbook*. University Park: Pennsylvania State University Press, 1989.

Secondary Sources

Aberth, John, ed. *The Black Death: The Great Mortality of 1348–1350; A Brief History with Documents*. Boston: Bedford St. Martin's, 2005.
Abulafia, David. *The Western Mediterranean Kingdoms, 1200–1500: The Struggle for Dominion*. London: Longman, 1997.
Agrimi, Jole, and Chiara Crisciani. "Charity and Aid in Medieval Christian Civilization." In *Western Medical Thought from Antiquity to the Middle Ages*, edited by Mirko Grmek. Cambridge, MA: Harvard University Press, 1998.
Albanés, Joseph-Hyacinth. *Gallia Christiana Novissima: Histoire des archevèchés, évèchés, et abbayes de France*. Vol. 1. Montbéliard: Société Anonyme d'Imprimerie Montbéliardaise, 1899.
Allmand, C. T. *The Hundred Years War: England and France at War c. 1300–c. 1450*. Cambridge: Cambridge University Press, 2001.
Amargier, Paul. "Dauphine de Puymichel et son entourage au temps de sa vie Aptésienne (1345–1360)." In *Le peuple des saints: Croyances et dèvotions en Provence et Comtat Venaissin à la fin du Moyen Âge*, 111–123. Avignon: Institut de Recherches et d'Études du Bas Moyen Âge Avignonnais, 1986.
——. "Pétrarque et ses amis au temps de la verte feuillée." *Cahier de Fanjeaux* 26 (1991): 127–140.
Amundsen, Darrel W. "Medieval Canon Law on Medical and Surgical Practice by the Clergy." *Bulletin of the History of Medicine* 52, no. 1 (1978): 22–44.

Andenna, Cristina. "Women at the Angevin Court between Naples and Provence: Sancia of Majorca, Delphine of Puimichel, and the 'Struggle' for a Female Franciscan Life." In *Queens, Princesses and Mendicants: Close Relations in a European Perspective*, edited by Nikolas Jaspert and Imke Just, 29–51. Zurich: LIT Verlag, 2019.

Archambeau, Nicole. "The 'First Mortality' as a Time Marker in 14th-Century Provence." In *Viral Networks: Connecting Digital Humanities and Medical History*, edited by E. Thomas Ewing and Katherine Randall, 157–184. Blacksburg, VA: VT Publishing, 2018.

——. "Healing Options during the Plague: Survivor Stories from a Fourteenth-Century Canonization Inquest." *Bulletin of the History of Medicine* 85 (2011): 531–559.

——. "'His Whole Heart Changed": Political Meanings of a Mercenary's Emotional Transformation." Micrologus 34 (2010): 169–190.

——. "Medical and Scientific Understandings." In *A Cultural History of the Emotions in the Medieval Age*, edited by Juanita Feros Ruys and Clare Monagle, 17–30. London: Bloomsbury, 2019.

——. "Miraculous Healing for the Warrior Soul: Transforming Fear, Violence, and Shame in the Canonization Inquest for Delphine de Puimichel, 1363." *Historical Reflections / Réflexions Historiques* 41 (2015): 14–27.

——. "Remembering Delphine's Books: Reading as a Means to Shape a Holy Woman's Sanctity." In *Writing Medieval Women's Lives*, edited by Amy Livingstone and Charlotte Newman Goldy, 33–49. New York: Palgrave, 2013.

Archimbaud, Gabrielle Démians d'. "Archéologie et villages désertés en Provence résultats de fouilles." In *Villages désertés et histoire economique, XIe–XVIIIe siècles*, 287–301. Paris: SEVPEN, 1965.

Armstrong-Partida, Michelle. "Conflict in the Parish: Antagonistic Relations between Clerics and Parishioners." In *A Companion to Pastoral Care in the Late Middle Ages (1200–1500)*, edited by Ronald Stansbury, 173–212. Leiden: Brill, 2010.

Arnold, John. "Inside and Outside the Medieval Laity: Some Reflections on the History of Emotions." In *European Religious Cultures: Essays Offered to Christopher Brooke on the Occasion of His Eightieth Birthday*, edited by Miri Rubin, 107–130. London: Institute of Historical Research, 2008.

Arrizabalaga, Jon. "Facing the Black Death: Perceptions and Reactions of University Medical Practitioners." In *Practical Medicine from Salerno to the Black Death*, edited by Luis García-Ballester et al., 237–288. Cambridge: Cambridge University Press, 1994.

Aurell, Martin, Jean-Paul Boyer, and Noël Coulet. *La Provence au Moyen Âge*. Aix-en-Provence: Publications de l'Université de Provence, 2005.

Bakhtin, M. M., Michael Holquist, and Caryl Emerson. *The Dialogic Imagination: Four Essays*. Austin: University of Texas Press, 1998.

Baratier, Édouard, Georges Duby, and Ernest Hildersheimer. *Atlas historique: Provence, Comtat Venaissin, Principaute de Monaco, Principaute d'Orange, Comte de Nice*. Paris: Librairie Armand Colin, 1969.

Barbero, Alessandro. "Letteratura e politica fra Provenza e Napoli." In *L'état Angevin: Pouvoir, culture et société entre XIIIe et XIVe siècle*, 159–171. Rome: École Française de Rome, 1998.

Barjavel, C. F. H. *Dictionnaire historique, biographique et bibliographique de Département de Vaucluse*. Vol. 1. Carpentras: de l. Devillario, 1841.

Barnel, Christine. "Town and Country in Provence: Toulon, Its Notaries, and Their Clients." In *Urban and Rural Communities in Medieval France: Provence and Languedoc, 1000–1500*, edited by Kathryn Reyerson and John Drendel. Leiden: Brill, 1998.

Barthélémy, Louis. *Histoire d'Aubagne: Chef-lieu de baronnie depuis son origine jusqu'en 1789*. Marseille: Barlatier et Barthelet, 1889.

——. *Inventaire chronologique et analytique des chartes de la maison de Baux*. Marseille: Barlatier-Feissat pere et fils, 1882.

Bartlett, Robert. *The Hanged Man: A Story of Miracle, Memory, and Colonialism in the Middle Ages*. Princeton, NJ: Princeton University Press, 2004.

——. "Symbolic Meanings of Hair in the Middle Ages." *Transactions of the Royal Historical Society* 4 (1994): 43–60.

——. *Trial by Fire and Water: The Medieval Judicial Order*. Oxford: Clarendon Press, 1988.

——. *Why Can the Dead Do Such Great Things? Saints and Worshippers from the Martyrs to the Reformation*. Princeton, NJ: Princeton University Press, 2013.

Barton, Richard. "'Zealous Anger' and the Renegotiation of Aristocratic Relationships in Eleventh- and Twelfth-Century France." In *Anger's Past: The Social Uses of an Emotion in the Middle Ages*, edited by Barbara Rosenwein, 153–170. Ithaca, NY: Cornell University Press, 1998.

Bautier, Robert Henri, ed. *Atlas Belfram*. Paris: Librarie Armand Colin, 1969.

Beattie, Blake. "*Coram Papa* Preaching and Rhetorical Community at Papal Avignon." In *Preacher, Sermon and Audience in the Middle Ages*, edited by Carolyn Muessig, 63–87. Leiden: Brill, 2002.

Bednarski, Steven. *Curia: A Social History of a Provençal Criminal Court in the Fourteenth Century*. Montpellier: Presses Universitaires de la Méditerranée, 2013.

Bell, Susan Groag. "Medieval Women Book Owners: Arbiters of Lay Piety and Ambassadors of Culture." *Signs* 7, no. 4 (1982): 742–768.

Benedictow, Ole. *The Black Death, 1346–1353: The Complete History*. Woodbridge, UK: Boydell Press, 2004.

Benham, Jenny. *Peacemaking in the Middle Ages: Principles and Practices*. Manchester, UK: Manchester University Press, 2011.

Bériou, Nicole. "La confession dans les écrits théologiques et pastoraux du XIII siècle: Médication de l'âme ou démarche judiciaire?" In *L'aveu, antiquité et Moyen Âge*, edited by Jean-Claude Maire Vigueur, 261–282. Rome: École Française de Rome, 1986.

——. "The Right of Women to Give Religious Instruction in the Thirteenth Century." In *Women Preachers and Prophets through Two Millennia of Christianity*, edited by Beverly Mayne Kienzle and Pamela J. Walker, 134–145. Berkeley: University of California Press, 1998.

Bériou, Nicole, and David D'Avray, eds. *Modern Questions about Medieval Sermons: Essays on Marriage, Death, History, and Sanctity*. Spoleto: Centro Italiano di Studi Sull'alto Medioevo, 1994.

Berlière, Ursmer. *Un ami de Pétrarque: Louis Heyligen de Beeringen*. Rome: Institute Historique Belge, 1905.

Biller, Peter. "Confession in the Middle Ages: Introduction." In *Handling Sin: Confession in the Middle Ages*, edited by Peter Biller and A. J. Minnis. York: York Medieval Press, 1998.

Biraben, Jean-Noël. *Les hommes et la peste en France et dans les pays européen et méditerranéens*. Vol. 2. Paris: Mouton, 1975–1976.

Blamires, Alcuin. "Women and Preaching in Medieval Orthodoxy, Heresy, and Saints' Lives." *Viator* 26 (1995): 135–152.

Boisard, Pierre. "La vie intellectuelle de la noblesse Angevine à la fin du XIVe siècle d'après *Le Chevalier de la Tour Landry*," In *La littérature Angevine médiévale*, 135–154. Paris: Honoré Champion, 1981.

Bolduc, Michelle. "The *Breviari d'Amor*: Rhetoric and Preaching in Thirteenth-Century Languedoc." *Rhetorica* 24 (2006): 403–425.

Bonnaud, Jean-Luc. *Un état en Provence. Les officiers locaux du comte de Provence au XIVe siécle (1309–1382)*. Rennes: Presses Universitaires de Rennes, 2007.

——."Les juges mages du comté de Provence et de Forcalquier à la fin du Moyen Âge (XIIIe–XVe siècle)." In *Les grands officiers dans les territoires Angevins: I grandi ufficiali nei territori angioini*, edited by Riccardo Rao, 189–206. Rome: École Française de Rome, 2017.

——. "L'origine géographique de clavaires et notaires de cour de l'administration comtale locale en Provence au XIVe siècle." In *La société rurale et les institutions gouvernementales au Moyen Âge*. Edited by John Drendel, 131–147. Montréal: Éditions CERES, 1995.

Boquet, Damien, and Piroska Nagy. *Medieval Sensibilities: A History of Emotions in the Middle Ages*. Medford, MA: Polity Press, 2018.

Botana, Federico. "Virtuous and Sinful Uses of Temporal Wealth in the *Breviari d'amor* of Matfre Ermengaud (MS BL Royal 19.C.I)." *Journal of the Warburg and Courtauld Institutes* 67 (2004): 49–80.

——. *The Works of Mercy in Italian Medieval Art (c. 1050–1400)*. Leiden: Brepols, 2011.

Bourdieu, Pierre. *Outline of a Theory of Practice*. Cambridge: Cambridge University Press, 1977.

Bowers, Barbara, and Linda Migl Keyser, eds. *The Sacred and the Secular in Medieval Healing: Sites, Objects, and Texts*. London: Routledge, 2016.

Boyer, Jean Paul, ed. "Les Baux et le modèle royal: Une oraison funèbre de Jean Régina de Naples (1334)." *Provence Historique* 181 (1995): 427–452.

——, ed. *La justice temporelle dans les territoires Angevins aux XIIIe et XIVe siècles: Théories et pratiques*. Rome: École Française de Rome, 2005.

——."Prêcher Marseille: Paroles franciscaines à l'aube du XIVe siècle." In *La Provence et Fréjus sous la première maison d'Anjou (1246–1382)*, edited by Jean-Paul Boyer and Thierry Pécout, 135–170. Aix-en-Provence: Publications de l'Université de Provence, 2010.

——. "La prédication de Robert de Sicile (1309–1343) et les communes d'Italie: Le cas de Gênes." In *Prêcher la paix et discipliner la société: Italie, France, Angleterre (XIIIe-XVe siècles)*, edited by R. M. Dessi, 382–411. Turnhout: Brepols, 2005.

——. "Contribution à la demographie de la Provence Savoyarde au XIVe siècle." *Provence Historique* 135 (1984): 35–53.

Boyer, Jean-Paul, and François-Xavier Emmanuelli, eds. *De Provence et d'ailleurs: Mélanges offerts à Noël Coulet*. *Provence Historique* 195–196 (1999).

Boyer, Jean-Paul, and Thierry Pécout. Introduction to *La Provence et Fréjus sous la première maison d'Anjou (1246–1382)*, edited by Jean-Paul Boyer and Thierry Pécout, 10–16. Aix-en-Provence: Publications de l'Université de Provence, 2010.

Boyle, Leonard. *Pastoral Care, Clerical Education, and Canon Law, 1200–1400*. London: Variorum Reprints, 1981.

Boze, Elzear. *Histoire de l'église d'Apt*. Apt: Jh. Trémollière, Imprimeur-Libraire, 1820.

Braet, Herman, and Verner Verbeke, eds. *Death in the Middle Ages*. Leuven: Leuven University Press, 1983.

Brown, Peter. *The Cult of Saints: Its Rise and Function in Latin Christianity*. Chicago: University of Chicago Press, 1981.

——. *The Ransom of the Soul: Afterlife and Wealth in Early Western Christianity*. Cambridge, MA: Harvard University Press, 2015.

Brundage, James. *The Medieval Origins of the Legal Profession: Canonists, Civilians, and Courts*. Chicago: University of Chicago Press, 2008.

Bruzelius, Caroline. "Queen Sancia of Mallorca and the Convent Church of Sta. Chiara in Naples." *Memoirs of the American Academy in Rome* 40 (1995): 69–100.

Butaud, Germain. "Aperçus sur la coseigneurie en Comtat Venaissin (XIIe–XVe siècles)." *Mélanges de l'École française de Rome* 122 (2010): 63–87.

Butaud, Germain, and Vincent Challet. "Guerre et transfert *intra muros* des monastères en Languedoc et en Comtat Venaissin (milieu XIVe–milieu XVe siècle)." *Cahiers de Fanjeaux* 44 (2009): 517–568.

Bylebyl, Jerome. "Galen on the Non-natural Causes of Variation in the Pulse." *Bulletin of the History of Medicine* 45 (1971): 482–485.

Bynum, Caroline Walker. *Christian Materiality: An Essay on Religion in Late Medieval Europe*. Cambridge, MA: MIT Press, 2015.

——. "Did the Twelfth Century Discover the Individual?" *Journal of Ecclesiastical History* 31 (1980): 1–17.

——. "The Female Body and Religious Practice." In *Fragmentation and Redemption: Essays on Gender and the Human Body in Medieval Religion*, edited by Caroline Walker Bynum, 181–238. New York: Zone Books, 1992.

——. *Holy Feast and Holy Fast: The Religious Significance of Food to Medieval Women*. Berkeley: University of California Press, 1987.

——. "Wonder." *American Historical Review* 102 (1997): 1–17.

Caciola, Nancy. "Wraiths, Revenants and Ritual in Medieval Culture." *Past and Present* 152 (1996): 3–45.

——. *Discerning Spirits: Divine and Demonic Possession in the Middle Ages*. Ithaca, NY: Cornell University Press, 2003.Caferro, William. *John Hawkwood: An English Mercenary in Fourteenth-Century Italy*. Baltimore: Johns Hopkins University Press, 2006.

Caferro, William. *John Hawkwood: An English Mercenary in Fourteenth-Century Italy*. Baltimore: Johns Hopkins University Press, 2006.

——. *Petrarch's War: Florence and the Black Death in Context*. Cambridge: Cambridge University Press, 2018.

Callahan, Daniel. "The Peace of God and the Cult of Saints in Aquitaine in the Tenth and Eleventh Centuries." In *The Peace of God: Social Violence and*

Religious Response in France around the Year 1000. Edited by Thomas Head and Richard Landes, 165–183. Ithaca, NY: Cornell University Press, 1992.

Cambell, Jacques. "Le sommaire de l'enquête pour la canonisation de S. Elzear de Sabran, T.O.F. (1323)." *Miscellanea Francescana* 73 (1973): 438–441.

Campbell, Anna Montgomery. *The Black Death and Men of Learning*. New York: AMS Press, 1996.

Campbell, Bruce. *The Great Transition: Climate, Disease, and Society in the Late-Medieval World*. Cambridge: Cambridge University Press, 2016.

Carmichael, Ann. *Plague and the Poor in Renaissance Florence*. Cambridge: Cambridge University Press, 1986.

——. "Universal and Particular: The Language of Plague, 1348–1500." In *Pestilential Complexities: Understanding Medieval Plague*, edited by Vivian Nutton, 17–52. London: Wellcome Trust Centre for the History of Medicine at UCL, 2008.

Carozzi, Claude. "Une béguine joachimite: Douceline, soeur d'Hugues de Digne." *Cahiers de Fanjeaux* 10 (1975): 169–201.

Carruthers, Mary. *The Book of Memory: A Study of Memory in Medieval Culture*. Cambridge: Cambridge University Press, 1990.

Casagrande, Carla. "'Motions of the Heart' and Sins: The *Specchio de' peccati* by Domenico Cavalca." In *In the Garden of Evil: The Vices and Culture in the Middle Ages*, edited by Richard Newhauser, 128–144. Toronto: Pontifical Institute of Mediaeval Studies, 2005.

Casteen, Elizabeth. *From She-Wolf to Martyr: The Reign and Disputed Reputation of Johanna I of Naples*. Ithaca, NY: Cornell University Press, 2015.

Catlos, Brian. "Mahomet Abenadalill: A Muslim Mercenary in the Service of the Kings of Aragon, 1290–1291." In *Jews, Muslims and Christians in and around the Crown of Aragon: Studies in Honour of Professor Elena Lourie*, edited by Harvey Hames, 257–302. Leiden: Brill, 2003.

Cazenave, Annie. "Aveu et contrition: Manuels de confesseurs et interrogatoires d'inquisition en Languedoc et en Catalogne (XIIIe–XIVe siècles)." In *La piété populaire au Moyen Age*, 333–352. Paris: Bibliothèque Nationale, 1977.

Chase, Melissa. "Fevers, Poisons, and Apostemes: Authority and Experience in Montpellier Plague Treatises." *Annals of the New York Academy of Sciences* 441 (1985): 153–170.

Chérest, Aimé. *L'archiprêtre: Épisodes de la Guerre de Cents Ans au XIVe siècle*. Paris: A. Claudin, 1879.

Chevalier, Ulysse. *Réportoire des sources historiques de Moyen Âge: Bio-Bibliographie*, vol. 1. Paris: Librairie de la Société Bibliographique, 1877.

Cheyette, Frederick. *Ermengarde of Narbonne and the World of the Troubadours*. Ithaca, NY: Cornell University Press, 2001.

——. "Some Reflections on Violence, Reconciliation, and 'The Feudal Revolution.'" In *Conflict in Medieval Europe: Changing Perspectives on Society and Culture*, edited by Warren Brown and Piotr Górecki, 243–264. Aldershot: Ashgate, 2003.

Chiffoleau, Jacques. *La comptabilité de l'au-dela: Les hommes, la mort et la religion dans la région d'Avignon à la fin du Moyen Âge*. Rome: École Français de Rome, 1980.

——. *Les justices du pape: Délinquance et criminalité dans la règion d'Avignon au quatorziéme siècle*. Paris: Publications de la Sorbonne, 1984.

Clanchy, Michael. *From Memory to Written Record: England, 1066–1307*. 2nd ed. Oxford: Blackwell, 1993.

Clark, Katherine. "Purgatory, Punishment, and the Discourse of Holy Widowhood in the High and Later Middle Ages." *Journal of the History of Sexuality* 16, no. 2 (2007): 169–203.

Clemens, Neal. "The Establishment of the Cult of Mary Magdalene in Provence, 1279–1543." PhD diss., Columbia University, 1997.

Coakley, John W. *Women, Men, and Spiritual Power: Female Saints and Their Male Collaborators*. New York: Columbia University Press, 2006.

Cohen, Esther. "Animated Pain of the Body." *American Historical Review* 105 (2000): 36–68.

Cohen, Jeremy. *Living Letters of the Law: Ideas of the Jew in Medieval Christianity*. Berkeley: University of California, 1999.

Cohen-Hanegbi, Naama. *Caring for the Living Soul: Emotions, Medicine, and Penance in the Late Medieval Mediterranean*. Leiden: Brill, 2017.

Constable, Giles. "The Ideal of Inner Solitude in the Twelfth Century." In *Horizons marins, itinéraires spirituels*, edited by Henri Dubois, Jean-Claude Hocquet, and Andre Vauchez, 27–34. Paris: Publications de la Sorbonne, 1987.

Contamine, Philippe. "Les companies d'aventure en France pendant la Guerre de Cent Ans." In *La France au XIVe et XVe siècles: Hommes, mentalités, guerre et paix*, chap. 7. London: Variorum Reprints, 1981.

——. "En guise de conclusion: Les villes de Languedoc et la chevauchée d'Édouard, prince de Galles (12 Octobre–28 Novembre 1355)." In *Défendre la ville dans les pays de la Méditerranée Occidentale au Moyen Âge*, edited by Daniel Le Blévec, 194–210. Montpellier: Centre historique de recherches et d'études sur la Méditerranée médiévale occidentale, 2002.

——. "L'idée de guerre à la fin du Moyen Âge: Aspects juridiques et éthiques." In *La France au XIVe et XVe siècles: Hommes, mentalités, guerre et paix*, chap. 8. London: Variorum Reprints, 1981.

——. *La vie quotidienne pendant la Guerre de Cent Ans: France et Angleterre, XIVe siècle*. New York: Hachette, 1978.

——. *War in the Middle Ages*. Translated by Michael Jones. Oxford: Basil Blackwell, 1984.

Cortez, Fernand. *Les Grands Officiers Royaux de Provence au Moyen Âge*. Aix-en-Provence: Société d'Études Provençales, 1921.

Coulet, Noël. "Aix, capitale de la Provence Angevine." In *L'état Angevin: Pouvoir, culture et société entre XIIIe et XIVe siècle*. Rome: École Française de Rome, 1998.

——. *Aix-en-Provence: Espace et relations d'une capitale (milieu XIVe s.–milieu XVe s.)*. Aix-en-Provence: Publications de l'Université de Provence, 1988.

——. "Un fragment de registre se la cour du juge mage de Provence à la fin du Moyen Âge." In *La justice temporelle dans les territoires Angevines*, edited by Jean-Paul Boyer, Anne Mailloux, and Laure Verdon, 189–206. Rome: École Française de Rome, 2005.

——. "Les mendiants à Aix-en-Provence, XIIIe–XVe siècle." *Cahiers de Fanjeaux* 44 (2009): 391–416.

——. "Les juifs en Provence au bas Moyen-Âge: Les limites d'une marginatlité?" In *Minorités et marginaux en France méridionale et dans le péninsule ibérique VIIe–XVIIIe siècles*, 203–219. Paris: Presses du CNRS, 1986.

——. " La désolation des églises de Provence à la fin du Moyen Age." *Provence Historique* 23 (1956): 34–52.

Coulet, Noël, and Jean-Michel Matz, eds. *La noblesse dans les territoires Angevins à la fin du Moyen Âge*. Rome: École Française de Rome, 2000.

Courtemanche, Andrée. "La rumeur de Manosque: Femmes et honneur au XIVe siècle." In *Normes et pouvoir à la fin du Moyen Âge*, edited by Marie-Claude Déprez-Masson, 128–144. Montreal: CERES, 1989.

Courtenay, William J. "Curers of Body and Soul: Medical Doctors as Theologians." In *Religion and Medicine in the Middle Ages*, edited by Peter Biller and Joseph Ziegler, 69–75. York: York Medieval Press, 2001.

Cox, Eugene. *The Eagles of Savoy: The House of Savoy in Thirteenth-Century Europe*. Princeton, NJ: Princeton University Press, 1974.

Christiakos, George, et al. "Recent Results on the Spatiotemporal Modeling and Comparative Analysis of Black Death and Bubonic Plague Epidemics." *Public Health* 121 (2007): 700–720.

Dalarun, Jacques. *La sainte et la cité: Micheline de Pesaro (1356) Tertiaire Franciscaine*. Rome: École Française de Rome, 1992.

Damasio, Antonio. *The Feeling of What Happens: Body and Emotion in the Making of Consciousness*. New York: Harcourt, Brace, 1999.

Davis, Natalie Zemon. *Fiction in the Archives: Pardon Tales and Their Tellers in Sixteenth-Century France*. Stanford: Stanford University Press, 1987.

Debby, Nirit Ben-Aryeh. "The Preacher as Women's Mentor." In *Preacher, Sermon, and Audience in the Middle Ages*, edited by Carolyn Muessig, 229–254. Leiden: Brill, 2002.

Delumeau, Jean. *Sin and Fear: The Emergence of a Western Guilt Culture 13th–18th Centuries*. New York: St. Martin's Press, 1990.

Demaitre, Luke E. *Doctor Bernard de Gordon: Professor and Practitioner*. Toronto: Pontifical Institute of Mediaeval Studies, 1980.

——. *Medieval Medicine: The Art of Healing from Head to Toe*. Santa Barbara: Praeger, 2013.

Denifle, Henri. La *désolation des églises, monastères et hopitaux en France pendant la Guerre de Cent Ans. Vol 2 La Guerre de Cent Ans jusqu'a la mort de Charles V*. Paris: Alphonse Picard et Fils, 1899.

Deploige, Jeroen. "Meurtre politique, émotions collectives et catharsis littéraire: Guibert de Nogent et Galbert de Bruges faces au révolts urbaines de Laon (1111–1112) et de Bruges (1127–1128)." In *Politiques des émotions au Moyen Âge*, edited by Damien Boquet and Piroska Nagy, 225–254. Florence: Sismel, 2010.

——. "Studying Emotions: The Medievalist as Human Scientist?" In *Emotions in the Heart of the City (14th–16th Century)*, edited by Anne Van Bruaene, 3–14. Turnhout: Brepols, 2005.

Dérens, Jean-Arnault. "La prédication et la ville: Practiques de la parole et 'religion civique' à Montpellier aux XIVe et XVe siècles." *Cahiers de Fanjeaux* 32 (1997): 335–362.

Desplenter, Youri, Jürgen Pieters, and Walter Melion, eds. *The Ten Commandments in Medieval and Early Modern Culture*. Leiden: Brill, 2017.

Devries, Kelly. "Medieval Mercenaries: Methodology, Definitions, and Problems." In *Mercenaries and Paid Men: The Mercenary Identity in the Middle Ages*, edited by John France, 43–60. Leiden: Brill, 2008.

Dormeier, Heinrich. "Saints as Protectors against Plague: Problems of Definition and Economic and Social Implications." In *Living with the Black Death*, edited by Lars Bisgaard and Leif Søndergaard, 161–186. Gylling: University of Southern Denmark, 2009.

Drendel, John. "The Institutions of Village Government in Later Medieval Provence and the Origins of the Council of Trets." *Historical Reflections/Réflexions Historiques* 19 (1993): 249–266.

——."Notarial Practice in Rural Provence in the Early Fourteenth Century." In *Urban and Rural Communities in Medieval France: Provence and Languedoc, 1000–1500*, edited by Kathryn Reyerson and John Drendel, 209–235. Leiden: Brill, 1998.

——. "Note sur l'exploitation de la terre gaste dans le finage de Brignoles au XIVe siècle." *Provence Historique* 256 (2014): 371–379.

Dubled, Henri. *Histoire du Comtat Venaissin*. Villaure: CREDEL, 1982.

Duffin, Jacalyn. *Medical Miracles: Doctors, Saints and Healing in the Modern World*. Oxford: Oxford University Press, 2009.

Duggan, Lawrence. "Fear and Confession on the Eve of the Reformation." *Archiv für Reformationsgeschichte* 75 (1984): 153–175.

Dulong, Marthe. "Les dernières années de sainte Delphine à Apt d'après les procès de canonisation." *Provence Historique* 6, special number (1956): 132–138.

——. "Édition critique de la vie provençale de sainte Delphine et l'étude comparée jointe à la vie du procès de canonisation. Doctoral dissertation. École des Chartres, 1928.

Dumas, Geneviève. *Santé et société à Montpellier à la fin du Moyen Âge*. Leiden: Brill, 2015.

Dunbabin, Jean. *The French in the Kingdom of Sicily, 1266–1305*. Cambridge: Cambridge University Press, 2011.

——.*Charles I of Anjou: Power, Kingship, and State-Making in Thirteenth-Century Europe*. London: Routledge, 1998.

Duranti, Alessandro, and Charles Goodwin. *Rethinking Context: Language as an Interactive Phenomenon*. Cambridge: Cambridge University Press, 1992.

Earenfight, Theresa. *Queenship in Medieval Europe*. London: Palgrave Macmillan, 2013.

Einbinder, Susan. *After the Black Death: Plague and Commemoration among Iberian Jews*. Philadelphia: University of Pennsylvania Press, 2018.

——. *No Place of Rest: Jewish Literature, Expulsion, and the Memory of Medieval France*. Philadelphia: University of Pennsylvania Press, 2009.

Eisen, Rebecca J., and Kenneth L. Gage. "Adaptive Strategies of *Yersinia pestis* to Persist during Inter-epizootic and Epizootic Periods." *Veterinary Research* 40 (2009): doi:10.1051/vetres:2008039.

Eisen, Rebecca J., et al. "Early-Phase Transmission of *Yersinia pestis* by Unblocked Fleas as a Mechanism Explaining Rapidly Spreading Plague Epizootics." *Proceedings of the National Academy of Sciences of the United States of America* 103 (2006): 15380–15385.

Elliott, Dyan. "Dress as Mediator between the Inner and Outer Self: The Pious Matron of the High and Later Middle Ages." *Mediaeval Studies* 53 (1991): 279–308.

——. *Proving Woman: Female Spirituality and Inquisitional Culture in the Later Middle Ages*. Princeton, NJ: Princeton University Press, 2004.

——. *Spiritual Marriage: Sexual Abstinence in Medieval Wedlock*. Princeton, NJ: Princeton University Press, 1993.

Emery, Richard. "The Black Death of 1348 in Perpignan." *Speculum* 42 (1967): 611–623.

Ernst, Waltraud, ed. *Plural Medicine, Tradition and Modernity, 1800–2000*. London: Routledge, 2002.

Everard, Judith. "Sworn Testimony and Memory of the Past in Brittany, c. 1100–1250." In *Medieval Memories: Men, Women and the Past, 700–1300*, edited by Elisabeth van Houts, 86–105. London: Longman, 2001.

Fancy, Hussein. *The Mercenary Mediterranean: Sovereignty, Religion, and Violence in the Medieval Crown of Aragon*. Chicago: University of Chicago Press, 2016.

Farmer, Sharon. "Book Review for *Capetian Women* by Kathleen Nolan." *Medieval Feminist Newsletter* 41 (2006): 103–106.

——. "Persuasive Voices: Clerical Images of Medieval Wives." *Speculum* 61 (1986): 517–543.

——. "Softening the Hearts of Men: Women, Embodiment, and Persuasion in the Thirteenth Century." In *Embodied Love: Sensuality and Relationship as Feminist Values*, edited by Paula Cooey, Sharon Farmer, and Mary Ellen Ross, 115–135. San Francisco: Harper and Row, 1987.

——. *Surviving Poverty: Gender, Ideology, and the Daily Lives of the Poor*. Ithaca, NY: Cornell University Press, 2002.

Faure, Claude. *Étude sur l'administration et l'histoire du Comtat Venaissin du XIIIe au XVe siècle (1229–1417)*. Paris: Honoré Champion, 1909.

Fenster, Thelma, and Daniel Lord Smail. Introduction to *Fama: The Politics of Talk and Reputation in Medieval Europe*, edited by Thelma Fenster and Daniel Lord Smail, 1–11. Ithaca, NY: Cornell University Press, 2003.

Finucane, Ronald C. *Miracles and Pilgrims: Popular Beliefs in Medieval England*. New York: St. Martin's Press, 1995.

Firnhaber-Baker, Justine. "Techniques of Seigneurial War in the Fourteenth Century." *Journal of Medieval History* 36 (2010): 90–103.

——. "Seigneurial War and Royal Power in Later Medieval Southern France." *Past and Present* 208 (2010): 37–76.

——. *Violence and the State in Languedoc, 1250–1400*. Cambridge: Cambridge University Press, 2014.

Fowler, Kenneth. *Medieval Mercenaries*. Vol. 1, *The Great Companies*. Oxford: Blackwell, 2001.

Frömark, Anders. "Telling the Miracle: The Meeting between Pilgrim and Scribe as Reflected in Swedish Miracle Collections." In *Miracles in Medieval Canonization Processes: Structures, Functions, and Methodologies*, edited by Christian Krötzl and Sari Katajala-Peltomaa, 131–155. Turnhout: Brepols, 2018.

Fulton, Rachel. *From Judgment to Passion: Devotion to Christ and the Virgin Mary, 800–1200*. New York: Columbia University Press, 2002.

Garcia-Ballester, Luis. "Changes in the *Regimina Sanitatis*: The Role of the Jewish Physicians." In *Health, Disease, and Healing in Medieval Culture*, edited by Sheila Campbell, Bert Hall, and David Klausner, 119–131. New York: St. Martin's Press, 1992.

——. "The Construction of a New Form of Learning and Practicing Medicine in Medieval Latin Europe," In *Galen and Galenism: Theory and Medical Practice from Antiquity to the European Renaissance*, chap. VII, edited by Jon Arrizabalaga, Monserrat Cabre, Lluis Cifuentes, and Fernando Salmon. Aldershot: Ashgate, 2002.

——. "Soul and Body: Disease of the Soul and Disease of the Body in Galen's Medical Thought." In *Atti del Terzo Colloquio Galenico Internazionale (Pavia: 10–12 Settembre 1986)*, edited by Paolo Manuli and Mario Vegetti, 117–152. Naples: Bibliopolis, 1988.

Geary, Patrick. *Furta Sacra: Thefts of Relics in the Central Middle Ages*. Princeton: Princeton University Press, 2011.

——. "The Saint and the Shrine: The Pilgrim's Goal in the Middle Ages." In *Living with the Dead in the Middle Ages*, 163–176. Ithaca, NY: Cornell University Press, 1994.

Geltner, Guy. *Roads to Health: Infrastructure and Urban Wellbeing in Later Medieval Italy*. Philadelphia: University of Pennsylvania Press, 2019.

——. "The Path to Pistoia: Urban Hygiene before the Black Death." *Past and Present* 246 (2020): 3–33.

——. "In Camp and on the March: Military Manuals as Sources for Studying Premodern Public Health." *Medical History* 63 (2019): 44–60.

Gendt, Anne Marie de. *"L'art d'éduquer les nobles damoiselles: Le livre de chevalier de la Tour Landry*. Paris: Honoré Champion, 2003.

Gescer, Otto. "Doctors and Preachers against the Plague: Attitudes toward Disease in Late Medieval Plague Tracts and Plague Sermons." In *The Sacred and the Secular in Medieval Healing: Sites, Objects, and Texts*, edited by Barbara Bowers and Linda Keyser, 78–102. London: Routledge, 2016.

Gil Sotres, Pedro. "Modelo Teorico y Observacion Clinica: Las Pasiones del Alma en la Psicologia Medica Medieval." In *Comprehendre et maitriser la nature au Moyen Âge: Melanges d'histoire des sciences offert à Guy Beaujouen*, 181–204. Geneva: Droz, 1994.

——. "The Regimens of Health." In *Western Medical Thought from Antiquity to the Middle Ages*, edited by Mirko Grmek, 291–318. Cambridge, MA: Harvard University Press, 1998.

Ginzburg, Carlo. "The Inquisitor as Anthropologist." In *Clues, Myths, and the Historical Method*, 156–165. Baltimore: Johns Hopkins University Press, 1989.

Giordanengo, Gérard. *"Arma legesque colo*: L'état et le droit en Provence (1246–1343)." In *La noblesse dans les territoires Angevins à la fin du Moyen Âge*, edited by Noël Coulet and Jean-Michel Matz, 35–80. Rome: École Française de Rome, 2000.

Glénisson, Jean. "La seconde peste: L'épidémie de 1360–1362 en France et en Europe." *Annuaire-Bulletin de la Société de l'Histoire de France* (1969): 27–38.

Goering, Joseph. "The Internal Forum and the Literature of Penance and Confession." *Traditio* 59 (2004): 175–227.

——. "Leonard E. Boyle and the Invention of *Pastoralia*." In *A Companion to Pastoral Care in the Late Middle Ages (1200–1500)*, edited by Ronald Stansbury, 7–20. Leiden: Brill, 2010.

Goffman, Erving. *Forms of Talk*. Philadelphia: University of Pennsylvania Press, 1981.

——. *Frame Analysis: An Essay on the Organization of Experience*. Boston: Northeastern University Press, 1974.

Good, Byron, and Arthur Kleinman, eds. *Culture and Depression: Studies in Anthropology and Cross-Cultural Psychiatry of Affect and Disorder*. Berkeley: University of California Press, 1985.

Goodich, Michael. "Canonization and the Hagiographical Text." In *Miracles and Wonders: The Development of the Concept of Miracle, 1150–1350*, edited by Michael Goodich, 88–95. Aldershot: Ashgate, 2007.

——. Introduction to *Voices from the Bench: The Narratives of Lesser Folk in Medieval Trials*, edited by Michael Goodich, 1–13. New York: Palgrave Macmillan, 2006.

——. "*Mirabilis Deus in sanctis suis*: Social History and Medieval Miracles." In *Signs, Wonders, Miracles: Representations of Divine Power in the Life of the Church*, edited by Kate Cooper and Jeremy Gregory, 135–156. Woodbridge: Boydell Press, 2005.

——. *The Other Middle Ages: Witnesses at the Margins of Medieval Society*. Philadelphia: University of Pennsylvania Press, 1998.

——. "Reason or Revelation? The Criteria for the Proof and Credibility of Miracles in Canonization Inquest Processes." In *Procès de canonisation au Moyen Âge: Aspects juridiques et religieux*, edited by Gábor Klaniczay, 181–197. Rome: École Française de Rome, 2004.

——. *Violence and Miracle in the Fourteenth Century: Private Grief and Public Salvation*. Chicago: University of Chicago Press, 1995.

Gouk, Penelope and Helen Hills. "Towards Histories of Emotions." In *Representing Emotions: New Connections in the Histories of Art, Music, and Medicine*, edited by Penelope and Helen Hills Gouk. Aldershot: Ashgate, 2005.

Grainger, Ian, Duncan Hawkins, Lynne Cowal, and Richard Mikulski. *The Black Death Cemetery, East Smithfield, London*. London: Museum of London Archaeology Service, 2008.

Green, Monica. Editor's introduction to *Pandemic Disease in the Medieval World: Rethinking the Black Death*. *Medieval Globe* 1 (2014).

——. "Integrative Medicine: Incorporating Medicine and Health into the Canon of Medieval European History." *History Compass* 7 (2009): 1218–1245.

Griffiths, Paul. *What Emotions Really Are: The Problem of Psychological Categories*. Chicago: University of Chicago Press, 1997.

Grmek, Mirko. "The Concept of Disease." In *Western Medical Thought from Antiquity to the Middle Ages*, edited by Mirko Grmek. Cambridge, MA: Harvard University Press, 1998.

——. "Influence of Avicenna on Western Medicine in the Middle Ages." *Salerno* 1 (1967): 7–21.

Guigue, Georges. *Les Tard-Venus en Lyonnais, Forez, et Beaujolais—1356–1369*. Lyon: Imprimerie Vitte et Perrussel, 1886.

Guillemain, Bernard. *La cour pontificale d'Avignon, 1309–1376*. Paris: Éditions E. de Boccard, 1966.

Hanawalt, Barbara. *The Ties That Bound: Peasant Families in Medieval England*. Oxford: Oxford University Press, 1989.

Harmening, Dieter. *Superstitio*. Berlin: Erich Schmidt Verlag, 1979.

Harre, Rom, ed. *The Social Construction of Emotions*. New York: Basil Blackwell, 1986.

Harris, Roy. "The Occitan Translations of John XII and XIII–XVIII from a Fourteenth-Century Franciscan Codex (Assisi, Chisea Nuova MS. 9)." *Transactions of the American Philosophical Society* 75 (1985): 1–149.

Hartnell, Jack. *Medieval Bodies: Life, Death, and Art in the Middle Ages*. London: Wellcome Collection, 2018.

Harvey, Ruth. *The Inward Wits: Psychological Theory in the Middle Ages and the Renaissance*. London: Warburg Institute, 1975.

Hasenohr, Geneviève. "Un donat de dévotion en Langue d'Oc du XIIIe siècle: Le *Liber divini amoris*." *Cahier de Fanjeaux* 35 (2000): 219–243.

Hasse, Dag Nikolaus. *Avicenna's "De Anima" in the Latin West*. London: Warburg Institute; Turin: Nino Aragno Editore, 2000.

Hayez, Anne-Marie. "La défense d'Avignon au temps des papes." In *Défendre la ville dans les pays de la Méditerranée Occidentale au Moyen Âge*, edited by Daniel le Blévec, 64–101. Montpellier: Université Paul-Valéry, 2002.

——. "L'entourage d'Urbain V: Parents, amis et familiers." *Annuaire de la Société des Amis du Palais de Papaes* (1988–1989): 31–45.

Hayez, Anne-Marie, and Michel Hayez. "Les saints honoré à Avignon aux XIVe siècle." In *Le peuple des saints: Croyances et dèvotions en Provence et Comtat Venaissin à la fin du Moyen Âge*, 199–222. Avignon: Institut de Recherches et d'Études du Bas Moyen Âge Avignonnais, 1986.

Hayez, Jérôme. "Practiques et discours de marchands migrants: Les Toscans d'Avignon au XIVe et XVe siècles." In *"Arriver" en ville: Les migrants en milieu urbain au Moyen Âge*, edited by Cédric Quertier, Roxane Chilà, and Nicolas Pluchot, 225–241. Paris: Publications de la Sorbonne, 2013.

Head, Thomas. "The Development of the Peace of God in Aquitaine (970–1005)." *Speculum* 74 (1999): 656–686.

Head, Thomas and Richard Landes, eds. *The Peace of God: Social Violence and Religious Response in France around the Year 1000*. Ithaca, NY: Cornell University Press, 1992.

Hébert, Michel. "Les assemblées représentatives dans le royaume de Naples et dans le Comté de Provence." In *L'état Angevin: Pouvoir, culture et société entre XIIIe et XIVe siècle*, 475–490. Rome: École Française de Rome, 1998.

——. "La cristallisation d'une identité: Les États de Provence, 1347–1360" In *Événement, Identité et Histoire*, edited by Claire Dolan, 151–164. Sillery: Les éditions du Septentrion, 1991.

——. "Du village à l'état: Les assemblées locales en Provence aux XIVe et XIVe siècles." In *La société rural et les institutions gouvernementales au Moyen Âge*, edited by John Drendel, 103–116. Montréal: Éditions CERES, 1995.

——. "Guerre, finance et administration: Les États de Provence de novembre 1359." *Revue d'Histoire de Philologie: Le Moyen Âge* 83 (1977): 103–130.

——. "La noblesse Provençale et les États de Provence." In *La noblesse dans le territoires Angevins à la fin du Moyen Âge*, edited by Noël Coulet and Jean-Michel Matz, 327–345. Rome: École Française de Rome, 2000.

——, ed. *Vie privée et ordre public à la fin du Moyen-Âge: Études sur Manosque, la Provence et le Piémont (1250–1450)*. Aix-en-Provence: Université de Provence, 1987.

Heller, Sarah-Grace. "Anxiety, Hierarchy, and Appearance in Thirteenth-Century Sumptuary Laws and the *Roman de la Rose*." *French Historical Studies* 27 (2004): 312–348.

Herlihy, David. *The Black Death and the Transformation of the West*. Cambridge, MA: Harvard University Press, 1997.

Hoffmann, Richard. *An Environmental History of Medieval Europe*. Cambridge: Cambridge University Press, 2014.

——. "Footprint Metaphor and Metabolic Realities: Environmental Impacts of Medieval European Cities." In *Nature's Past: The Environment and Human History*, edited by Paolo Squatriti, 288–325. Ann Arbor: University of Michigan Press, 2006.

Horden, Peregrine. "Household Care and Informal Networks: Comparisons and Continuities from Antiquity to the Present." In *The Locus of Care: Families, Communities, Institutions, and the Provision of Welfare since Antiquity*, edited by Peregrine Horden and Richard Smith, 21–67. London: Routledge, 1998.

——. "A Non-natural Environment: Medicine without Doctors and the Medieval European Hospital." In *The Medieval Hospital and Medical Practice*, edited by Barbara Bowers. Aldershot: Ashgate, 2007.

——. "Ritual and Public Health in the Early Medieval City." In *Histories of Urban Public Health*, edited by Sally Sheard and Helen Power, 17–40. Aldershot: Ashgate, 2000.

Horden, Peregrine, and Nicholas Purcell. *The Corrupting Sea: A Study of Mediterranean History*. Oxford: Blackwell, 2000.

Housley, Norman. "Indulgences for Crusading, 1417–1517." In *Promissory Notes on the Treasury of Merits: Indulgences in Late Medieval Europe*, edited by R. N. Swanson, 277–307. Leiden: Brill, 2006.

——. "The Mercenary Companies, the Papacy, and the Crusades, 1356–1378." *Traditio: Studies in Ancient and Medieval History, Thought, and Religion* 38 (1982): 253–280.

Houts, Elisabeth van. "Gender and Authority of Oral Witnesses in Europe (800–1300)." *Transactions of the Royal Historical Society* 9 (1999): 201–220.

Huizinga, Johan. *The Autumn of the Middle Ages*. Translated by Rodney J. Payton and Ulrich Mammitzsch. Chicago: University of Chicago Press, 1996.

Iancu-Agou, Danièle. *Provincia judaica: Dictionnaire de géographie historique des Juifs en Provence médiévale*. Paris: Peeters, 2010.

Izbicki, Thomas M. "The Origins of the *De Ornatu Mulierum* of Antoninus of Florence." *MLN* 119, Supplement (2004): s142–s161.

Jackson, Stanley W. "Acedia the Sin and Its Relationship to Sorrow and Melancholia." In *Culture and Depression: Studies in the Anthropology and Cross-Cultural Psychiatry of Affect and Disorder*, edited by Arthur and Byron Good Kleinman, 43–62. Berkeley: University of California Press, 1985.

——. "Unusual Mental States in Medieval Europe I: Medical Syndromes of Mental Disorder." *Journal of the History of Medicine and Allied Sciences* 27 (1972): 262–297.

Jacquart, Danielle. "Medical Explanations of Sexual Behavior in the Middle Ages." In *Homo Carnalis: The Carnal Aspect of Medieval Human Life*, edited by Helen Rodnite Lemay, 1–21. Binghamton: State University of New York at Binghamton, 1990.

———. "Medical Practice in Paris in the First Half of the Fourteenth Century." In *Practical Medicine from Salerno to the Black Death*, edited by Luis Garcia Ballester et al., 196–210. Cambridge: Cambridge University Press, 1994.

Jacquart, Danielle, and Claude Alexandre Thomasset. *Sexuality and Medicine in the Middle Ages*. Princeton, NJ: Princeton University Press, 1988.

Jacques, Paul. "Témoignage historique et hagiographie dans le procès de canonisation de Louis d'Anjou." *Provence Historique* 23 (1973): 305–317.

Jacquin, Gérard. "Éducation et culture de la noblesse en Anjou au XIVe siècle." In *La noblesse dans les territoires Angevins à la fin du Moyen Âge*, edited by Noël Coulet and Jean-Michel Matz, 677–688. Rome: École Française de Rome, 2000.

Jansen, Katherine Ludwig. *The Making of the Magdalen: Preaching and Popular Devotion in the Later Middle Ages*. Princeton, NJ: Princeton University Press, 2000.

———. "Mary Magdalen and the Mendicants: The Preaching of Penance in the Late Middle Ages." *Journal of Medieval History* 21 (1995): 1–25.

———. *Peace and Penance in Late Medieval Italy*. Princeton, NJ: Princeton University Press, 2018.

Jansen, Philippe. "Les influences italiennes dans l'administration de la Provence orientale sous les comtes de la dynastie angevine." In *La Provence et Fréjus sous la première maison d'Anjou (1246–1382)*, edited by Jean-Paul Boyer and Thierry Pécout, 183–201. Aix-en-Provence: Publications de l'Université de Provence, 2010.

Jarcho, Saul. "Galen's Six Non-naturals: A Bibliographic Note and Translation." *Bulletin of the History of Medicine* 44 (1970): 372–377.

Jaritz, Gerhard, ed. *Oral History of the Middle Ages: The Spoken Word in Context*. Krems: Medium Aevum Quotidianum, 2001.

Johnson, Timothy ed. *Franciscans and Preaching: Every Miracle from the Beginning of the World Came about through Words*. Leiden: Brill, 2012.

Jordan, Mark. "The Fortune of Constantine's Pantegni." In *Constantine the African and 'Ali Ibn Al-'Abbas Al-Magusi*, edited by Charles Burnett and Danielle Jacquart, 286–302. Leiden: Brill, 1994.

Jordan, William C. *The Great Famine*. Princeton, NJ: Princeton University Press, 1996.

Katajala-Peltomaa, Sari. *Gender, Miracles, and Daily Life: The Evidence of Fourteenth-Century Canonization Processes*. Turnhout: Brepols, 2009.

———. "Narrative Strategies in the Depositions: Gender, Family, and Devotion." In *Miracles in Medieval Canonization Processes: Structures, Functions, and Methodologies*, 227–256. Turnhout: Brepols, 2018.

Keen, Maurice Hugh. *The Laws of War in the Middle Ages*. London: Routledge, 1965.

———. *Nobles, Knights, and Men-at-Arms in the Middle Ages*. London: Hambledon Press, 1996.

Keil, Gundolf. "Die Frau als Artzin und Patientin in der Medizinishcen Fachprosa des Deutschen Mittelalters." Paper presented at the Frau und Spatmittelalterlicher Alltag, Krems an der Donau, 1986.

Kelleher, Marie. "'The Sea of Our City': Famine, Piracy, and Urban Sovereignty in Medieval Barcelona." *Mediterranean Studies* 24 (2016): 1–22.

Kelley, Emily. "For the Hope of Salvation and the Honor of Family: Merchant Devotional Concerns in Early Sixteenth-Century Burgos." In *Saints as Intercessors between the Wealthy and the Divine: Art and Hagiography among the Medieval Merchant Classes*, edited by Emily Kelley and Cynthia Turner Camp, 89–109. London: Routledge, 2019.

Kelly, Samantha. *The New Solomon: Robert of Naples (1304–1343) and Fourteenth-Century Kingship*. Leiden: Brill, 2003.

——. "Noblesse de robe et noblesse d'esprit à la cour de Robert de Naples: La question d''Italianisation.'" In *La noblesse dans les territoires Angevins à la fin du Moyen Âge*, edited by Noël Coulet and Jean-Michel Matz, 347–361. Rome: École Française de Rome, 2000.

Kemp, E. W. *Canonization and Authority in the Western Church*. New York: AMS Press, 1980.

Kennedy, Angus. "Christine de Pizan's *Epistre a la reine*: A Woman's Perspective on War and Peace?" War and Peace: *Critical Issues in European Societies and Literature, 800–1800*. Edited by Albrecht Classen and Nadia Margolis, 395–423. Berlin: De Gruyter, 2011.

Kieckhefer, Richard. *Magic in the Middle Ages*. Canto ed. Cambridge: Cambridge University Press, 1990.

——. "The Specific Rationality of Medieval Magic." *American Historical Review* 99, no. 3 (1994): 813–836.

——. *Unquiet Souls: Fourteenth-Century Saints and Their Religious Milieu*. Chicago: University of Chicago Press, 1984.

Kinch, Ashby. *Imago Mortis: Meditating Images of Death in Late Medieval Culture*. Leiden: Brill, 2013.

——, ed. *Procès de canonisation au Moyen Âge: Aspects juridiques et religieux*. Rome: École Française de Rome, 2004.

Klaniczay, Gábor. "Hagiography and Historical Narrative." In *Chronicon: Medieval Narrative Sources*, edited by Janos Bak and Ivan Jurkovic, 111–118. Leiden: Brepols, 2013.

——. *Holy Rulers and Blessed Princesses: Dynastic Cults in Medieval Central Europe*. Translated by Éva Pálmai. Cambridge: Cambridge University Press, 2002.

——. "The Inquisition of Miracles in Medieval Canonization Processes." In *Miracles in Medieval Canonization Processes: Structures, Functions, and Methodologies*, edited by Christian Krötzl and Sari Katajala-Peltomaa, 43–73. Turnhout: Brepols, 2018.

——. "La noblesse et le culte des saints dynastiques sous les rois Angevins." In *La noblesse dans les territoires Angevins à la fin du Moyen Âge*, edited by Noël Coulet and Jean-Michel Matz, 511–526. Rome: École Française de Rome, 2000.

——. "Speaking about Miracles: Oral Testimony and Written Record in Medieval Canonization Trials." In *The Development of Literate Mentalities in East Central Europe*, edited by Anna Adamska and Marco Mostert, 365–395. Turnhout: Brepols, 2004.

——. "Legends as Life Strategies for Aspirant Saints in the Later Middle Ages." *Journal of Folklore Research* 26 (1989): 151–171.

Klaniczay, Gábor, Karen Margolis, and Susan Singerman. *The Uses of Supernatural Power: The Transformation of Popular Religion in Medieval and Early-Modern Europe*. Cambridge: Polity, 1990.

Klapisch-Zuber, Christiane. "Plague and Family Life." In *The New Cambridge Medieval History*, vol. 6, 124–154. Cambridge: Cambridge University Press, 2000.

Kleinberg, Aviad M. *Prophets in Their Own Country: Living Saints and the Making of Sainthood in the Later Middle Ages*. Chicago: University of Chicago Press, 1992.

Kleinman, Arthur. *The Illness Narratives: Suffering, Healing, and the Human Condition*. New York: Basic Books, 1988.

——. *Patients and Healers in the Context of Culture*. Berkeley: University of California Press, 1980.

Kleinman, Arthur, and Byron Good, eds. *Culture and Depression: Studies in the Anthropology and Cross-Cultural Psychiatry of Affect and Disorder*. Berkeley: University of California Press, 1985.

Klibansky, Raymond, Erwin Panofsky, and Fritz Saxl. *Saturn and Melancholy: Studies in the History of Natural Philosophy, Religion, and Art*. New York: Basic Books, 1964.

Knuuttila, Simo. *Emotions in Ancient and Medieval Philosophy*. Oxford: Clarendon Press, 2004.

Koopmans, Rachel. *Wonderful to Relate: Miracle Stories and Miracle Collecting in High Medieval England*. Philadelphia: University of Pennsylvania Press, 2011.

Korte, Anne-Marie, ed. *Women and Miracle Stories: A Multidisciplinary Approach*. Leiden: Brill, 2001.

Kosmer, Ellen. "Gardens of Virtue in the Middle Ages." *Journal of the Warburg and Courtauld Institutes* 41 (1987): 302–307.

Koziol, Geoffrey. "Monks, Feuds, and the Making of Peace in Eleventh-Century Flanders." In *The Peace of God: Social Violence and Religious Response in France around the Year 1000*. Edited by Thomas Head and Richard Landes, 239–258. Ithaca, NY: Cornell University Press, 1992.

Krötzl, Christian. "*Miracula Post Mortem*: On Function, Content, and Typological Changes." In *Miracles in Medieval Canonization Processes: Structures, Functions, and Methodologies*, 157–175. Turnhout: Brepols, 2018.

——. "Prokuratoren, Notare, und Dolmetscher: Zu Gestaltung und Ablauf der Zeugeneinvernahmen bei spätmittelalterlichen Kanonisationsprozessen." *Hagiographica* 5 (1998): 119–140.

——. "Vulgariter sibi exposito: Zu Übersetzung und Sprachbeherrschung im Spätmittelalter am Biespiel von Kanonisationsprozessen." *Das Mittelalter* 2, no. 1 (1997): 111–118.

Krötzl, Christian and Sari Katajala-Peltomaa. "Approaching Twelfth- to Fifteenth-Century Miracles: Miracle Registers, Collections, and Canonization Processes as Source Material." In *Miracles in Medieval Canonization Processes: Structures, Functions, and Methodologies*, edited by Christian Krötzl and Sari Katajala-Peltomaaa, 1–39. Turnhout: Brepols, 2018.

Krueger, Haven C. *Avicenna's Poem on Medicine*. Springfield, IL: Charles C Thomas, 1963.

Kuuliala, Jenni. "Heavenly Healing or Failure of Faith? Partial Cures in Later Medieval Canonization Processes." In *Church and Belief in the Middle Ages: Popes, Saints, and Crusaders*, edited by Kirsi Salonen and Sari Katajala-Peltomaa, 171–198. Amsterdam: Amsterdam University Press, 2016.

Labande, Léon-Honoré. "L'occupation de Pont-Saint-Esprit par les Grandes Compagnies." *Revue Historique de Provence* (1901): part 1, 79–95, and part 2, 146–164.

Labov, William. "The Transformation of Experience in Narrative Syntax." In *Language in the Inner City: Studies in the Black English Vernacular*, edited by William Labov, 354–396. Philadelphia: University of Pennsylvania Press, 1972.

Lakoff, George, and Mark Johnson. *Metaphors We Live By*. Chicago: University of Chicago Press, 1980.

Lansing, Carol. *Passion and Order: Restraint of Grief in the Medieval Italian Communes*. Ithaca, NY: Cornell University Press, 2008.

Lavoie, Rodrigue. "Medecine et gynecologie au Moyen Âge: Un example Provençal." *Razo cahiers du Centre d'Études medieavales de Nice* (1984): 135–143.

Leavitt, John. "Meaning and Feeling in the Anthropology of Emotions." *American Ethnologist* 23, no. 3 (1996): 514–539.

Le Blevec, Daniel. "Un medècine face au miracle: Jean de Tournemire (1390)." In *Le peuple des saints: Croyances et dèvotions en Provence et Comtat Venaissin à la fin du Moyen Âge*, 125–136. Avignon: Institut de Recherches et d'Études du Bas Moyen Âge Avignonnais, 1986.

Lees, Claire, ed. *Medieval Masculinities: Regarding Men in the Middle Ages*. Minneapolis: University of Minneapolis Press, 1994.

Lenoble, Clément. *L'exercice de la pauvreté: Économie et religion chez les franciscains d'Avignon (XIIIe–XVe siècles)*. Rennes: Presses Universitaires de Rennes, 2013.

Léonard, Émile-Guillaume. "Un ami de Petrarque, senechal de Provence: Giovanni Barrili." *Études Italiennes* 9 (1927): 109–142.

——. *Les Angevins de Naples*. Paris: Presses Universitaires de France, 1954.

——. *Histoire de Jeanne 1re, reine de Naples, comtesse de Provence (1343–1382)*. 3 vols. Monaco: Imprimerie de Monaco, 1936.

——. *La jeunesse de Jeanne Ire: Reine de Naples, comtesse de Provence*. Paris: Librairie Auguste Picard, 1932.

——. "Niccolò Acciaiuoli victime de Boccacce." *Mélanges de philologique, d'histoire, et littérature offerts à Henri Hauvette*, 139–148. Paris: Presses Françaises, 1934.Lett, Didier. *Un procès de canonisation au Moyen Âge: Essai d'histoire sociale, Nicolas de Tolentino, 1325*. Paris: Presses Universitaires de France, 2008.

Lindberg, David C. "Medieval Science and Its Religious Context." *Osiris*, 2nd ser. 10, (1995): 60–79.

Little, Katherine. *Confession and Resistance: Defining the Self in Late Medieval England*. South Bend, IN: University of Notre Dame Press, 2006.

Little, Lester. "Pride Goes before Avarice: Social Change and the Vices in Latin Christendom." *American Historical Review* 76 (1971): 23.

——. "Les techniques de la confession et la confession comme technique." In *Faire croire: Modalités de la diffusion et de la réception des messages religieux du XIIe au XVe siècle*, 87–99. Rome: École Française de Rome, 1981.

Lobrichon, Guy. *La religion des laïcs en Occident: XIe–XVe siècles*. Paris: Hachette, 1994.

Luttrell, Anthony. "Juan Fernandez de Heredia at Avignon." In *El cardenal Albornoz y el Colegio de España*, edited by Evelio Verdera y Tuells, 287–316. Zaragoza: Real Colegio de España en Bolonia, 1972–1973.

Lutz, Catherine. "Depression and the Translation of Emotional Worlds." In *Culture and Depression*, edited by Arthur Kleinman and Byron Good, 63–100. Berkeley: University of California Press, 1985.

——. "Moral Discourse and the Rhetoric of Emotion." In *Language and Politics of Emotion*, edited by Lila Abu-Lughod and Catherine Lutz, 46–68. New York: Cambridge University Press, 1990.

Lutz, Catherine, and Lila Abu-Lughod. "Introduction: Emotion, Discourse, and the Politics of Everyday Life." In *Language and the Politics of Emotion*, edited by Catherine Lutz and Lila Abu-Lughod, 1–23. Cambridge: Cambridge University Press, 1990.

Magou-Nortier, Elisabeth. "The Enemies of the Peace: Reflections on a Vocabulary, 500–1100." In *The Peace of God: Social Violence and Religious Response in France around the Year 1000*, edited by Thomas Head and Richard Landes, 58–79. Ithaca, NY: Cornell University Press, 1992.

Maguire, Henry. "Magic and Money in the Early Middle Ages." *Speculum* 72, no. 4 (1997): 1037–1054.

Mansfield, Mary C. *The Humiliation of Sinners: Public Penance in Thirteenth-Century France*. Ithaca, NY: Cornell University Press, 1995.

Martin, Dennis. "Popular and Monastic Pastoral Issues in the Later Middle Ages." *Church History* 56, no. 3 (1987): 320–332.

Mate, Mavis. *Daughters, Wives and Widows after the Black Death: Women in Sussex, 1350–1535*. Woodbridge, UK: Boydell Press, 1998.

Maufras, Odile. "Les castrum des Baux-de-Provence: Histoire d'un site fortifié médiéval." *Provence Historique* 159 (1990): 79–95.

Maurel, Christian. "Pouvoir royal et pouvoir municipal (XIVe–Xve siècle)." In *Marseille au Moyen Âge: Les horizons d'une ville portuaire*, edited by Thierry Pécout, 225–231. Paris: Éditions Désiris, 2009.

Mazel, Florian. "Affaire de foi et affaire de famille en haute Provence au XIVe siècle, autour de saint Elzéar (1323) et de sainte Dauphine (1360)." *Provence Historique* 49 (1999): 353–366.

——. *La noblesse et l'Église en Provence, fin Xe–début XIVe siècle: L'exemple des familles d'Agoult-Simiane, de Baux et de Marseille*. Paris: Èditions du CTHS, 2002.

——. "La noblesse Provençal face à la justice souveraine (1245–1320): L'âge du pragmatism." In *La noblesse dans les territoires Angevins à la fin du Moyen Âge*, edited by Noël Coulet and Jean-Michel Matz, 343–370. Rome: École Française du Rome, 2000.

McCleery, Iona. "Multos ex Medicinae Arte Curaverat, Multos Verbo et Oratione: Curing in Medieval Portuguese Saints' Lives." *Studies in Church History* 41 (2006): 192–202.

McDonough, Susan Alice. *Witnesses, Neighbors, and Community in Late Medieval Marseille*. New York: Palgrave Macmillan, 2013.

McNeill, John T. "Medicine for Sin as Prescribed in the Penitentials." *Church History* 1, no. 1 (1932): 14–26.

McVaugh, Michael. "Arnald of Villanova's *Regimen Almarie (Regimen castra sequentium)* and Medieval Military Medicine." *Viator* 23 (1992): 201–214.

——. "The Experimenta of Arnald of Villanova." *Journal of Medieval and Renaissance Studies* 1 (1971): 107–118.

——. *Medicine before the Plague: Practitioners and Their Patients in the Crown of Aragon, 1285–1345*. Cambridge: Cambridge University Press, 1993.

Methuen, Charlotte. "'Virgin Widow': A Problematical Social Role for the Early Church?" *Harvard Theological Review* 90, no. 3 (1997): 285–298.

Meyer, Paul. "La traduction Provençale de la Légende Dorée." *Romania* 27 (1898): 93–137.

Michaud, Francine. "Le pauvre transformé: Les hommes, les femmes et la charité à Marseille, du XIIe siècle jusqu'à la Peste noire." *Revue Historique* 311, no. 2 (2009): 243–290.

——. "La peste, la peur et l'espoir: Le pèlerinage jubilaire de romeux marseillais en 1350." *Le Moyen Âge* 104 (1998): 399–434.

Michaud-Quantin, Pierre. "Textes pénitentiels Languedociens au XIIIe siècle." In *Le Crédo, la morale et l'Inquisition*, 151–172. Toulouse: Édouard Privat, Éditeur, 1971.

Michetti, Raimondo, ed. *Notai, miracoli e culto dei santi: Pubblicità e autenticazione del sacro tra XII e XV secolo*. Milan: Dott. A. Giuffrè Editore, 2004.

Millet, Hélene. "Les chanoines de cathédrals du Midi." In *La cathédrale (XIIe–XIVe)*, 121–144. Toulouse: Éditions Privat, 1994.

Mollat, Guillaume. *The Popes at Avignon, 1305–1378*. Translated by Janet Love. London: Thomas Nelson and Sons, 1963.

Mooney, Catherine M. "Voice, Gender, and the Portrayal of Sanctity." In *Gendered Voices: Medieval Saints and Their Interpreters*, edited by Catherine M. Mooney, 1–15. Philadelphia: University of Pennsylvania Press, 1999.

Mowbray, Donald. *Pain and Suffering in Medieval Theology*. Suffolk: Boydell Press, 2009.

Muessig, Carolyn, ed. *Preacher, Sermon and Audience in the Middle Ages*. Leiden: Brill, 2002.

——. "Sermon, Preacher, and Society in the Middle Ages." *Journal of Medieval History* 28 (2012): 73–91.

——. "Prophecy and Song: Teaching and Preaching by Medieval Women." In *Women Preachers and Prophets through Two Millennia of Christianity*, edited by Beverly Mayne Kienzle and Pamela J. Walker, 146–158. Berkeley: University of California Press, 1998.

——. "What Is Medieval Monastic Preaching?" In *Medieval Monastic Preaching*, edited by Carolyn Muessig, 1–16. Leiden: Brill, 1998.

Murray, Alexander. "Counseling in Medieval Confession." In *Handling Sin: Confession in the Middle Ages*, edited by Peter Biller and A. J. Minnis. York: York Medieval Press, 1998.

Nagy, Piroska. *Le don des larmes au Moyen Âge*. Paris: Albin Michel, 2000.

Neaman, Judith. *Suggestion of the Devil: The Origins of Madness*. New York: Anchor Books, 1975.

Newhauser, Richard, ed. *In the Garden of Evil: The Vices and Culture in the Middle Ages*. Toronto: Pontifical Institute of Mediaeval Studies, 2005.

——, ed. *The Seven Deadly Sins: From Communities to Individuals*. Leiden: Brill, 2007.

——. "The Treatise on Vices and Virtues in Latin and the Vernacular." *Typologie des Sources du Moyen Âge Occidental* 68. Turhout: Brepols, 1993.

Newhauser, Richard, and Susan Ridyard, eds. *Sin in Medieval and Early Modern Culture: The Tradition of the Seven Deadly Sins*. York: York University Press, 2012.

Niccoli, Ottavia. "Rinuncia, pace, perdono: Rituali di pacificazione della prima età moderna." *Studi Storici* 40 (1999): 219–261.

Nichols, Eljenholm. "The Etiquette of Pre-Reformation Confession in East Anglia." *Sixteenth Century Journal* 17 (1986): 145–163.

Niebyl, Peter H. "The Non-naturals." *Bulletin of the History of Medicine* 45 (1971): 468–492.

Nutton, Vivian. "God, Galen and the Depaganization of Ancient Medicine." In *Religion and Medicine in the Middle Ages*, edited by Peter Biller and Joseph Ziegler, 16–32. York: York Medieval Press, 1999.

Oakley, Thomas. "The Penitentials as Sources for Medieval History." *Speculum* 15, no. 2 (1940): 210–223.

Oberman, Heiko. *The Harvest of Medieval Theology: Gabriel Biel and Late Medieval Nominalism*. Cambridge, MA: Harvard University Press, 1963.

O'Boyle, Cornelius. *The Art of Medicine: Medical Teaching at the University of Paris, 1250–1400*. Leiden: Brill, 1998.

Ochs, Elinor, and Lisa Capps. *Living Narrative: Creating Lives in Everyday Storytelling*. Cambridge, MA: Harvard University Press, 2001.

——. "Narrating the Self." *Annual Review of Anthropology* 25 (1996): 19–43.

O'Neill, Ynez Viole. *Speech and Speech Disorders in Western Thought before 1600*. London: Greenwood Press, 1980.

Oro, Guido Guerri dall'. Les mercenaires dans le campagnes Napolitaines de Louis le Grand, Roi de Hongrie, 1347–1350. In *Mercenaries and Paid Men: The Mercenary Identity in the Middle Ages*, edited by John France, 61–88. Leiden: Brill, 2008.

Otchakovsky-Laurens, François. *La vie politique à Marseille sous la domination Angevine (1348–1385)*. Rome: École Française de Rome, 2017.

Ottoson, Per-Gunnar. *Scholastic Medicine and Philosophy*. Naples: Bibliopolis, 1982.

Paladilhe, Dominique. *La reine Jeanne Comtesse de Provence*. Paris: Perrin, 1997.

Palanque, Jean-Rémy. *Le diocèse d'Aix-en-Provence*. Paris: Éditions Beauchesne, 1975.

Park, Katherine. "Medicine and Magic: The Healing Arts." In *Gender and Society in Renaissance Italy*, edited by Judith C. Brown and Robert C. Davis. London: Longman, 1998.

Passerat, Georges. "Douceline, Delphine et las autres ou la sainteté feminine en Occitaine à la fin du Moyen Âge." *Bulletin de littérature ecclésiastique* 98 (1997): 235–250.

Paul, Jacques. "Expression et perception du temps d'après l'enquête sur les miracles de Louis d'Anjou." In *Temps, memoire, tradition, au Moyen Âge*, edited by Bernard Guillemain. Aix-en-Provence: Université de Provence, 1983.

——. "'Les frères Prêcheurs de la province de Provence." *Cahiers de Fanjeaux* 36 (2001): 19–59.

Payen, Jean-Charles. *Le motif du repentire dans la literature française medieval (des origens à 1230)*. Geneva: Librairie Droz, 1967.

Payer, Pierre. *The Bridling of Desire: Views of Sex in the Later Middle Ages*. Toronto: University of Toronto Press, 1993.

Pécout, Thierry, ed. *Quand gouverner c'est enquêter: Les practiques politiques de l'enquête princière (occident, XIIIe–XIVe siècles)*. Paris: De Boccard, 2010.

——. "Marseille et la reine Jeanne." In *Marseille au Moyen Âge: Les horizons d'une ville portuaire*, edited by Thierry Pécout, 215–224. Paris: Éditions Désiris, 2009.

Pennington, Kenneth. "Peace and Concord in Medieval Society and Thought." In *Peace and Concord*, edited by Francesco Borghesi. Cambridge: Cambridge University Press, forthcoming.

Perroy, Edouard. "At the Origin of a Contracted Economy: The Crises of the 14th Century." In *Essays in French Economic History*, edited by Rondo Cameron, Franklin Mendels, and Judith Ward, 91–105. Homewood, IL: Richard D. Irwin, 1970.

Peters, Edward. "*Vir inconstans*: Moral Theology as Paleopsychology." In *In the Garden of Evil: The Vices and Culture in the Middle Ages*, edited by Richard Newhauser, 59–73. Toronto: Pontifical Institute of Mediaeval Studies, 2005.

Peters, Greg. "Religious Orders and Pastoral Care in the Late Middle Ages." In *A Companion to Pastoral Care in the Late Middle Ages (1200–1500)*, edited by Ronald Stansbury, 263–284. Leiden: Brill, 2010.

Petkov, Kiril. *The Kiss of Peace: Ritual, Self, and Society in the High and Late Medieval West*. Leiden: Brill, 2003.

Petroff, Elizabeth Alvilda, ed. *Medieval Women's Visionary Literature*. New York: Oxford University Press, 1986.

Piron, Sylvain. "Mouvements et dissidences Spirituels XIIIe–XIVe siècles." *Oliviana* 3 (2009).

——. "Les studia Franciscains de Provence et d'Aquitaine." In *Philosophy and Theology in the Studia of the Religious Orders at the Papal and Royal Courts. Acts of the XVth International Colloquium of the Société Internationale pour l'Étude de la Philosophie Médiévale, University of Notre Dame, 8–10 October, 2008* (2012): 303–358.

Poëzévara, Sandra, and Yann Codou. *Saintetés Aptesiennes: Trésors, architecture et dévotions dans une cité épiscopal*. Apt: Ville d'Apt Éditions, 2019.

Pollock, Linda A. *With Faith and Physic: The Life of a Tudor Gentlewoman, Lady Grace Mildmay, 1552–1620*. New York: St. Martin's Press, 1995.

Porter, Roy. *Patients and Practitioners: Lay Perceptions of Medicine in Pre-industrial Society*. Cambridge: Cambridge University Press, 1985.

——. "Western Medicine and Pain: Historical Perspectives." In *Religion, Health and Suffering*, edited by John R. Hinnells and Roy Porter. London: Kegan Paul International, 1999.

Pryds, Darleen. *The King Embodies the Word: Robert d'Anjou and the Politics of Preaching*. Leiden: Brill, 2000.

Pryor, John H. *Business Contracts of Medieval Provence: Selected Notulae from the Cartulary of Giraud Amalric of Marseilles, 1248*. Toronto: Pontifical Institute of Mediaeval Studies, 1981.

Rather, L. J. "The 'Six Things Non-natural': A Note on the Origins and Fate of a Doctrine and Phrase." *Clio Medica* 3 (1968): 337–347.

Rawcliffe, Carole. *Urban Bodies: Communal Health in Late Medieval English Towns and Cities*. Woodbridge: The Boydell Press, 2013.

Reinburg, Virginia. "Hearing Lay People's Prayer." In *Culture and Identity in Early Modern Europe (1500–1800)*, edited by Barbara Diefendorf and Carla Hesse, 19–39. Ann Arbor: University of Michigan Press, 1993.

Reyerson, Kathryn. *Women's Networks in Medieval France: Gender and Community in Montpellier, 1300–1350*. New York: Palgrave Macmillan, 2016.

——. "Medieval Walled Space: Urban development vs. defense." In *City Walls: The Urban Enceinte in Global Perspective*, edited by James D. Tracy, 88–116. Cambridge: Cambridge University Press, 2000.

Reyerson, Kathryn, and John Drendel, eds. *Urban and Rural Communities in Medieval France: Provence and Languedoc, 1000–1500*. Leiden: Brill, 1998.

Richards, Graham. "Emotions into Words—or Words into Emotions?" In *Representing Emotions: New Connections in the Histories of Art, Music, and Medicine*, edited by Penelope Gouk and Helen Hills, 49–67. Aldershot: Ashgate, 2005.

Richter, Michael. "The Search for Spoken Language in Medieval Texts: Mission Impossible? The Case of Italy in the Ninth Century." In *La fabrique du signe: Linguistique de l'émergence entre micro- et macro-structures*, edited by Michel Banniard and Dennis Philps, 106–113. Toulouse: Presses Universitaires du Mirail, 2010.

Rigaudière, Albert. "Le financement des fortifications urbaines en France du milieu de XIVe siècle à la fin du XVe siècle." *Revue Historique* 273 (1985): 19–95.

Ritchey, Sara. "Health, Healing, and Salvation: Hagiography as a Source for Medieval Healthcare." In *Hagiography and the History of Latin Christendom, 500–1500*, edited by Samantha Herrick, 417–436. Leiden: Brill, 2019.

Rohr, Christian. "Writing a Catastrophe: Describing and Constructing Disaster Perception in Narrative Sources from the Late Middle Ages." *Historical Social Research* 32 (2007): 88–102.

Roncière, Charles M. de la. "L'état Angevin 1265–1340: Pouvoir et sociétés dans le Royaume et la Comté, Bilan d'un colloque." In *L'état Angevin: Pouvoir, culture, et société entre XIIIe et XIVe siècle*, 649–664. Rome: École Française de Rome, 1998.

Rosenwein, Barbara, ed. *Anger's Past: The Social Uses of an Emotion in the Middle Ages*. Ithaca, NY: Cornell University Press, 1998.

——. *Emotional Communities in the Early Middle Ages*. Ithaca, NY: Cornell University Press, 2006.

——. "Emotion Words." In *La sujet des émotions au Moyen Âge*, edited by Damien Boquet and Piroska Nagy, 93–106. Paris: Éditions Beauchesne, 2009.

——. "Worrying about Emotions in History." *American Historical Review* 107, no. 3 (2002): 821–845.

Ross, Michael, and Anne E. Wilson. "Constructing and Appraising Past Selves." In *Brain, Memory, and Belief*, edited by Daniel L. Schacter and Elaine Scarry, 231–258. Cambridge, MA: Harvard University Press, 2000.

Roux, Augustin A. *Apt: Quelques aspects de son histoire*. Apt: Imprimerie Reboulin, 1967.

Ruggiero, Guido. *Binding Passions: Tales of Magic, Marriage and Power at the End of the Renaissance*. New York: Oxford University Press, 1993.

Rusconi, Roberto. "De la prédication à la confession: Transmission et contrôle de modèles de comportement au XIIIe siècle." In *Faire croire: Modalités de la diffusion et de la réception des messages religieux du XIIe au XVe siècle*, 67–85. Rome: École Française de Rome, 1981.

———. "Per mano di notario: Immagini e santi." In *Notai, miracoli e culto dei santi: Pubblicità e autenticazione del sacro tra XII e XV secolo*, edited by Raimondo Michetti, 185–202. Milan: Dott. A. Giuffrè Editore, 2004.

Saarinin, Risto. *Weakness of the Will in Medieval Thought*. New York: E. J. Brill, 1994.

Sautel, Joseph. "Catalogue descriptif des manuscrits liturgiques de l'église d'Apt." *Annales d'Avignon et du Comtat Venaissin* (1919): 53–111.

Sauve, Fernand. *Les épidémies de pest à Apt, notamment en 1588 et 1720–1721*. Aix: Typographie et Lithographie B. Niel, 1905.

———. "Une vielle cité Provençale: Les rues et les quartiers d'Apt, essai de restitution topographique et toponymique." Congrès des Sociétés savantes de Provence, 1906.

Sauze, Élisabeth. "L'habitat castral au bas Moyen Âge en Provence." In *La Provence et Fréjus sous la première maison d'Anjou (1246–1382)*, edited by Jean-Paul Boyer and Thierry Pécout, 53–70. Aix-en-Provence: Publications de l'Université de Provence, 2010.

Saxer, Victor. "Un bréviaire d'Apt du XIVe siècle retrouvé à Toulon." *Provence Historique* 21 (1971): 109–127.

———. "Le culte et la tradition de Sainte-Marie Magdalene en Provence." In *Le peuple des saints: Croyances et dèvotions en Provence et Comtat Venaissin à la fin du Moyen Âge*, 41–56. Avignon: Institut de Recherches et d'Études du Bas Moyen Âge Avignonnais, 1986.

———. "Philippe Cabassole et son *Libellus hystorialis* Marie beatissime Magdalene." In *L'état Angevin: Pouvoir, culture, et société entre XIIIe et XIVe siècle*, 193–204. Rome: École Française de Rome, 1998.

Schiffrin, Deborah. *Approaches to Discourse*. Oxford: Blackwell, 1994.

Schmitt, Jean Claude. *Ghosts in the Middle Ages: The Living and the Dead in Medieval Society*. Chicago: University of Chicago Press, 1998.

Schopfer, Jean. "Documents relatif à l'art du moyen âge contenus dans les manuscrits de N.-C. Fabri de Peiresc à la Bibliothèque de la ville de Carpentras." *Bulletin archéologique du Comité des travaux historiques et scientifiques* (1899): 330–395.

Shaffern, Robert. *g5*. Scranton: University of Scranton Press, 2007.

———. "The Medieval Theology of Indulgences." In *Promissory Notes on the Treasury of Merits: Indulgences in Late Medieval Europe*, edited by R. N. Swanson, 11–36. Leiden: Brill, 2006.

Shatzmiller, Joseph. *Jews, Medicine, and Medieval Society*. Berkeley: University of California Press, 1994.

———. *Médecine et justice en Provence médiévale: Documents de Manosque, 1262–1348*. Aix-en-Provence: Université de Provence, 1989.

Shatzmiller, Joseph, and Rodrigue Lavoie. "Medicine et gynocologie au Moyen Âge: Un example Provençal." *Razo: Cahiers du Centre d'Études Medievales de Nice* 4 (1984): 135–143.

Shaw, Judith. "Corporeal and Spiritual Homicide, the Sin of Wrath, and the Parson's Tale." *Traditio* 38 (1982): 281–300.

Shirk, Melanie. "The Black Death in Aragon, 1348–1351." *Journal of Medieval History* 7 (1981): 357–367.

Sibon, Juliette. "Échanges de practiques de savoirs entre médecins juifs et chrétiens à Marseille au XIVe siècle." In *Acteurs de transferts culturels en Méditerranée médiévale*, edited by Raina Abdellatif, Yassir Benhima, Daniel König, and Elisabeth Ruchaud, 157–167. Paris: Ateliers des Deutchen Historischen Instituts Paris, 2012.

Sigal, Pierre-André. *L'homme et le miracle dans la France médiéval (XIe–XIIe siècle)*. Paris: Les Éditions du CERF, 1985.

——. "Les temoins et les temoignages au procès de canonisation de Dauphine de Puimichel (1363)." *Provence Historique* 195–196 (1999): 461–471.

Siraisi, Nancy G. "Avicenna and the Teaching of Practical Medicine." In *Medicine and the Italian Universities, 1250–1600*, edited by Nancy G. Siraisi. Leiden: Brill, 2001.

——. *Medieval and Early Renaissance Medicine: An Introduction to Knowledge and Practice*. Chicago: University of Chicago Press, 1990.

——. *Taddeo Alderotti and His Pupils: Two Generations of Italian Medical Learning*. Princeton, NJ: Princeton University Press, 1981.

Smail, Daniel Lord. "Common Violence: Vengeance and Inquisition in Fourteenth-Century Marseille." *Past and Present* 151 (1996): 28–59.

——. *The Consumption of Justice: Emotions, Publicity, and Legal Culture in Marseille, 1264–1423*. Ithaca, NY: Cornell University Press, 2003.

——. "Hatred as a Social Institution in Late-Medieval Society." *Speculum* 76 (2001): 90–126.

——. *Imaginary Cartographies: Possession and Identity in Late Medieval Marseille*. Ithaca, NY: Cornell University Press, 1999.

——. "The General Taille of Marseille, 1360–1361: a social and demographic study." *Provence Historique* 165–166 (1999): 473–485.

——. "Notaries, Courts, and the Legal Culture of Late Medieval Marseille." In *Urban and Rural Communities in Medieval France*, edited by Kathryn Reyerson and John Drendel, 23–50. Leiden: Brill, 1998.

——. "Telling Tales in Angevin Courts." *French Historical Studies* 20, no. 2 (1997): 183–215.

——."Accommodating Plague in Medieval Marseille." Continuity and Change 11 (1996): 11–41.

Smoller, Laura. "Choosing Miracles for Vincent Ferrer." In *Miracles in Medieval Canonization Processes: Structures, Functions, and Methodologies*, 75–104. Turnhout: Brepols, 2018.

——. "Miracle, Memory, and Meaning in the Canonization of Vincent Ferrer, 1453–1454." *Speculum* 73 (1998): 429–454.

——. *The Saint and the Chopped-Up Baby: The Cult of Vincent Ferrer in Medieval and Early Modern Europe*. Ithaca, NY: Cornell University Press, 2014.

Søndergaard, Lief. "Imagining Plague: The Black Death in Medieval Mentalities." In *Living with the Black Death*, edited by Lars Bisgaard and Lief Søndergaard, 207–233. Gylling: University Press of Southern Denmark, 2009.

Sponsler, Claire. "Medieval Ethnography: Fieldwork in the European Past." *Assays: Critical Approaches to Medieval and Renaissance Texts* 7 (1992): 1–30.

Stansbury, Ronald. "Preaching and Pastoral Care in the Middle Ages." In *A Companion to Pastoral Care in the Late Middle Ages (1200–1500)*, edited by Ronald Stansbury, 23–40. Leiden: Brill, 2010.

Stouff, Louis. "Alimentation et démographie en Provence aux XIVe et XVe siècles." *Annales de démographie historique* (1976): 61–69.

——. "Une enquête économique en Provence au XIVe siècle." *Le Moyen Âge* 3–4 (1968): 507–542.

——. "Notaires et registres de notaires en Provence et à Arles XIIIe–XVe siècles." In *Le Médiéviste devant ses sources: Questions et méthodes*, edited by Claude Carozzi and Huguette Taviani-Carozzi, 249–269. Aix-en-Provence: Presses Universitaires de Provence, 2004.

——. "Les Provençaux et la mort dans les testaments (XIIIe–XVe siècle)." *Cahiers de Fanjeaux* 33 (1998): 199–222.

Sumption, Jonathan. *Trial by Fire*. Vol. 2 of *The Hundred Years War*. Philadelphia: University of Pennsylvania Press, 1999.

Sweeney, Eileen. "Aquinas on the Seven Deadly Sins: Tradition and Innovation." In *Sin in Medieval and Early Modern Culture: The Tradition of the Seven Deadly Sins*, edited by Richard Newhauser and Susan Ridyard, 85–106. York: York Medieval Press, 2012.

Taylor, Andrew. "Chivalric Conversation and the Denial of Male Fear." In *Conflicted Identities and Multiple Masculinities*, edited by Jacqueline Murray, 169–199. New York: Garland Publishing, 1999.

Temkin, Owsei. *Galenism: Rise and Decline of a Medical Philosophy*. Ithaca, NY: Cornell University Press, 1973.

Tentler, Thomas N. *Sin and Confession on the Eve of the Reformation*. Princeton, NJ: Princeton University Press, 1977.

Thayer, Anne. *Penitence, Preaching, and the Coming of the Reformation*. Aldershot: Ashgate, 2006.

Thayer, Anne and Katharine Lualdi. Introduction to *Handbook for Curates: A Late Medieval Manual on Pastoral Ministry*. Washington, DC: Catholic University of America Press, 2011.

Theis, Valérie. "Jean XXII et l'expulsion des juifs du Comtat Venaissin." *Annales. Histoire, Science Sociales* 67 (2012): 41–77.

Théolas, Henri. *Le vitrail d'Apt et le retour de la Papauté d'Avignon à Rome*. Avignon: Imprimerie D. Seguin, 1924.

Tocco, Francesco Paolo. "La conquista di Messina nell'immaginario soggettivo e nella politica d'e immagine di Niccolò Acciaiuoli." *Archivio Storico Italiano* 589 (2001): 527–546.

Toubert, Pierre. "Le Peste Noire dans les Abruzzes (1348–1350)." *Le Moyen Âge* 120 (2014): 11–26.

Toynbee, Margaret. *S. Louis of Toulouse and the Process of Canonisation in the Fourteenth Century*. Manchester, UK: Manchester University Press, 1929.

Varlik, Nükhet. *Plague and Empire in the Early Modern Mediterranean World*. Cambridge: Cambridge University Press, 2015.

Vauchez, André. "Aux origines de la 'Fama Sanctitatis' d'Elzéar (d. 1323) et de Dauphine de Sabran (d. 1360): Le marriage virginal." In *Le peuple des saints:*

Croyances et dèvotions en Provence et Comtat Venaissin à la fin du Moyen Âge, 153–66. Avignon: Institut de Recherches et d'Études du Bas Moyen Âge Avignonnais, 1986.

——. "La religion populaire dans la France Méridionale au XIVe siècle d'après les procès de canonisation." In *La religion populaire en Languedoc du XIIIe siècle à la moitié du XIVe siècle*, 91–108. Toulouse: Édouard Privat, 1976.

——. *Sainthood in the Later Middle Ages*. Translated by Jean Birrell. Cambridge: Cambridge University Press, 1997.

——. "Two Laypersons in Search of Perfection: Elzear de Sabran and Delphine of Puimichel." In *The Laity in the Middle Ages: Religious Beliefs and Devotional Practices*, edited by Daniel Bornstein, 73–82. Translated by Margery Schneider. London: University of Notre Dame Press, 1993.

——. "The Virginal Marriage of Elzear and Delphine." In *The Laity in the Middle Ages: Religious Beliefs and Devotional Practices*, edited by Daniel Bornstein, 191–203. Translated by Margery Schneider. Notre Dame, IN: University of Notre Dame Press, 1993.

Vauchez, André, and Daniel Ethan Bornstein. *The Laity in the Middle Ages: Religious Beliefs and Devotional Practices*. Translated by Margery Schneider. Notre Dame, IN: University of Notre Dame Press, 1993.

Vecchio, Silvana. "Peccatum Cordis." *Micrologus* 11 (2003): 325–342.

Verdon, Laure. "La notion d'*userpatio* et ses usages: Apports de la legislation et des enquêtes à la construction de la souveraineté en Provence (1250–1335)." In *Quand gouverner c'est enquêter: Les practiques politiques de l'enquête princière (Occident, XIIIe–XIVe siècles)*, 317–328. Paris: De Boccard, 2010.

Veyssière, Gérard. *Vivre en Provence au XIVe siècle*. Paris: Éditions d'Harmattan, 1998.

Voaden, Rosalynn. "A Marriage Made for Heaven: The Vies Occitan of Elzear of Sabran and Delphine of Puimichel." In *Framing the Family: Narrative and Representation in the Medieval and Early Modern Periods*, edited by Rosalynn Voaden and Diane Wolfthal. Tempe: Arizona Center for Medieval and Renaissance Studies, 2005.

Vodola, Elisabeth. *Excommunication in the Middle Ages*. Berkeley: University of California Press, 1986.

Volpato, Antonio. "Pubblicità del miracolo e certificazione delle testimonianze (secoli XIII–XIV)." In *Notai, miracoli e culto dei santi: Pubblicità e autenticazione del sacro tra XII e XV secolo*, edited by Raimondo Michetti. Milan: Dott. A. Guiffrè Editore, 2004.

Wack, Mary Frances. *Lovesickness in the Middle Ages: The Viaticum and Its Commentaries*. Philadelphia: University of Pennsylvania Press, 1990.

Ward, Benedicta. *Miracles and the Medieval Mind: Theory, Record, and Event 1000–1215*. London: Scholar Press, 1982.

Waters, Claire M. *Angels and Earthly Creatures: Preaching, Performance and Gender in the Later Middle Ages*. Philadelphia: University of Pennsylvania Press, 2004.

Watts, John. *The Making of Polities, 1300–1500*. Cambridge: Cambridge University Press, 2009.

Weinstein, Donald, and Rudolph Bell. *Saints and Society: The Two Worlds of Western Christendom, 1000–1700*. Chicago: University of Chicago Press, 1982.

Wenzel, Siegfried. "Preaching the Seven Deadly Sins." In *In the Garden of Evil*, edited by Richard Newhauser, 145–169. Toronto: Pontifical Institute of Mediaeval Studies, 2005.

——. *The Sin of Sloth: Acedia in Medieval Thought and Literature*. Chapel Hill: University of North Carolina Press, 1960.

Wetzstein, Thomas. *Heilige vor Gericht: Das Kanonisationsverfahren im europäischen Spätmittelalter*. Cologne: Böhlau, 2004.

White, Steven D. "The Politics of Anger." In *Anger's Past: The Social Uses of an Emotion in the Middle Ages*. Edited by Barbara Rosenwein, 127–152. Ithaca, NY: Cornell University Press, 1998.

Wickham, Chris. "*Fama* and the Law in Twelfth-Century Tuscany." In *Fama: The Politics of Talk and Reputation in Medieval Europe*, edited by Thelma Fenster and Daniel Lord Smail, 15–26 Ithaca, NY: Cornell University Press, 2003.

Wilkins, Ernest. "Philippe de Cabassoles on Petrarch." *Speculum* 35 (1960): 69.

Willmott, Hugh, et al. "A Black Death Mass Grave at Thonrton Abbey, Lincolnshire: The Discovery and Examination of a 14th-Century Rural Catastrophe." *Antiquity* 94 (2020): 179–196.

Wilson, Stephen, ed. *Saints and Their Cults: Studies in Religious Sociology, Folklore and History*. Cambridge: Cambridge University Press, 1983.

Wolf, Kenneth Baxter. *The Poverty of Riches: St. Francis of Assisi Reconsidered*. Edited by David Steinmetz. Oxford: Oxford University Press, 2003.

Wray, Shona Kelly. "Boccaccio and the Doctors: Medicine and Compassion in the Face of Plague." *Journal of Medieval History* 30 (2004): 301–322.

——. *Communities and Crisis: Bologna during the Black Death*. Leiden: Brill, 2009.

Zacour, Norman. "Talleyrand: The Cardinal of Périgord (1301–1364)." *Transactions of the American Philosophical Society* 50 (1960): 1–83.

Zanella, Gabriele. "La peste del 1348: Italia, Francia, et Germania." In *La Peste Nera: Dati di una realtà ed elementi di una interpretazione*, 49–135. Spoleto: Centro Italiano de Studi sull'alto Medio, 1994.

Zarri, Gabriella. "Places and Gestures of Women's Preaching in Quattro- and Cinquecento Italy." In *Charisma and Religious Authority: Jewish, Christian, and Muslim Preaching, 1200–1500*, edited by Katherine Jansen and Miri Rubin, 177–196. Turnhout: Brepols, 2010.

Zerner, Monique: "Une crise mortalité au XVe siècle a travers les testaments et le rôles d'impostion." *Annales, Histoire, Science Sociales* 34 (1979): 566–589.

Ziegler, Joseph. "Bodies, Diseases, and the Preservation of Health as Foci of Inter-religious Encounters in the Middle Ages." In *Médecine et religion: Compétition, collaboration, conflit; Cas de figures*, edited by L. Berlivet et al. Rome: École française de Rome, 2013.

——. *Medicine and Religion c. 1300*. Oxford: Clarendon Press, 1998.

——. "Practitioners and Saints: Medical Men in Canonization Processes in the Thirteenth to Fifteenth Centuries." *Social History of Medicine* 12 (1999): 191–225.

Index

Page numbers in *italics* indicate illustrations.

CPSIA information can be obtained
at www.ICGtesting.com
Printed in the USA
LVHW091113041121
702424LV00009B/276/J

9 781501 753664